SURGICAL
ATTENDING
ROUNDS
2nd Edition

SURGICAL ATTENDING ROUNDS

2nd Edition

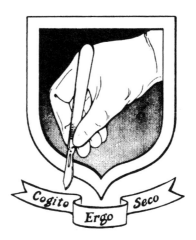

K. FRANCIS LEE, MD

Assistant Professor
Tufts University School of Medicine
Chief, Trauma/General Surgery
Baystate Medical Center
Springfield, Massachusetts

CORNELIUS M. DYKE, MD

The Sanger Clinic, PA
Carolinas Heart Institute
Carolinas Medical Center
Charlotte, North Carolina

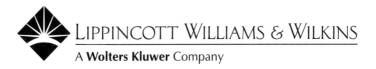

LIPPINCOTT WILLIAMS & WILKINS
A **Wolters Kluwer** Company

Editor: Lisa McAllister
Manager of Development Editing: Jane Velker
Development Editor: Beth Goldner
Managing Editor: Danielle Hagan
Marketing Manager: Justin Mayhew
Production Editor: Jennifer D. Weir

351 West Camden Street
Baltimore, Maryland 21201-2436 USA

227 East Washington Square
Philadelphia, PA 19106

The publisher is not responsible (as a matter of product liability, negligence, or otherwise) for any injury resulting from any material contained herein. This publication contains information relating to general principles of medical care that should not be construed as specific instructions for individual patients. Manufacturers' product information and package inserts should be reviewed for current information, including contraindications, dosages, and precautions.

Printed in Canada

First Edition, 1992

Library of Congress Cataloging-in-Publication Data

Surgical attending rounds / [edited by] K. Francis Lee, Cornelius M. Dyke. — 2nd ed.
    p.   cm.
    Includes bibliographical references and index.
    ISBN 0-683-30585-9
    1. Surgery—Examinations, questions, etc. I. Lee, K. Francis, 1929– . II. Dyke, Cornelius M.
    [DNLM: 1. Surgery examination questions. 2. Surgical procedures, operative examination questions.
       WO 18.2 S9617 1999]
    RD37.2.S9745 1999
    617'.0076—dc21
    DNLM/DLC   98-45984
    for Library of Congress   CIP

The publishers have made every effort to trace the copyright holders for borrowed material. If they have inadvertently overlooked any, they will be pleased to make the necessary arrangements at the first opportunity.

To purchase additional copies of this book, call our customer service department at **(800) 638-3030** or fax orders to **(301) 824-7390**. International customers should call **(301) 714-2324**.

99 00 01 02 03
1 2 3 4 5 6 7 8 9 10

Dedicated to the surgical housestaff and students at Baystate Medical Center, and to Arnie Salzberg, who taught me the art of surgical thinking.
(KFL)

Dedicated to Melanie, Mary Caroline, Katherine, and Peter, who make it all worthwhile.
(CMD)

Preface—Second Edition

The second edition of *Surgical Attending Rounds* builds upon the success of the original formula. We have preserved the Socratic question-and-answer format within the setting of realistic clinical cases. As each clinical scenario unfolds, the reader encounters important questions pertinent to the care of the patient. In the clinical setting, knowing what to ask is half the battle in the learning process. *Surgical Attending Rounds,* 2nd edition, strives to teach both the critical questions and the correct answers.

Based on feedback from our readers, several new features have been added to this edition. The index at the end of the book will facilitate selective readings. Chapters were completely rewritten by the authors to include recent medical advances such as minimally invasive surgery. We have expanded the number of figures, tables, and drawings from the original edition to help clarify topics that words cannot fully describe.

Most importantly, we have included at least one clinical management algorithm in each chapter. It is always dangerous to reduce a complex decision-making process into a simple algorithm; however, the clinical algorithm is quite useful as a framework for decision making and serves to highlight branch points on the decision tree; we felt the benefits far outweighed the shortcomings. Parts of the algorithms may be controversial and, by their very nature, may appear to represent subjective interpretation of incomplete or conflicting scientific data. But the algorithms remain a very efficient way of teaching the surgical thought process and summarizing a clinical topic. The logo on the title page depicts our intent: *Cogito ergo seco. I think, therefore I cut*—as we believe strongly that surgery is a cognitive discipline. It is our hope that this edition helps students at all levels think through the critical decision points in clinical surgery.

Preface—First Edition

As any medical student or resident on a clinical service knows, the experience of being unsure about an answer to a direct question from the attending physician is unpleasant. However, responses to questions asked in this situation are not easily forgotten. Attending surgeons and clinicians have used this Socratic method of teaching on their rounds to focus the discussion, emphasize key points, and evaluate residents since the inception of student surgical programs. *Surgical Attending Rounds* follows the same question-and-answer format. Each chapter is based on a particular patient presentation, as are rounds in the hospital. Using questions and answers, the reader is drawn throughout the patient's presentation and diagnostic evaluation to treatment and outcome. As on teaching rounds, important pathophysiological points are emphasized by specific, focused questions.

Surgical Attending Rounds is not a replacement for the classic surgical textbooks well known to all physicians; we have aimed to make it a teaching tool that complements these core textbooks. *Surgical Attending Rounds* attempts to fill a real need among residents and students with multiple demands on their time: namely, a succinct presentation of relevant material presented in an accessible manner. It is our hope that by using a case-oriented format, *Surgical Attending Rounds* will be able to present essential surgical information in a way that enhances retention and arouses interest in surgery.

Acknowledgments

We would like to extend our deep gratitude to Dr. Hunter McGuire, Jr., Professor of Surgery at the Medical College of Virginia and Chief Surgeon at the Hunter McGuire Veterans Administration Hospital in Richmond, Virginia. A master surgeon, as well as a perceptive artist, he has graciously supplied the artwork for the logo on the title page.

Joy Marlowe also deserves our sincere gratitude for her elegant and clean artwork.

We would also like to thank the editorial staff at Lippincott Williams & Wilkins for their support, encouragement, and skillful management, especially Carroll Cann, Danielle Hagan, and Beth Goldner. Allison Flaherty and Cathy Cole provided vital assistance with communication and typing.

Finally, we would like to acknowledge our deep sense of communion with our colleagues in surgery, students, and teachers alike. The strength of our specialty lies with its practitioners. It is our hope that *Surgical Attending Rounds,* 2nd edition, will aid and encourage tomorrow's surgeons as they prepare today.

Contributors

Nicholas P.W. Coe, MD
Professor of Surgery
Tufts University School of Medicine
Chief, Division of Endocrine and Metabolic Surgery
Director, Office of Surgical Education
Baystate Medical Center
Springfield, Massachusetts

Eric J. DeMaria, MD
Professor of Surgery
Chief, Section of General and Endoscopic Surgery
Director, MCV Center for Minimally Invasive Surgery
Medical College of Virginia
Virginia Commonwealth University
Richmond, Virginia

André Duranceau, MD
Professor of Surgery
Chief, Division of Thoracic Surgery
Université de Montréal
Montréal, Quebec, Canada

Cornelius M. Dyke, MD
The Sanger Clinic, PA
Carolinas Heart Institute
Carolinas Medical Center
Charlotte, North Carolina

Timothy Emhoff, MD
Assistant Professor of Surgery
Tufts University School of Medicine
Trauma/General Surgery
Baystate Medical Center
Springfield, Massachusetts

Pasquale Ferraro, MD
Assistant Professor of Surgery
Surgical Director, Lung Transplant Program
Université de Montréal
Montréal, Quebec, Canada

Viriato M. Fiallo, MD
Assistant Professor of Surgery
Tufts University School of Medicine
General Surgeon
Pioneer Valley Surgical Associates, PC
Ware, Massachusetts

James L. Frank, MD
Assistant Professor of Surgery
Tufts University School of Medicine
Attending Surgical Oncologist
Baystate Medical Center
Springfield, Massachusetts

James S. Gammie, MD
Fellow, Division of Cardiothoracic Surgery
University of Pittsburgh Medical Center
Pittsburgh, Pennsylvania

D. Lee Gorden, MD
Clinical Fellow, Department of Surgery
Veterans Administration Medical Center
University of Minnesota Medical School
Minneapolis, Minnesota

Jeffrey L. Kaufman, MD
Associate Professor of Surgery
Tufts University School of Medicine
Division of Vascular Surgery
Baystate Medical Center
Springfield, Massachusetts

K. Francis Lee, MD
Assistant Professor
Tufts University School of Medicine
Chief, Trauma/General Surgery
Baystate Medical Center
Springfield, Massachusetts

D. Scott Lind, MD
Associate Professor
Department of Surgery
University of Florida College of Medicine
Gainesville, Florida

Robert L. Madden, MD
Assistant Professor of Surgery
Tufts University School of Medicine
Director of Pancreas Transplantation
Baystate Medical Center
Springfield, Massachusetts

Richard Maley, MD
Chief Resident
Cardiothoracic Surgery
University of Pittsburgh Medical Center
Pittsburgh, Pennsylvania

Bruce A. Mast, MD
Assistant Professor of Surgery
Division of Plastic and Reconstructive Surgery
Director
Shands Wound Clinic
University of Florida
Chief, Section of Plastic and
  Reconstructive Surgery
Gainesville Veterans Affairs Medical Center
Gainesville, Florida

Andrew W.J. McFadden, MD
Associate Professor of Surgery
Division of General Surgery
Department of Surgery
Royal University Hospital
University of Saskatchewan
Saskatoon, Saskatchewan, Canada

Janette C. McGrath, MD
Chief Resident, Anesthesiology
Department of Anesthesiology
Allegheny University of the Health Sciences
Pittsburgh, Pennsylvania

Michael McGrath, MD
Chief Resident, Cardiothoracic Surgery
University of Pittsburgh Medical Center
Pittsburgh, Pennsylvania

Prashant K. Narain, MD
Resident, General Surgery
MCV Hospital
Medical College of Virginia
Virginia Commonwealth University
Richmond, Virginia

Marc Norris, MD
Assistant Professor of Surgery
Tufts University School of Medicine
Division of Vascular Surgery
Baystate Medical Center
Springfield, Massachusetts

David Page, MD
Associate Clinical Professor of Surgery
Tufts University School of Medicine
General Surgery
Baystate Medical Center
Springfield, Massachusetts

Andrew B. Peitzman, MD
Professor of Surgery
Director, Trauma and Surgical Critical Care
University of Pittsburgh
Pittsburgh, Pennsylvania

William P. Reed, MD
Professor of Surgery
Tufts University School of Medicine
Chief, Surgical Oncology
Baystate Medical Center
Springfield, Massachusetts

Jason J. Rosenberg, MD
Resident and Surgical Research Fellow
Division of Plastic and Reconstructive Surgery
Department of Surgery
University of Florida College of Medicine
Gainesville, Florida

Daniel A. Saltzman, MD
Fellow in Pediatric Surgery
Arkansas Children's Hospital
University of Arkansas for Medical Sciences
Little Rock, Arkansas

Jeannie F. Savas, MD
Assistant Professor of Surgery
Division of General/Trauma Surgery
Program Director of Surgery
Medical College of Virginia
Virginia Commonwealth University
Richmond, Virginia

Larry L. Shears II, MD
Resident
Department of Surgery
University of Pittsburgh Medical Center
Pittsburgh, Pennsylvania

Bruce J. Simon, MD
Assistant Professor of Surgery
Tufts University School of Medicine
Trauma/General Surgery
Baystate Medical Center
Springfield, Massachusetts

W. Charles Sternbergh III, MD
Staff Vascular Surgeon
Ochsner Clinic
Clinical Assistant Professor of Surgery
Tulane University School of Medicine
New Orleans, Louisiana

Todd M. Tuttle, MD
Surgical Oncology
Park Nicollet Clinic
Instructor, Surgery
University of Minnesota
Minneapolis, Minnesota

Ciaran J. Walsh, MB, BSc, FRCSI, MCh
Consultant Surgeon and Coloproctologist
Wirral Hospital
NHS Trust
United Kingdom

Jeffrey H. Widmeyer, MD
General and Vascular Surgeon
Lynchburg, Virginia

Jan Wojcik, MD
Assistant Professor of Surgery
Tufts University School of Medicine
Chief, Colorectal Surgery
Baystate Medical Center
Springfield, Massachusetts

Contents

Preoperative Assessment of the Surgical Patient

Janette C. McGrath

Mrs. Barr is a 65-year-old woman whom the anesthesiologist is called to see before surgery. She presented to the emergency department with abdominal pain and bilious emesis of 2 days' duration. After evaluation by the general surgery service, she is scheduled for an exploratory laparotomy for a presumed small bowel obstruction. Further medical history reveals hypertension, non–insulin-dependent diabetes mellitus, and severe degenerative joint disease, which limits her ability to walk. She has not seen her primary physician for 2 years. She has a 30-pack-year history of smoking.

Mrs. Barr's surgical history includes an aortofemoral bypass graft 8 years ago and a right femoropopliteal bypass graft 3 years ago. She takes a β-blocker and diuretic for hypertension, a nonsteroidal anti-inflammatory for joint pain, and glucophage for diabetes. She has no medical allergies.

What is Mrs. Barr's American Society of Anesthesiologists (ASA) status?
The ASA physical status is a means of classifying patients according to the extent of their systemic disease (Table 1.1). To determine ASA status, each patient's chart should have a thorough review; then each patient should undergo a thorough history and physical examination with evaluation of appropriate ancillary studies. Open-ended questions should be used for the history and should be asked in nonmedical terminology. Emergency surgery is associated with a high rate of morbidity and mortality.

Why is it important to ask the patient when he or she last had anything to eat or drink?
Determination of the patient's NPO (nil per os; nothing by mouth) status is important to assess the likelihood that there is food in the patient's stomach. Patients with normal gastric motility may require more than 4 hours to empty the

Table 1.1. AMERICAN SOCIETY OF ANESTHESIOLOGISTS (ASA) STATUS

Classification	Systemic Disease
ASA I	No organic disease
ASA II	Mild or moderate systemic disease without functional impairment
ASA III	Organic disease with definite functional impairment
ASA IV	Severe disease that is life-threatening
ASA V	Moribund patient, not expected to survive
ASA VI	Donor patient for organ harvesting

Note: An "E" classification added to the above denotes an emergency case. (Reprinted with permission from Ross AF, Tinker JH. Preoperative Evaluation of the Healthy Patient. In: Rogers MC, Tinker JH, Covino BG, et al., eds. Principles and Practice of Anesthesiology. St. Louis: Mosby-Year Book, 1993:4.)

stomach of solid matter (1). However, patients with decreased gastric motility must be treated as if they had a full stomach and undergo endotracheal intubation with a rapid-sequence technique.

What patients are considered to have a full stomach?
Patients with gastric outlet obstructions or any intestinal obstruction are considered to have a full stomach, as are all trauma patients, obese patients, gravid women, and patients with diabetes mellitus or electrolyte abnormalities.

What is rapid-sequence intubation?
Rapid-sequence intubation is a technique used for patients at risk for aspiration. It is performed as follows: The patient is preoxygenated with 100% oxygen, and an intravenous anesthetic agent is administered, followed rapidly by intravenous succinylcholine. Cricoid pressure is applied to occlude the esophagus in the event of passive regurgitation (Figure 1.1) and is maintained until tracheal intubation is confirmed by measuring end-tidal carbon dioxide, documenting bilateral breath sounds, and inflating the endotracheal tube cuff.

Why is a patient's anesthetic history important?
In simple terms, history repeats itself. If old charts are available, they should be reviewed to determine ease of laryngoscopy and intubation, type of anesthetic used, and any complications associated with anesthesia. If old charts are not available, the physician should ask the patient what types of anesthetics the patient has had (e.g., regional versus general). Details of the previous anesthetics should be sought; the patient should be asked whether he or she has ever been told that the anesthesiologist had difficulty placing a breathing tube or whether he or she required prolonged postoperative ventilation.

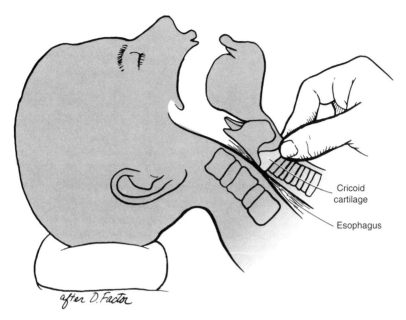

after D.Factor

Figure 1.1.   Use of the Sellick maneuver. Pressure is applied to the cricoid cartilage to occlude the esophagus. Cricoid pressure prevents aspiration of gastric contents during the administration of anesthesia. (Reprinted with permission from Stehling LC. Management of the airway. In: Barash PG, Cullen BF, Stoelting RK, eds. Clinical Anesthesia. Philadelphia: Lippincott, 1992:695.)

Why is a family history of problems with anesthetics important?
A family history of problems with anesthetics may indicate inherited risks (e.g., malignant hyperthermia). Many patients have not had prior surgery, but the anesthesiologist should be made aware of inherited conditions that may threaten life.

Mrs. Barr states that she had general anesthesia for her aortobifemoral bypass graft and had no problems. However, her sister almost died of an intraoperative "fever."

What is malignant hyperthermia?
Malignant hyperthermia is an autosomal dominant trait that causes severe fevers and massive catabolism. It is triggered by the induction of general anesthesia. Initially, it manifests as tachycardia and cardiac dysrhythmia, which can result in complete cardiac collapse. The manifestation may not occur until 24 hours after exposure. The physiologic mechanism is believed to be an excessive release of calcium from the sarcoplasmic reticulum in skeletal muscle, which results in severe muscle contractures. Anesthetic agents known to trigger malignant hyperthermia are the volatile anesthetics (e.g., halothane, desflurane, isoflurane),

succinylcholine, and decamethonium (2). Total intravenous anesthesia and regional anesthesia are generally considered safe for these patients. Malignant hyperthermia is associated with other disorders, such as Duchenne's muscular dystrophy and King-Denborough syndrome (3).

Once a complete history is obtained, a thorough physical examination should be performed with particular attention paid to the airway and cardiovascular, pulmonary, and neurologic systems. Any other pertinent organ systems should also be assessed.

Why is an examination of the airway important?
Examination of the airway allows the anesthesiologist to assess how easy it will be to intubate the patient and to anticipate any difficulty with the airway. Considerations during examination include the Mallampati classification, extent of mouth opening, hyomental distance, and neck range of motion.

What is the Mallampati classification?
The Mallampati classification system assesses the size of the tongue relative to the oropharyngeal cavity (Figure 1.2). It is performed with the patient sitting upright and the head in a neutral position. The patient maximally opens his or her mouth and maximally protrudes his or her tongue. The patient should not phonate because this falsely raises the soft palate and gives an erroneous classification. The airway is classified by what structures are visualized:

• Class I: the soft palate, fauces, uvula, and anterior and posterior tonsillar pillars
• Class II: the soft palate, fauces, and uvula
• Class III: the soft palate and base of the uvula
• Class IV: the soft palate not visible

There is a significant correlation between Mallampati class and ease of laryngoscopy. Class I patients are expected to be relatively easy to intubate, whereas class IV patients are expected to be difficult to intubate.

Why does the anesthesiologist want to know the patient's height and weight?
Most drugs used in the operating room are dosed on body weight (milligrams per kilogram). This allows precise dosing. Spinal and epidural anesthesia dosing is based on height. Also, in the event that a pulmonary artery catheter is placed, body surface area (BSA) is used for such calculations as cardiac index and systemic vascular resistance index.

How is BSA calculated?

$BSA = \sqrt{[height\ (cm) \times weight\ (kg) \div 3600]}$. *Units are in meters squared (m^2).*

Mrs. Barr is unable to provide information about exercise tolerance because degenerative joint disease limits her mobility.

Class I   Class II

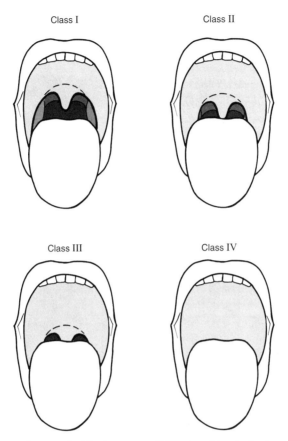

Class III   Class IV

Figure 1.2.   Mallampati classification system. Difficulty of intubation increases from Class I to Class IV. (Reprinted with permission from Cooper SD, Benumof JL, Reisner LS. The difficult airway: risk, prophylaxis, and management. In: Chestnut DH, ed. Obstetric Anesthesia. St. Louis: Mosby–Year Book, 1994:581.)

Why is exercise status important?
Mrs. Barr has several risk factors for coronary artery disease, including advanced age, hypertension, peripheral vascular disease, obesity, diabetes mellitus, and a history of smoking. Roberts and Tinker have provided indicators of high-risk patients needing a thorough evaluation (Table 1.2).

If a patient's surgery is elective, a thorough cardiac workup is warranted. It may include an electrocardiogram, dobutamine stress test, echocardiogram, and possibly cardiac catheterization. Because Mrs. Barr's surgery is an emergency, a thorough cardiac workup is not feasible. However, an electrocardiogram should be obtained as a preoperative baseline because of her high-risk status.

Table 1.2.   INDICATORS OF HIGH-RISK PATIENTS
WHO NEED A THOROUGH EVALUATION

Cardiovascular	Pulmonary	Neurologic
Third heart sound gallop	Chronic lung disease	Central nervous system injury
Jugular venous distention	FEV$_1$ <2.0 L	Carotid bruit
MI within 6 months	Obesity	
Dysrhythmias	Hypercapnia at rest	
Age >70 years	Age >70 years	
Emergency operation	Site of operation	
Important aortic stenosis	Smoking history	
Poor general health		

FEV$_1$ = forced expiratory volume in 1 second. MI = myocardial infarction. (Reprinted with permission from Roberts SL, Tinker JH. Perioperative Myocardial Infarction. In: Gravenstein N, Kirby RR, eds. Complications in Anesthesiology. Philadelphia: Lippincott-Raven, 1996:339.)

For example, evidence of prior myocardial infarction might prompt the use of invasive hemodynamic monitoring (e.g., pulmonary artery catheter, arterial line) or alter the choice of anesthetic agents. Depending on the procedure to be performed, a regional technique may be used.

What, if any, intraoperative monitoring would be appropriate in this patient's case?
Mrs. Barr should have a large-bore (14- to 18-g) intravenous catheter in place for fluid administration. She would benefit from an arterial line because of her history of hypertension. A pulmonary artery catheter is beneficial for evaluation of her intravascular volume status because there is a potential for massive third-space fluid losses in this type of surgery.

How are maintenance intravenous fluid requirements and intraoperative requirements calculated?
Maintenance intravenous fluids are calculated according to body weight for both children and adults. The initial 10 kg of a person's body weight is allotted at 4 mL/kg; the second 10 kg is allotted at 2 mL/kg; and any remaining weight is allotted at 1 mL/kg. Calculation of the patient's fluid deficit should be based on maintenance volume and the number of hours he or she has been NPO. Half of this fluid should be replaced during the first hour of surgery, and 25% of the volume should be replaced during each of the subsequent 2 hours. Additional intraoperative fluid requirements are calculated according to third-space fluid losses anticipated in the operating room, which are also based on the patient's weight. Operations without much fluid loss, such as eye surgery, have third-space losses of 2 mL/kg per hour. Operations with moderate fluid losses, such as ventral hernia repair, are replaced at 6 mL/kg per hour. Large operations with

much exposed viscera, such as abdominal aorta resection or exploratory laparotomy, have large fluid shifts, and the patients are given an additional 10 to 15 mL/kg per hour. The overall determinant of adequate fluid resuscitation should be urine output, which should be at least 0.5 mL/kg per hour.

What are this patient's options for postoperative pain control?
The three most commonly employed techniques for control of pain after abdominal surgery are intermittent intravenous opioid administration, intravenous patient-controlled analgesia (PCA), and epidural catheter.

What is intravenous PCA?
PCA is a device attached to the patient's maintenance intravenous line that allows programing of administration of opioids. A baseline infusion of opioids may be ordered, and the patient controls how often additional boluses are given. PCA devices have a lockout period that prevents overdosing. Most hospitals have printed PCA order forms. A typical order includes a loading dose, a maintenance dose with lockout interval, and a 4-hour maximum dose limit. Antiemetics and antipruritics should be routinely ordered, because the most common side effects of PCA are pruritis and nausea or emesis.

What is epidural anesthesia?
An epidural catheter is placed, usually preoperatively, into the epidural space. The level of required anesthesia helps to determine the spinal level at which the catheter is placed. The catheter is attached to an infusion pump that can continuously infuse a local anesthetic or opioid. Epidural PCA operates along the same principles as intravenous PCA. Contraindications to epidural catheter placement include refusal by the patient, uncorrected coagulopathy, local infection at the sight of the puncture, uncorrected hypovolemia, and anticipated major blood loss (4). Main risks associated with epidural catheter placement include blood vessel puncture, dural puncture, backache, and severe hypotension. Spinal headache is caused by inadvertent entry into the cerebrospinal fluid (dural puncture). The risks range from blood vessel puncture (2.8%) to permanent paralysis (0.02%) (5).

After the epidural anesthetic is placed but prior to the procedure, the anesthesiologist notes that the patient is very lethargic and has facial twitching.

Why should the anesthesiologist be concerned?
Although it is very unlikely with spinal anesthesia, the anesthesiologist must be concerned about a toxic local reaction to the anesthetic. These reactions may also occur when concurrent local anesthesia is used by the surgeon or when a large dose of local anesthetic is inadvertently given in the vascular system instead of the subcutaneous tissue.

What is the maximum amount of lidocaine or bupivacaine that should be administered to a patient?
In adults, the maximum dose of lidocaine is approximately 500 mg, and the maximum dose of bupivacaine (Marcaine) is about 200 mg. The route of administration affects the rate of uptake. Intercostal blocks result in the highest plasma levels of local anesthetics, followed by brachial plexus blocks. Spinal anesthesia results in extremely low levels of anesthesic in the plasma.

How are lidocaine and bupivacaine toxicity manifested?
Local anesthesia toxicity manifests primarily through the cardiac and central nervous systems, with bupivacaine having more cardiac disturbances than lidocaine. The patient may exhibit tinnitus, perioral dysesthesias, seizures, or unconsciousness. Hypercarbia decreases the seizure threshold significantly, so opioids must be used with caution. Cardiac manifestations of bupivacaine are primarily conduction abnormalities, dysrhythmia, and cardiac arrest (8).

Mr. Jackson, an 80-year-old man, presents for a transurethral resection of the prostate (TURP) for a slowly bleeding prostate tumor. His hematocrit is 39%. His medical history is significant for rheumatoid arthritis and a few episodes of congestive heart failure. Further questioning reveals that the patient's father had to be on a ventilator after general anesthesia for a small inguinal hernia repair because he "could not breathe."

What is pseudocholinesterase deficiency?
Pseudocholinesterase, or plasma cholinesterase, deficiency is an inherited disorder that results in varying levels of plasma cholinesterase. Plasma cholinesterase is the enzyme responsible for the metabolism of succinylcholine, mivacurium (a nondepolarizing neuromuscular relaxant), and ester anesthetics (e.g., cocaine, procaine, chloroprocaine, tetracaine). Patients with this disorder are typically asymptomatic; however, they may exhibit prolonged apnea after administration of succinylcholine or mivacurium. This condition may be exacerbated by ectothiophate eye drops or by severe liver dysfunction. Neuromuscular blockade may last 120 to 300 minutes or longer (6).

Mr. Jackson's physical examination is remarkable for decreased neck extension, a short hyoid mental distance, and a Mallampati III airway. The patient is alert and well oriented.

What is the optimal type of anesthesia for this patient?
Two major factors specifically make spinal anesthesia the optimal choice for this patient: his cardiac status and the type of surgery he is having. His family history of presumed pseudocholinesterase deficiency and his difficult airway preclude the use of succinylcholine or mivacurium for rapid-sequence intubation, and his airway makes the use of longer-acting muscle relaxants undesirable. An

awake intubation with general anesthesia is another option for this patient, and it may be considered ideal by some anesthesiologists because it allows the airway to be secured early.

What is TURP syndrome?

TURP syndrome occurs when the patient undergoing transurethral resection of the prostate absorbs large quantities of hypotonic irrigation solution used during surgery, resulting in volume overload and hyponatremia. Symptoms include altered mental status, cyanosis, pulmonary edema, and eventual cardiac collapse from congestive heart failure. Glycine toxicity also manifests as altered mental status due to hyperammonemia. TURP syndrome is related to the length of surgery, the irrigating pressure of solution, and the extent of resection (7). Spinal anesthesia allows continual assessment of the patient's mental status and pulmonary status.

What is spinal anesthesia?

Also known as subarachnoid block, spinal anesthesia is local anesthesia delivered directly into the subarachnoid space. Any of several types of local anesthetic can be used depending on the anticipated duration of the surgery. The most commonly used anesthetics are lidocaine, bupivacaine, and tetracaine. The subarachnoid entry for TURP is usually performed at the L4-L5 or L3-L4 interspace. The level, or height, of anesthesia depends primarily on the volume instilled.

What are the risks of spinal anesthesia?

The main risks are pruritis, urinary retention, bleeding, infection, risk of spinal headache, intravascular absorption of medication, and a "high spinal." Pruritis is common after intrathecal (spinal) opioid administration. Bleeding abnormalities must be ruled out by a thorough history before subarachnoid anesthesia is attempted because a hematoma may have permanent neurologic sequelae. Infection is rare but can result in meningitis. Subarachnoid block should never be performed if there is evidence of infection where the block is to be placed, and strict sterile technique should be used. Spinal, or post dural puncture, headache is more common with subarachnoid blocks than with epidural catheter placement, occurring in approximately 11% of patients undergoing spinal anesthesia. Factors associated with a high incidence of postdural puncture headache are female gender, pregnancy, young age, large needle size, needle orientation, and multiple attempts (9). Postdural puncture headache is usually treated conservatively with intravenous fluid hydration and analgesics.

What is a "high spinal"?

When the level of anesthesia is too high on the spinal cord, higher cord function may be impaired (most serious being the inhibition of respiration). As the level of anesthesia rises cephalad above T2, the patient subjectively feels dyspneic, with upper limb parasthesias and weakness. The patient has difficulty

speaking because of the inability to exchange air. In extreme cases, consciousness is lost. The treatment for a high spinal is early recognition and prompt institution of mechanical ventilation until the spinal anesthesia regresses (10).

Mr. Jackson is a good candidate for a subarachnoid block, so the surgical team
must be prepared for a difficult airway in the event that the block fails or results in a high spinal. Preparations for a difficult airway (e.g., laryngeal mask airway, lighted stylet, fiberoptic laryngoscope) should be available in case of a
complication, such as a failed subarachnoid anesthesia, a toxic reaction, or a
high subarachnoid anesthesia.

**A 40-year-old man, Mr. McMahon, presents for thoracotomy and left
pneumonectomy for cancer. He has an extensive smoking history (75
pack-years) and easily becomes dyspneic. He is 6'2" tall and weighs
80 kg. The remainder of his medical and surgical history is unremarkable. Physical examination is unremarkable except for bilateral
distant breath sounds with wheezing throughout.**

What preoperative studies are necessary for this patient?
Basic laboratory work for Mr. McMahon should include a complete blood
count with quantitative platelet count, blood type, crossmatch for 2 units of
packed red blood cells, basic chemistry, liver function testing, chest radiograph,
and electrocardiogram.

What information can an arterial blood gas measurement provide?
A preoperative measurement of arterial blood gas on room air provides the
physician with the baseline values for this patient. It allows assessment of the
extent of any hypoxemia and hypercarbia. Patients with baseline compensated
respiratory acidosis (i.e., $PaCO_2$ above 45 mm Hg) are at particular risk (11).

What are the types of acid-base abnormalities, and what can be expected with each?
There are four basic types of abnormalities: respiratory acidosis, respiratory alkalosis, metabolic acidosis, and metabolic alkalosis. They are commonly found
in combination, and the combinations are usually compensatory (12).

To simplify the assessment of arterial blood gases, pH is checked first. Normal
pH is 7.35 to 7.45; a pH below 7.35 is considered acidotic, and a pH above
7.45 is considered alkalotic. A normal pH implies either no abnormality (if the
carbon dioxide and bicarbonate levels are normal) or a compensated disorder.
The pH is never overcompensated; that is, in the presence of respiratory acidosis, the bicarbonate level never overcompensates to make the pH alkalotic.
Metabolic compensation occurs at a much slower rate (over many hours to
days) than does respiratory compensation. The four possible acid-base abnormalities are summarized here and in Table 1.3:

Table 1.3.   DETERMINING ACID–BASE ABNORMALITY THROUGH pH AND ARTERIAL BLOOD GASES

Acid–Base Abnormality	pH	Carbon Dioxide (CO_2)	Bicarbonate (HCO_3^-)
Acute respiratory acidosis	↓	↑	–
Chronic respiratory acidosis (compensated)	↓/–	↑	↑
Acute respiratory alkalosis	↑	↓	–
Chronic respiratory alkalosis (compensated)	↑/–	↓	↓
Acute metabolic alkalosis	↑	–/↑	↑
Chronic metabolic alkalosis (compensated)	↑/–	↑	↑
Acute metabolic acidosis	↓	–/↓	↓
Chronic metabolic acidosis (compensated)	↓/–	↓	↓

- The patient who is acidotic or has a carbon dioxide level greater than 45 (normal carbon dioxide level is 35 to 45 mm Hg) has *respiratory acidosis*. If the bicarbonate level is high (normal bicarbonate level is 22 to 26 mmol/L), one can expect that the acidosis is compensated. If the bicarbonate level is low, one can assume that the patient has a mixed primary respiratory and metabolic acidosis.
- The patient who is alkalotic with a low carbon dioxide level has *respiratory alkalosis*. If the bicarbonate level is low, it is compensated; if it is high, the patient can be assumed to have mixed primary respiratory and metabolic alkalosis.
- The patient who is alkalotic with a high bicarbonate level has *metabolic alkalosis*. If the carbon dioxide level is high, it is compensated; if it is low, it is a *mixed primary metabolic and respiratory alkalosis*.
- The patient who is acidotic with a low bicarbonate level has *metabolic acidosis*. If the carbon dioxide level is low, it is compensated; if it is high, it is a *mixed primary metabolic and respiratory acidosis*.

What is anion gap acidosis and what are its major causes?
Anion gap acidosis cannot be accounted for by the major cations and anions in the body (i.e., sodium, chloride, bicarbonate) (12). It primarily arises from an excess of minor anions (e.g., lactate, ketones, organic acids). The human body normally has an anion gap of less than 12, which is typically calculated by subtracting the major plasma anions from the major plasma cations (Na^+) $-$ [(Cl^-) $+$ (HCO_3^-]. Common causes of metabolic acidosis with an anion gap include diabetic ketoacidosis, lactic acidosis, aspirin toxicity, methanol ingestion, uremia, and ethylene glycol ingestion.

Management Algorithm for the Preoperative Patient

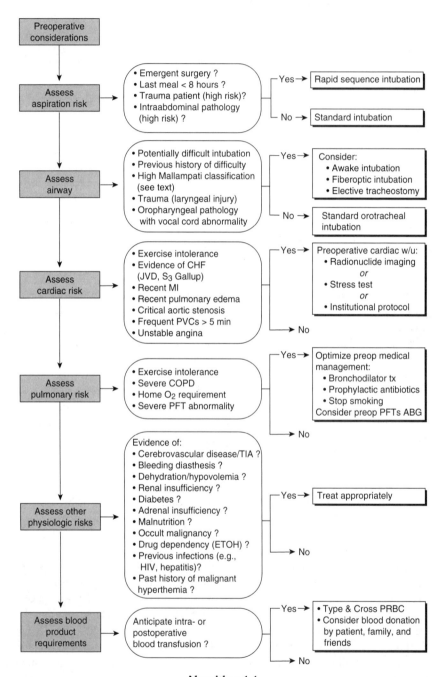

Algorithm 1.1.

REFERENCES

1. James CF. Pulmonary aspiration of gastric contents. In: Gravenstein N, Kirby RR, eds. Complications in Anesthesiology. Philadelphia: Lippincott-Raven, 1996:176.

2. Malignant hyperthermia. In: Gravenstein N, Kirby RR, eds. Complications in Anesthesiology. Philadelphia: Lippincott-Raven, 1996:149.

3. Brownell AKW. Malignant hyperthermia: relationship to other diseases. Br J Anaesth 1988;60:303.

4. Covino BG, Lambert DH. Epidural and spinal anesthesia. In: Barash PG, Cullen BF, Stoelting RK, eds. Clinical Anesthesia. Philadelphia: Lippincott, 1992:815.

5. Dawkins CLM. Anatomy of the complications of extradural and caudal block. Anaesthesia 1969;24:554.

6. Rosenberg H, Fletcher J, Seitman D. Pharmacogenetics. In: Barash PG, Cullen BF, Stoelting RK, eds. Clinical Anesthesia. Philadelphia: Lippincott, 1992:603–605.

7. Mazze RI, Fujinaga M, Wharton RS. Fluid and electrolyte problems. In: Gravenstein N, Kirby RR, eds. Complications in Anesthesiology. Philadelphia: Lippincott-Raven, 1996:470.

8. Covino BG. Pharmacology of local anesthetic agents. In: Rogers MC, Tinker JH, Covino BG, et al., eds. Principles and Practice of Anesthesiology. St. Louis: Mosby–Year Book, 1993:1247–1249.

9. Brown DL. Spinal, epidural, and caudal anesthesia. In: Miller RD, ed. Anesthesia. New York: Churchill Livingstone, 1994:1521.

10. Vandam LD. Complications of spinal and epidural anesthesia. In: Gravenstein N, Kirby RR, eds. Complications in Anesthesiology. Philadelphia: Lippincott-Raven, 1996:567.

11. Benumof JL, Alfrey DD. Anesthesia for thoracic surgery. In: Miller RD, ed. Anesthesia. New York: Churchill Livingstone, 1994:1666–1667.

12. Shapiro BA, Peruzzi WT. Interpretation of blood gases. In: Ayres SM, Grenvik A, Holbrook PR, et al., eds. Textbook of Critical Care. Philadelphia: Saunders, 1995:279.

Wound Healing and Repair

Jason J. Rosenberg and Bruce A. Mast

An explosion of an underground steam line being serviced by a public works crew causes injuries to several people, who are being treated at the local emergency department. Burn and trauma teams are standing by.

The first patient is a 27-year-old construction worker with thermal steam burns over his face, arms, and anterior torso. An appropriate advanced cardiac life support trauma evaluation reveals no other injuries.

What are the functions of normal skin, and how does the initial and short-term care of a patient with burn injury address each function?

The skin serves three primary purposes: fluid maintenance, thermoregulation, and protection against bacterial infections. Disruption of the continuity of the skin, as a result of either trauma or disease, presents several challenges (1). An immediate concern is fluid maintenance. There are several formulas for calculating the size of the burn wound and the method of fluid replacement in the initial phases of burn treatment. In addition, burn patients are hypermetabolic and often hyperthermic as their bodies respond to the stress of injury, so close attention must be paid to thermoregulation throughout healing. Finally, topical antimicrobial treatment is an important part of initial and continued burn care until the body is able to reestablish this important antibacterial barrier (2).

The next patient to arrive has a 6-cm laceration to the anterior left thigh because he was hit by a piece of flying sheet metal. This appears to be his only injury.

How is this injury managed?

The first step in treatment, after a careful total assessment of the patient, is evaluation of the severity of the wound. Full-thickness wounds penetrating the dermis usually require sutures. More superficial wounds confined to the epidermis often heal with local wound care. All wounds heal by a combination of three processes: epithelialization, connective tissue deposition, and contraction. The depth and extent of the wound dictate which process predominates.

Which are the most important types of dermal collagen in wound healing, and what are their functions?
Collagen is a protein that primarily provides structure to the extracellular matrix. To date, 13 genetically distinct types of collagen have been identified, each with the characteristic triple-helix conformation (3). Among these, collagen types I through IV have been studied and their roles in wound healing and tissue repair have been characterized. Types I and III collagen are found primarily in the dermis; type II is associated with hyaline cartilage; and type IV is found in the basement membrane.

Type I collagen, which first appears in the healing wound 72 hours after the injury, is associated with the appearance of mature wound fibroblasts. Type III collagen, the first type to appear in the wound, as early as 24 to 48 hours after injury, is thought to provide the initial framework for healing. Type IV collagen forms the framework of the basement membrane; restoration of the type IV collagen network is a hallmark of normal epidermal wound healing. Type II collagen, which is seen in hyaline cartilage and cartilagelike tissues, acts under the influence of certain bone growth factors to promote bone and cartilaginous healing.

What are the principles of wound closure and what are the surgical options for closing wounds, both traumatic and surgical?
The goal of wound closure regardless of the mechanism of injury is to coapt the skin edges so as to promote normal healing without compromising the blood flow to the injured tissues. Wounds treated within 8 hours can be cleaned and closed surgically, hence heal by primary intention. After this time, bacterial contamination of the wound leads to a high risk of infection if the wound is closed primarily. This type of wound is treated with frequent dressing changes and heals by contraction of the defect. Such wounds are said to heal by secondary intention. Alternatively, delayed primary closure can be employed: A wound that is initially left open (usually because of contamination) is treated with wet-to-dry dressing changes for some period to debride the wound mechanically. When the wound is thought to be suitably clean, the edges are coapted, and the wound is thus closed. If inspection of the wound alone is insufficient to assess contamination, tissue biopsies can reveal the bacterial content. Wounds with fewer than 10^5 organisms per gram of tissue are suitable for closure.

How does contraction occur, and what is its role in wound healing?
Contraction is the process by which the area of an open wound decreases concentrically; it heals from the edges in. This process is thought to be mediated by myofibroblasts, specialized fibroblasts that contain the contractile protein actin

(4). An alternative theory is that the predominant cells in the wound undergoing contraction are quiescent fibroblasts (5) and that contraction occurs as fibroblasts reorganize the extracellular matrix within the wound. Contraction must not be confused with wound contracture, which is the scar deformity resulting from wound and scar contraction across mobile planes. Many contractures are perpendicular to the movement axis of joints, and they impair function (6).

The next patient to arrive is a 67-year-old woman who saw the explosion while driving, ran off the road, and struck a tree. She was wearing a seatbelt. There was severe front-end damage to the car, and the air bags were deployed. An initial trauma evaluation reveals the patient to be persistently hypotensive after fluid challenge, and an ultrasound evaluation demonstrates 250 mL of fluid in the peritoneum. Trauma laparotomy reveals a ruptured spleen, which is removed without complication. The midline fascia is closed with a running prolene suture, and the skin is closed with surgical staples.

What are the four phases of wound healing for this patient?
For descriptive purposes, wound healing comprises four phases—hemostasis, inflammation, proliferation, and remodeling (7). These phases actually occur in a continuum and are not separated temporally.

Hemostasis is achieved through a combination of clot and thrombus formation and reactive vasospasm. Clot formation is also important as a physical barrier to bacterial contamination and fluid loss. A secondary vasodilation, increased capillary permeability, chemoattraction, and activation of leukocytes follow this initial vasoconstriction. Platelets, the first cells to enter the wound, do so during this stage. The alpha granules within the platelets contain cytokines and polypeptide growth factors that promote healing (8).

Inflammation is the second phase in wound healing. Neutrophils are the first leukocytes to enter the wound. They serve several functions: they amplify the inflammatory response via tumor necrosis factor-α and interleukins; they help control local bacterial contamination and prevent infection; and they remove damaged and denatured extracellular matrix components and debride devitalized tissues. The neutrophil response peaks 24 hours after the injury (9). Monocytes, the next cells to enter the wound, are attracted by bacterial products and extracellular matrix breakdown products along with transforming growth factor-β, which is secreted by platelets, neutrophils, and monocytes. These cells amplify and control the immune response. Monocytes are activated into macrophages, which destroy bacteria and further debride the devitalized tissue. Macrophages also provide a prolonged and abundant supply of growth factors, which modulate the healing response. Active macrophages persist in the wound for about 5 days.

Proliferation is predominated by cellular proliferation and extracellular matrix deposition. Fibroblast proliferation at the wound site is followed by collagen and noncollagen matrix protein synthesis and deposition. As collagen is produced within the wound, the healing tissue regains integrity and tensile strength. Angiogenesis also occurs as endothelial cell proliferation coordinates with capillary budding and new blood vessel formation. Epithelial cell migration and proliferation are usually complete at this phase of healing for primarily closed wounds.

Remodeling, the final and longest phase in the wound healing process, entails the dynamic remodeling of collagen and the formation of mature scar. It is this phase that is responsible for the gain in strength of the mature scar because of the structural modification of collagen. Full maturation of a wound may take up to a year as the extracellular matrix is remodeled and as hypercellularity and hypervascularity recede.

What is the role of growth factors in wound healing?
The primary regulatory proteins within wounds are the polypeptide growth factors. More than 20 growth factors that modulate wound healing have been described. These proteins influence one or more of the following:

1. Chemotaxis for various cells important to the healing process
2. Cellular proliferation
3. Matrix protein production
4. Modulation of the inflammatory response
5. Angiogenesis

Growth factors are secreted by a variety of cells throughout the healing process. Furthermore, their activities are multiple and often overlap. For example, transforming growth factor-β is secreted by platelets, macrophages, and fibroblasts. It stimulates fibroblast proliferation and collagen production while inhibiting epithelialization. Fibroblast growth factor is elicited from macrophages and fibroblasts; it stimulates fibroblast proliferation but also promotes angiogenesis. There is a considerable overlap in growth factor source and function within wounds. The predominant source of growth factors is the macrophage; depletion of these cells from the wound results in profound deficiencies in healing.

Which medications impede wound healing, and which phase of healing do they affect?
A number of pharmacologic agents can affect the healing process. Corticosteroids, used commonly in a number of inflammatory disorders, can impair the inflammatory phase of healing (10). Similarly, immunosuppressive drugs used in patients with solid organ transplants can be troublesome. Cytotoxic agents, such as those used in chemotherapy regimens, can impair the proliferative phase of wound healing.

When should the first dressing be changed?
Epithelialization, or reconstitution of the disrupted epithelial covering, occurs
within the first 24 to 48 hours, and therefore the sterile surgical dressing is left
in place for the first 48 hours.

How does age affect wound healing?
A number of well-described changes in healing occur with age. The rate of contraction of open traumatic wounds slows as age increases. The decreased healing rate stems from a variety of factors. Experimental studies have shown that
cellular activity in wounds from older animals is diminished (11). Epithelialization also is slow in the elderly. Connective tissue deposition is similarly retarded.
Blunted fibroblast contractility is implicated in decreasing the contraction rate.
A weak immune response, often seen in the elderly, slows the inflammatory
phase of healing. However, these changes in healing have minimal clinical significance in uncomplicated wounds in otherwise healthy patients.

**On postoperative day 3, the wound edges in the splenectomy patient
are noted to be erythematous, and a small amount of serous fluid is
expressed from the inferior aspect of the wound.**

How should this complication be treated?
The erythema and fluid are hallmarks of a superficial wound infection. The involved portion of the wound should be opened by removing the surgical staples. All collected fluid should be drained, and a sample should be sent to the
laboratory for bacterial culture. An avenue for spontaneous drainage of any un-
seen fluid should also be provided. The underlying fascia should be examined
to rule out fascial dehiscence.

How does bacterial infection affect wound healing?
Bacterial infection delays or reverses healing in two ways: (*a*) by secondary protein degradation within the wound as the result of bacterial proteolytic action
and (*b*) by prolongation of the inflammatory phase. It is important to distinguish between bacterial contamination and infection. Controlled contamination (e.g., with *Staphylococcus aureus*), the presence of bacteria in quantities insufficient to overwhelm the host immune response, may actually accelerate
wound healing. Bacterial infection, which is uniformly detrimental, occurs
when either bacterial count or bacterial virulence overwhelms host defenses.
The bacterial count required to overwhelm host defenses depends on the competency of the host's immune system; elderly and immunocompromised patients are at higher risk than the general population.

How is the wound managed after surgical drainage?
The wound has been converted from a primarily closed wound to one that must
heal by secondary intention. Daily dressing changes are needed to debride the

wound as it granulates. Granulation tissue, which is not seen in primarily closed wounds, is beefy red tissue rich with capillary loops that develop in open healing wounds. Angiogenesis is responsible for the formation of new blood vessels in healing wounds.

What type of dressing should be used for wounds?
The optimal dressing to be used largely depends on the type of wound being treated. An absorbent dressing, such as cotton gauze, is selected for exudative wounds. The goal of this dressing is to prevent bacterial overgrowth and maceration of the tissue. Exudative properties of the wound must be considered during selection of the dressing. Acute wounds are maximally exudative 24 hours after injury, whereas in chronic wounds after debridement, exudation peaks between 48 and 72 hours. Dressings containing calcium alginate are effective for chronic exudative wounds because they absorb many times their mass in fluid.

In less exudative wounds, nonadherent dressings (e.g., commercial gauze impregnated with petroleum jelly or water-based jelly) may be applied to prevent trauma to the healing wound during dressing changes. These dressings should be covered by a second dressing that seals the edges of the nonadherent dressing to prevent the influx of bacteria and protect the surrounding normal skin from maceration.

Wet-to-dry dressings are often used on contaminated wounds. An absorbent dressing such as cotton gauze is moistened with isotonic saline, placed in the wound, and covered with a dry dressing. As the moist dressing dries, it adheres to the wound, and when it is removed, it mechanically debrides the wound. Care must be taken to avoid soaking the dressing and macerating the wound. Furthermore, prolonged debridement removes healing tissue along with contaminants and delays healing.

Occlusive dressings are used for clean, minimally exudative wounds. These dressings are permeable to air and water vapor but not to water and microbes. They not only promote an optimal healing environment for the wound bed but also protect normal skin that surrounds the wound. These dressings are frequently used for skin graft donor sites. Hydrocolloids and gels combine the characteristics of occlusion and absorbency. These gumlike dressings display both wet and dry tack that allows them to adhere to noninjured skin while absorbing exudate. Removal of this type of dressing is atraumatic; these dressings are well suited for use on chronic wounds.

A variety of solutions and substances are applied to wounds to enhance or facilitate healing. Most should be mentioned only to be condemned. Saline is useful, as mentioned previously, with wet-to-dry dressings to facilitate debridement. Mild acetic acid is used with frequent dressing changes in wounds superficially infected with *Pseudomonas*. However, other solutions may hinder healing. Dakin's solution has been shown to kill fibroblasts, impair neutrophil migration, and impair wound healing in experimental models. Similarly, Betadine can actually increase the likelihood of infection and delay healing by damaging normal wound cells. Its use in contaminated wounds should be for a limited duration in selective circumstances.

How does angiogenesis occur?
Angiogenesis leads to the formation of new blood vessels in healing tissues. Both direct and indirect factors guide this process. Direct factors act on endothelial cell migration and/or proliferation. These include β-fibroblast growth factor, α-fibroblast growth factor, transforming growth factor-α, and tumor necrosis factor-α. Indirect factors, such as transforming growth factor-α, platelet-derived growth factor, vascular endothelial growth and prostaglandins exert their actions via recruitment of cellular components that release direct angiogenic factors. New blood vessel formation is directed at the region of the wound with the lowest oxygen tension (12, 13).

How strong is scar tissue relative to uninjured tissue?
Although the amount of collagen deposited in the wound after an injury may approximate or even exceed that of normal skin, the healing wound is unable to regenerate a completely normal organization of collagen. Even though the strength of scar tissue never equals that of undamaged skin, under normal circumstances, approximately 3 months after injury the tensile strength of the wound reaches 80% of its preinjury state (14).

What systemic conditions most frequently impair wound healing?
The systemic conditions that most frequently hinder wound healing are bacterial infection, malnutrition, diabetes, peripheral vascular disease, and tissue irradiation.

How does malnutrition affect wound healing?
Malnutrition, commonly seen in cancer patients, impairs the ability of the body to synthesize and deposit connective tissue during proliferative healing. Accompanying deficiencies in vitamins and trace elements can impair various stages of healing. Absence of vitamin C results in abnormal amino acid sequence in procollagen, so that the molecules are rapidly degraded within the cell. Minerals are required for proper cross-linking of collagen during the remodeling phase.

How does irradiation affect wound healing?
Tissue irradiation has several effects on healing. Acute radiation changes include erythema, inflammation, edema, desquamation, and ulceration, which make the tissues difficult to handle surgically. The chronic effects include changes in

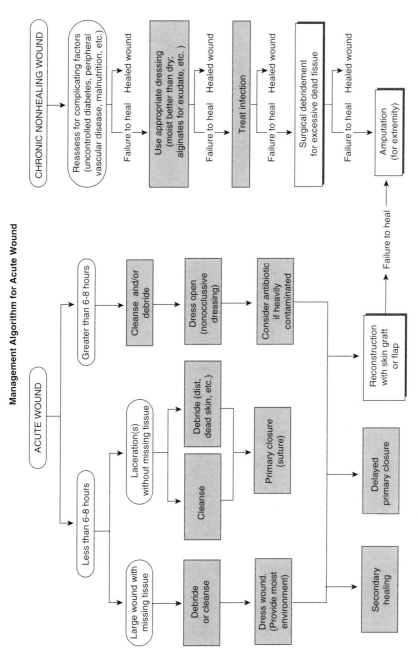

Algorithm 2.1.

pigmentation, atrophy of the epithelium and dermis, decreased local vascularity associated with fibrosis, telangiectasia, sebaceous and sweat gland dysfunction, and necrosis and neoplasia. Together, these effects of radiation decrease oxygen in the wound bed, impair angiogenesis, increase susceptibility to infection, and diminish deposition of extracellular matrix.

Why is wound healing impaired in diabetic patients?
Diabetic patients have impaired sensation, usually seen in the stocking-glove distribution as a result of diabetic neuropathy. This decreased sensation leads to repeated minor trauma that is often not detected by the patient. The impairment of immune response in diabetic patients reduces the ability to fight infection and respond appropriately during the inflammatory phase of wound healing. These patients also have poor connective tissue deposition. A confounding variable in diabetes is the coexistence of peripheral vascular disease. Vascular examination is indicated to distinguish an ischemic wound from a diabetic wound. Ischemic wounds result from deficient oxygen delivery and unavailability of metabolic substrates to support cellular activity; they can be recognized by the absence of palpable pulses in the affected extremities. In contrast to a diabetic wound without a vascular component, an ischemic wound may heal solely after a revascularization procedure.

REFERENCES

1. Mast BA, Cohen IK. Normal wound healing. In: Achauer BM, Eriksson EF, Guyuron B, et al., eds. Plastic Surgery: Indications, Operations, Outcomes. Mosby–Year Book, in press.
2. Sabiston DC, ed. Textbook of Surgery: The Biological Basis of Modern Surgical Practice. 14th ed. Philadelphia: Saunders, 1991.
3. Peacock EE. Collagenolysis: the other side of the equation. World J Surg 1980;4: 297–302.
4. Andersen L, Attstrom R, Feferskov O. Effect of experimental neutropenia on oral wound healing in guinea pigs. Scand J Dent Res 1978;86:237–247.
5. Simpson DM, Ross R. The neutrophilic leukocyte in wound repair: a study with anti-neutrophilic serum. J Clin Invest 1972;51:2009–2023.
6. Knighton DR, Hunt TK, Scheunstuhl H, et al. Oxygen tension regulates expression of angiogenesis factor by macrophages. Science 1983;221:1283–1285.
7. Mast BA. Healing in other tissues. Surg Clin North Am 1997;77:529–547.
8. Jackson DS. Development of fibrosis: cell proliferation and collagen formation in rats and rabbits. Acta Chir Scand 1963;126:187–196.
9. Ruberg RL. Role of nutrition in wound healing. Surg Clin North Am 1984;64: 705–714.
10. Wahl LM, Wahl SM. Inflammation. In: Cohen IK, Diegelmann RF, Lindblad WJ, eds. Wound Healing: Biochemical and Clinical Aspects. Philadelphia: Saunders, 1992: 40–62.
11. Mast BA. The skin. In: Cohen IK, Diegelmann RF, Lindblad WJ, eds. Wound Heal-

ing: Biochemical and Clinical Aspects. Philadelphia: Saunders, 1993:344–355.

12. Phillips C, Wenstrup RJ. Biosynthetic and genetic disorders of collagen. In: Cohen IK, Diegelmann RF, Lindblad WJ, eds. Wound Healing: Biochemical and Clinical Aspects. Philadelphia: Saunders, 1993:152–176.

13. Stenenson TR, Mathes SJ. Wound healing. In: Miller TA, Towland BJ, eds. Physiologic basis of modern surgical care. St. Louis: Mosby, 1988:1010–1013.

14. Diegelmann RF, Rothkipf LC, Cohen IK. Measurement of collagen biosynthesis during wound healing. J Surg Res 1975;19:239–243.

CHAPTER
3

Breast Cancer

Andrew W.J. McFadden

Mrs. Murphy is a healthy 55-year-old woman who has a cluster of microcalcifications on her annual screening mammogram. She is advised to have a biopsy. Mrs. Murphy has no previous breast problems. She is past menopause and has no breast symptoms. On physical examination there is no lymphadenopathy, and her breasts are normal.

What are the mammographic signs of malignancy?
Mammographic signs of malignancy include stellate or dominant masses, architectural distortion, and skin or nipple thickening or retraction. Some types of microcalcifications are also associated with malignancy. The size, shape, number, density, and extent of microcalcifications help to determine the risk of a malignancy being present.

How is it determined that Mrs. Murphy needs a biopsy?
To this point in Mrs. Murphy's care, all that exists is a radiologic finding; more information is needed. Previous mammograms should be compared. Additional coned or compression mammograms may be needed to define the calcifications. It also is very important to discuss the findings with the radiologist. The American College of Radiology has proposed a classification system to help management decisions. Not all radiologists use this system, but consulting with the radiologist should help to classify the risk. If there is any doubt, the opinion of a second radiologist should be obtained (1).

After review of the mammograms, the radiologist believes Mrs. Murphy's abnormality is new and moderately suspicious.

What is the best way to sample this lesion for biopsy?
Because this lesion is not palpable, the physician must continue to consult with the radiologist. The standard biopsy technique for such a lesion is a wire-localized breast biopsy. The radiologist places a long wire through the skin to the microcalcifications, using stereotactic guidance. During surgery, the wire is followed to the lesion; then a wide excision is done around the tip of the wire. To ensure that

24

the microcalcifications are in the specimen, a radiograph of the specimen is taken. The procedure is complete only after the calcifications in the specimen are seen to be the same as those in the mammogram (2).

What is the role of stereotactic core biopsy?
Stereotactic core biopsy is a new technique. As with wire placement, stereotactic guidance is used with biopsy to take tissue samples with large-gauge needles. The technique is most accurate if the mammographic abnormality is a mass; it has a higher false-negative rate when used to diagnose calcifications. The overall false-negative rate is not yet known; therefore, if the findings are benign, the woman must be followed carefully (3).

Mrs. Murphy undergoes a stereotactic core biopsy. The pathologist confirms the presence of the microcalcifications in the specimen and makes a diagnosis of ductal carcinoma in situ (DCIS).

What is DCIS?
Almost 30% of breast neoplasms diagnosed by mammography are DCIS, a precancerous lesion characterized by malignant cells in the ducts but showing no evidence of invasion through the basement membrane. However, these lesions may progress to invade the basement membrane. It is thought that if untreated, 20 to 30% of these patients develop invasive ductal carcinoma. This is a demanding diagnosis for the pathologist. As many as 10% of these lesions may be reclassified as benign or malignant on review by a second pathologist (4).

Does this patient need any other procedures?
Only a biopsy has been performed up to this point. Invasive cancer is found in 30% of microcalcific lesions after excision; therefore, this patient should have a wire-localized excisional biopsy.

Mrs. Murphy undergoes an excisional biopsy. The final pathology indicates there is a single focus of DCIS smaller than 1 cm. It is completely excised.

Does Mrs. Murphy require any further treatment? Does she need an axillary node dissection?
Without further treatment, 2.6% of cases of DCIS recur per year; 50% of these recurrences are invasive. Death among patients with recurrent DCIS is very unusual. The addition of radiotherapy may reduce the rate of recurrence to 1.3% per year. Mastectomy is the other option to reduce the rate of recurrence. This can be a very difficult choice for a woman. To help make this decision, review and consultation by radiologists, oncologists, and plastic surgeons may provide further information.

As for the role of axillary node dissection, fewer than 1% of axillary node dissections performed for DCIS show metastatic disease. Obviously, in these cases, an area of invasion was not seen by the pathologist. Axillary node dissection is not recommended for the treatment of patients with DCIS.

Mrs. Gaudet is 60-year-old woman with a 4-month history of a left breast mass that is asymptomatic. During this time, the mass has enlarged. She is otherwise healthy, and a review of systems does not reveal any concerns. She has never had a mammogram. On examination, there is no supraclavicular or infraclavicular lymphadenopathy. With the patient sitting with her hands above her head, a skin retraction at the upper outer quadrant is clearly visible. Palpation of the left breast reveals a 2-cm irregular, partially mobile mass in the same quadrant. There also are several enlarged nodes in the left axilla.

What is the differential diagnosis of this lump?
Breast cancer is a disease of aging. The risk of developing breast cancer between the ages of 20 and 30 years is 0.04%. The risk of developing breast cancer at age 65 to 75 years is 3.2%. A woman who lives 110 years has a 10% risk of developing breast cancer. Therefore, as a woman ages, the likelihood of a new breast mass being cancer increases. This means the differential diagnosis varies among age groups. For women older than 50 years, this mass may be a malignancy, fibrocystic change (especially if she is taking hormone replacement therapy), or fat necrosis (5).

How should the physician proceed to a diagnosis?
A diagnostic mammogram would be useful. This provides more information about the characteristics of the mass and any other suspicious lesions, and it allows evaluation of the contralateral breast.

What should be done if the mammogram does not show a mass?
"A suspicious lump is a suspicious lump" until there is a histologic diagnosis. Mammograms miss 10 to 15% of cancers. Options for obtaining tissue for diagnosis are a fine-needle aspiration biopsy (FNAB), a core biopsy, and an open biopsy. FNAB is an excellent first test. Interpreting the result requires a pathologist skilled in cytology. The final pathology should provide a reasonable explanation for the mass; unfortunately, a diagnosis of benignancy does not rule out cancer.

Mrs. Gaudet undergoes FNAB, and the cytologist reports finding atypical cells suspicious for malignancy.

How should Mrs. Gaudet now be treated?
At this point there still is no diagnosis. A repeat FNAB or open biopsy should now be performed. If an open biopsy is performed, a rim of normal tissue

should be excised around the mass to obtain pathologically negative margins. If the cancer is completely excised, there may be no need for further surgical treatment of the primary lesion.

Mrs. Gaudet undergoes an excisional biopsy. The finding is invasive ductal cancer, 1.8 cm when completely excised.

If the lesion is completely excised, is any further treatment necessary?
There are two main issues in the treatment of breast cancer: local control and treatment of systemic disease. Local recurrence rates after lumpectomy alone approach 30%. The best local control of this cancer is obtained by the addition of radiotherapy to the affected breast or by a mastectomy. The mortality related to breast cancer is the same after either of these options; deaths occur because of metastatic disease. Therefore, physicians must try to determine who is at greatest risk for developing or harboring metastasis, which is called staging the disease (6).

The TNM (tumor, nodes, metastasis) system is the standard staging system for breast cancer (Table 3.1). The size of Mrs. Gaudet's tumor is now known. A thorough history and physical examination combined with a chest radiograph stages the patient for metastasis, but there is no information about the lymph node status. This requires an axillary node biopsy as a separate operation or as part of a modified radical mastectomy.

So what exactly are the options available to Mrs. Gaudet?
Mrs. Gaudet may choose to do nothing. This choice is associated with the highest local recurrence rate. The decision to give adjuvant or postoperative chemotherapy is very much based on the tumor status of the lymph nodes. If Mrs. Gaudet does not have an axillary node dissection, she may be denying herself the

Table 3.1.   TNM STAGING FOR BREAST CANCER

Stage	Tumor	Nodes (regional)	Metastasis
0	in situ	No metastasis	None
I	<2 cm	No metastasis	None
II	≤2 cm	Moveable ipsilateral	None
	2–5 cm	No metastasis or movable ipsilateral	None
	>5 cm	No metastasis	None
III	Any size	Fixed ipsilateral or internal mammary	None
	Direct invasion of chest wall or skin	Any	None
IV	Any tumor	Any	Distant metastasis

benefits of this chemotherapy. The addition of radiotherapy to the affected breast reduces local recurrence rates about as much as a mastectomy, but again there is no information about the status of her lymph nodes. The ideal choice is axillary node dissection with radiation therapy or modified radical mastectomy.

Mrs. Gaudet chooses to have a modified radical mastectomy.

What are the anatomic landmarks used in a mastectomy?
The breast sits on the anterior chest wall lateral to the sternum and extending to the mid-axillary line. The tail of Spence is an extension of the breast to the axilla. In the vertical axis, the breast extends from the second to the sixth ribs.

A modified radical mastectomy entails an axillary node dissection. What is the rationale for this, and what are the surgical principles for this part of the operation?
The axilla is the site of the main lymph node basin draining the breast. The status of the lymph nodes is one of the principle factors of staging patients with breast cancer. At least 10 lymph nodes are needed to make sure nodal metastasis are not missed. The axilla has level I, level II, and level III nodes that are lateral to, under, and medial to the pectoralis minor muscle, respectively. The standard operation is dissection and removal of level I and II lymph nodes.

What anatomic structures are at risk with this operation?
The operation entails the dissection and identification of the axillary vein, which may sustain damage. The major risk is to adjacent nerves. The intercostal brachial nerve is a sensory nerve to the posteromedial aspect of the upper arm. It is frequently damaged, and patients may have postoperative pain or numbness. The long thoracic nerve lies on the chest wall and innervates the serratus anterior muscle. Damage to this nerve results in a winged scapula. Finally, the thoracodorsal nerve can be damaged, resulting in weakness in the latissimus dorsi muscle.

What complications may occur?
Early complications include skin flap necrosis, bleeding, and infection. Long-term complications include numbness and pain, shoulder stiffness, and lymphedema.

Mrs. Gaudet undergoes an uneventful operation. The final pathology does not show any residual tumor. Of 20 lymph nodes, 3 are positive for metastasis. The pathologist also determines that the tumor is estrogen receptor positive.

Should Mrs. Gaudet receive adjuvant chemotherapy?
Mrs. Gaudet is past menopause and has an estrogen receptor–positive tumor and node-positive disease. Therefore, she has a 50 to 60% chance of develop-

ing metastatic disease. The recommendation is that she begin a 5-year course of tamoxifen, an antiestrogen drug.

If Mrs. Gaudet were still menstruating, what would be her adjuvant therapy?
The recommendations for adjuvant chemotherapy depend on menopausal status and the patient's risk of recurrence (7). The risk of recurrence is categorized as low, intermediate, or high according to the size and grade of the tumor, the presence or absence of estrogen receptors, and any lymphatic or vascular invasion. The expression of many new prognostic markers, such as p53 and erb-2, are being studied, but few have yet been used prospectively to treat patients. If Mrs. Gaudet were still menstruating, she would be offered multiagent chemotherapy. There are two recommended regimens; Mrs. Gaudet should have either six cycles of cyclophosphamide, methotrexate, and 5-fluorouracil (CMF) or four cycles of doxorubicin (Adriamycin) and cyclophosphamide (AC).

Mrs. Gaudet's 35-year-old daughter, Marie Gaudet, attends your clinic. She is worried about her risk of developing breast cancer. Findings of a complete history and physical examination are normal. A thorough review of the family history determines that Mrs. Gaudet's sister was diagnosed with breast cancer at age 45 years, and Mrs. Gaudet's mother died of breast cancer at age 40 years.

What percentage of breast cancers are inherited?
As many as 5 to 10% of breast cancers may be inherited. Breast cancer may be divided into three categories:

1. Sporadic (no relatives with breast cancer for two generations)
2. Familial (breast cancer in one or more first- or second-degree relatives
3. Hereditary (the same as familial but the cancers occur at a younger age, are frequently bilateral, are associated with other primary tumors, and appear to inherited in an autosomal dominant pattern)

What hereditary syndromes are associated with an increased risk of breast cancer?
The BRAC1 gene, or hereditary breast–ovary cancer syndrome, may account for 40 to 50% of hereditary breast cancer. As many of 80% of women who inherit this gene develop breast cancer, and 40% develop ovarian cancer. The BRAC2 gene has also been identified with an increased risk of breast cancer. Other less common syndromes include Li-Fraumeni syndrome, ataxia, telangiectasia, Cowden's disease, and Bloom's syndrome.

How should the physician deal with Ms. Gaudet's problem?
Ms. Gaudet should be offered genetic testing. Although testing for BRAC1 and BRAC2 is commercially available, it should not be done as a blood test. Genetic

counseling before and after such testing is required. It is possible that Ms. Gaudet will refuse testing after considering many of the social and ethical problems that arise with a positive test.

Ms. Gaudet goes for genetic counseling and testing and is found to be positive for the BRAC1 gene. She returns to discuss a plan of management.

What options are available to Ms. Gaudet?
Intense follow-up and prophylactic mastectomy are the two choices. Follow-up entails biannual physical examinations and annual mammograms beginning immediately for Ms. Gaudet, who is 35 years old (annual mammograms start at age 20 years for BRAC1-positive women). Also, because of the risk of ovarian cancer, screening pelvic and transvaginal ultrasounds are used. There is no evidence that this protocol reduces cancer deaths in this group of patients. Studies are needed to determine the best method of follow-up.

Intuitively, prophylactic mastectomy should reduce the risk of cancer because the breast tissue is removed, and there is some scientific evidence to support this. However, a mastectomy is able to remove only approximately 90% of breast tissue, and some degree of risk remains. Surveys of women who have had this operation performed report a very high rate of dissatisfaction. The best management plan has not yet been determined, but careful communication with geneticists and early involvement of a plastic surgeon is advisable (8).

Ms. Cromwell is a 25-year-old woman with painful breasts. She is a jogger, and it has become difficult for her to run. On examination, both breasts are found to be tender, particularly in the upper outer quadrants. Both breasts are nodular and firm. There is no lymphadenopathy.

What is fibrocystic change of the breast?
Fibrocystic change is a benign process that is present to some degree in all women. It is usually asymptomatic, but women may notice breast nodules or have mastalgia or nipple discharge. Biopsies may show cysts, fibrosis, sclerosing adenosis, or epithelial hyperplasia (Table 3.2).

What other information is needed to manage Ms. Cromwell's case?
More information about the characteristics of the pain is needed. For example, is the pain related to her menstrual cycle, or is it cyclic? The physician should elicit any history of trauma and identify aggravating and relieving factors, such as movement.

Table 3.2. DIFFERENTIAL DIAGNOSIS OF BREAST PAIN

True Breast Pain
  Cyclical
  Noncyclical trigger spot
Musculoskeletal
  Tietze's syndrome
  Cervical root syndrome
  Rib injury
  Thoracic spine osteoarthritis
Inflammatory
  Breast abscess
  Mammary duct ectasia
Miscellaneous
  Pregnancy
  Mondor's syndrome
  Trauma
  Psychologic
  Psychosexual
Breast Cancer
  5% have pain
  0.5% of patients with breast pain have cancer

Ms. Cromwell describes the pain as a dull, achy pain that is at its worst 7 to 10 days prior to menses. At that time, the pain radiates into her axilla. There is no history of trauma. Anything that causes pressure or movement of her breast is uncomfortable.

How should the physician proceed?
It is important to determine why Ms. Cromwell has now sought medical attention. Many patients worry that pain is a sign of cancer. Although 5 to 10% of patients with cancer have breast pain, only 0.5% of patients with reported breast pain have cancer. In women older than 35 years, a mammogram may be suggested to rule out a mass. There is spontaneous resolution of the pain in 20 to 50% of patients; 10 to 20% of women seek further help (9).

What is the treatment of this pain?
For the majority of women, simple reassurance is all that is needed. First-line treatment is analgesics and heat. Reduction in caffeine intake and dietary fat may be beneficial. Evening primrose oil is a dietary supplement that has been found to be effective. Hormone agonists (e.g., danazol) and antagonists (e.g., tamoxifen) are effective but have a significant number of side effects. These agents should be reserved for unresponsive patients and those with severe pain.

Is mastectomy an option for patients with intractable pain?
Surgery does not guarantee relief of pain. Many patients continue to have pain; painful scars may develop; and the end result may be dissatisfying. Surgery is not recommended as a treatment for mastalgia.

Mrs. Gomez is a 30-year-old mother of a 5-year-old boy. She has a 2-month history of bloody discharge from her right nipple. She notices some blood on her nightgown every morning and is able to express a small amount of blood. She does monthly breast examinations and has not noticed any masses. There is no family history of breast cancer. Physical examination reveals no masses, and the physician cannot express any blood from the nipple.

How can the diagnosis be confirmed?
The first step is to ask Mrs. Gomez to try to express blood. If she is unable to do so, she should be asked not to examine herself for a few days, and a return appointment should be arranged. The hope is that sufficient blood will accumulate to demonstrate the problem.

Mrs. Gomez returns a week later, and the physician is able to express blood from a duct at the 2 o'clock position on the right breast.

What investigations are indicated?
The obvious concern is that there is cancer. Other causes of bloody discharge include ductal papilloma, Paget's disease of the nipple, and fibrocystic change (Table 3.3). Mammography may identify an occult mass and therefore is the best first test. A galactogram may identify a lesion in the duct. This is done by cannulation of the affected duct and injection of contrast.

Mrs. Gomez has a normal mammogram, but a galactogram reveals a small growth consistent with a duct papilloma.

What is a papilloma?
A papilloma is a benign lesion; however, the problem is that 0.5% of these lesions are papillary cancers. The association of a breast mass and calcifications constitute a stronger indication of cancer. Excisional biopsy of the affected duct is the next best investigation and is also the treatment for this problem in the majority of women.

Mrs. Smith is a 52-year-old woman who is referred to surgery because of a breast abscess. Mrs. Smith has noticed that her left breast gradually has enlarged and become uncomfortable during the past month. The breast became red and mildly tender 2 weeks ago. She sought

Table 3.3.   CAUSES OF NIPPLE DISCHARGE

Bloodstained
  Duct papilloma
  Intraduct cancer (30%)
  Paget's disease of nipple
  Fibrocystic change
Serous
  Duct hyperplasia
  Cancer
  Pregnancy
Greenish-brown
  Mammary duct ectasia
  Fibrocystic change
Purulent
  Breast abscess
Creamy
  Duct ectasia
Milky
  Postlactation
  Drug induced (O.C.P.)
  Prolactinoma

medical attention and was prescribed antibiotics. Despite this treatment, the problem has become worse.

During examination, the patient is afebrile. Her left breast is obviously very much enlarged. The skin over the breast is red, tense, and dimpled. No discrete mass can be identified. There is no lymphadenopathy.

Why have the antibiotics not worked?
The bacteria associated with breast abscesses in Mrs. Smith's age group differ from those associated with lactation, and they may be caused by gram-negative anaerobes. Therefore, it is possible that the wrong antibiotics were chosen. It also is possible that the abscess will need surgical drainage. The diagnosis also may be wrong. Mrs. Smith has the classic features of an inflammatory carcinoma of the breast.

How can a diagnosis be determined for Mrs. Smith?
Mrs. Smith should have an immediate breast ultrasound to look for an abscess.

An ultrasound is done, and no abscess is seen.

Management Algorithm for Image Guided Biopsies

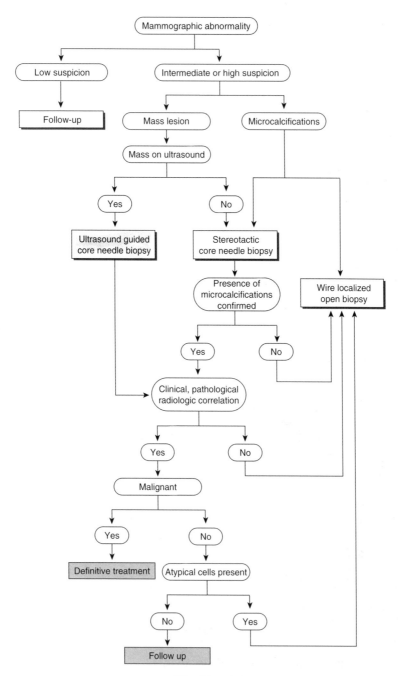

Algorithm 3.1.

Management Algorithm for Breast Cancer - Adjuvant Chemotherapy

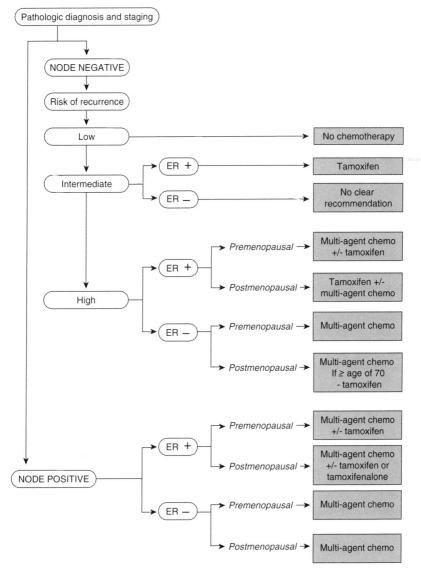

Note: (1) Risk: There is no perfect model to define the risk of recurrence based on primary tumor factors. Currently used factors include: size, lymphatic or vascular invasion, histologic and nuclear grade, and estrogen receptor status. Many other such as p52 or c-erB-2 expression are being investigated.

(2) Multi-agent chemotherapy: The standard regimens are: 6 cycles—cyclophosphamide, methotrexate, and 5-fluorouracil or 4 cycles—adriamycin and cyclophosphamide.

Algorithm 3.2.

Should the antibiotics be changed?
No. Mrs. Smith should have a mammogram.

What is inflammatory cancer of the breast?
Inflammatory cancer of the breast is the most aggressive form of breast cancer.
It accounts for 1 to 3% of breast cancers. The classic presentation is an enlarging breast, erythema, and skin edema resulting in characteristic dimpling of the skin resembling the skin of an orange (peau d'orange). In most cases, the cancer is widely infiltrating, so that no mass is palpable. Invasion of the dermal lymphatics is common.

It is very important to make a quick diagnosis and not delay treatment any further. A mammogram may show a mass or demonstrate the extent of infiltration. A punch biopsy of affected skin and a core biopsy of the breast should be sufficient for diagnosis, but if there is any doubt, an incisional biopsy should be performed.

Mrs. Smith's skin biopsy does not show invasion of the dermal lymphatics, but the core biopsy of the breast reveals a poorly differentiated adenocarcinoma.

Does the negative skin biopsy mean this is not an inflammatory carcinoma?
No. Inflammatory carcinoma is a constellation of clinical signs associated with an aggressive breast cancer. Mrs. Smith has those clinical signs and now has a biopsy finding of cancer.

Should Mrs. Smith be scheduled for surgery?
Inflammatory carcinoma of the breast is not treated with surgery, at least not at first. Historically, when surgery or radiation therapy or both were the primary treatments, the local recurrence rates were 50 to 80%, and metastasis occurred in more than 90% of patients. Multiagent chemotherapy is now the first treatment of choice, followed by radiation and surgery. This change in management has reduced local recurrence rates to 10 to 20% and has improved 5-year survival from 5 to 50% (10). Mrs. Smith should be sent to a medical oncologist to begin treatment.

REFERENCES

1. Clinical practice guidelines for the care and treatment of breast cancer. Can Med Assoc J 1998;158(3 Suppl).
2. D'Orsi C, Kopans DB. Mammography interpretation: the BI-RADS method. Am Fam Phys 1997;55:1548–1552.
3. Liberman L, et al. Analysis of cancers not diagnosed at stereotactic core breast biopsy. Radiology 1997;203:151–157.

4. Eusebi V, Feudale E, Foschini M, et al. Long-term follow-up of in situ carcinoma of the breast. Semin Diagn Pathol 1994;11:223.
5. Henderson IC. Risk factors for breast cancer development. Cancer 1993;71(Suppl): 2127.
6. Fisher B, Anderson S, Redmond CK, et al. Reanalysis and results after 12 years of follow-up in a randomized clinical trial comparing total mastectomy with lumpectomy with or without irradiation in the treatment of breast cancer. N Engl J Med 1995; 333:1456.
7. Early Breast Cancer Trialists Collaborative Group. Systemic treatment of early breast cancer by hormonal, cytotoxic, or immune therapy: 133 randomized trials involving 31,000 recurrences and 24,000 deaths among 75,000 women. Lancet 1992;339:1–15.
8. Lynch HT, Lynch JF. Breast cancer genetics: family history, heterogeneity, molecular genetic diagnosis and genetic counseling. Curr Probl Cancer 1996;20:329–365.
9. Klimberg VS. Etiology and management of breast pain. In: Harris JR, ed. Diseases of the breast. Philadelphia: Lippincott-Raven, 1996:99–106.
10. Buzdar AU, Singletary E, Booser DJ, et al. Combined modality treatment of stage III and inflammatory breast cancer. Surg Oncol Clin North Am 1995;4:715–734.

Thyroid and Parathyroid Disease

Nicholas P.W. Coe

THYROID DISEASE

Patricia Arnold is a 35-year-old woman with an asymptomatic neck mass, which she first noticed 3 weeks ago. Her history is unremarkable except for childhood tonsillectomy and adenoidectomy. She is taking birth control pills and has no known drug allergies. A family history reveals that a maternal aunt had Graves' disease; no other members had thyroid disease. The patient has a 20-pack-year smoking history and has one to two alcoholic drinks per week. A review of various other systems does not reveal any significant findings.

The physical examination reveals a healthy-looking woman in no acute distress. Her vital signs are normal: temperature, 36.5°C; blood pressure, 135/70 mm Hg; pulse rate 80 beats per minute; respiratory rate, 18 breaths per minute. The head and neck examination reveals no exophthalmos, lid lag, or intraoral lesions; the neck mass is not associated with any cervical adenopathy. The lungs are clear to auscultation; the heart rate and rhythm are regular and without murmurs; and the abdominal examination is normal. Neurologic function is intact, and findings are nonfocal.

What is the differential diagnosis for a neck mass?
Approximately 50% of neck masses that persist beyond 3 to 4 weeks originate from the thyroid gland. Inflammatory lesions, nonthyroidal malignant lesions, and congenital lesions account for the remaining 50%. Malignant lesions, such as lymphoma, carcinoma of the thyroid, and metastatic tumor from another head and neck site, are most common in adults, whereas inflammatory lesions are most common in children. Congenital lesions, such as thyroglossal duct and branchial cleft cysts, are also very common in children.

The 3-cm mass, which appears to be originating from the right thyroid lobe, is firm and not tender. There is no associated fever, chills, pressure, or symptoms of thyrotoxicity.

What are the symptoms of thyrotoxicity?
Heat intolerance, weight loss with increased appetite, tachycardia (sleeping pulse rate faster than 80 beats per minute), atrial arrhythmias, congestive heart failure (especially in the elderly), hyperkinetic behavior, emotional instability, insomnia, fatigue, muscle weakness, amenorrhea, and diarrhea are all symptoms of thyrotoxicity.

What does thyroid mean and where is the thyroid gland?
The word thyroid is derived from the Greek *thyreos,* or shield. The thyroid gland originates from two sites. The tuberculum impar at the base of the vallate papillae of the tongue forms the foramen cecum. The thyroid tissue descends into the neck along the line of the thyroglossal duct. The lateral component, which contributes the calcitonin-producing C cells, is derived from the fourth pharyngeal pouch.

The mature thyroid gland, which weighs about 20 g, drapes over the anterolateral aspect of the upper trachea just below the cricoid cartilage. The two lobes, connected by the isthmus, lie along the sides of the larynx and trachea, extending up to the level of the middle of the thyroid cartilage. The pyramidal lobe is a diverticulum extending upward from the isthmus. These lobes are between the trachea medially and the carotid sheaths and sternocleidomastoid muscles laterally; the strap muscles lie anterior to the thyroid lobes. The parathyroid glands and the recurrent laryngeal nerves are on the posterior surface of the lateral lobes of the thyroid gland. The nerves are typically found in the tracheoesophageal groove. A thin, fibrous capsule surrounds the thyroid gland.

What are the risk factors for thyroid malignancy?
A careful personal and family history helps determine whether a patient has any special risk factors for thyroid malignancy. Low-dose radiation exposure (300 to 1000 cGy) is associated with well-differentiated thyroid cancer (1). Low doses of radiation were commonly used between 1945 and 1955 to treat an enlarged thymus. Radiation was also used from the 1930s to the 1960s to treat diseases such as ringworm, keloids, capillary hemangiomata, and tubercular lymphadenopathy. In more recent times, exposure to radiation from the Chernobyl nuclear accident in April 1986 placed residents of the Ukraine, the Gomel region of Belorussia, and possibly other widespread areas of central Europe at high risk for developing thyroid malignancy.

A higher incidence of malignancy is also found in patients younger than 20 years, patients older than 60 years, and men than in the general population. A family history of thyroid disease is often present, especially in female relatives; this has little bearing on the treatment of the patient, but the possibility of the familial form of thyroid carcinoma should always be kept in mind.

Significant findings on physical examination include a mass with poorly defined borders, cervical adenopathy adjacent to the thyroid or in the posterior triangle, fixation of the gland, and vocal cord paralysis.

How should a thyroid mass be evaluated?
The main features that have to be determined are (*a*) whether the mass is malignant and (*b*) whether it is hyperfunctioning.

If a patient has no symptoms or signs of thyrotoxicosis, the simplest and most economical way to begin the workup is to determine the thyroid-stimulating hormone (TSH) level and obtain a fine-needle aspirate (FNA) of the thyroid with a 21- to 25-gauge needle. If the TSH level is normal, the patient is not likely to be thyrotoxic; if there is any doubt, thyroxine (T_4) and triiodothyronine (T_3) levels should be determined. Ultrasonography may be helpful in a patient whose neck is difficult to examine, but ultrasonography has largely been superseded by FNA for distinguishing between cystic and solid lesions. Radioactive scanning with ^{123}I- or ^{99m}Tc-labeled compounds can differentiate between cold lesions (those with low or no radioisotope uptake), warm lesions (those that take up the radioisotope but show no evidence of thyrotoxicosis), and hot lesions (those that concentrate the isotope to a greater degree than the remaining thyroid). Cold lesions should raise suspicion of malignancy and should always be evaluated with FNA. Warm and hot lesions are only rarely malignant.

What are the advantages and disadvantages of needle biopsy in the evaluation of a thyroid nodule?
FNA biopsy is safe, fast, sensitive, and cost effective, and it can be performed on an outpatient basis. Papillary, medullary, and anaplastic carcinomas can be diagnosed with this method. Certain elements, such as atypia and a microfollicular pattern, suggest malignancy, whereas a macrofollicular pattern or abundant colloid is more consistent with a benign lesion. However, this technique does not allow differentiation between malignant and benign follicular tumors because the distinction is made on the basis of vascular and/or capsular invasion, features that cannot be determined from an FNA.

What is the therapeutic approach if the FNA indicates that the lesion is benign?
If an experienced thyroid cytopathologist considers the aspirate to be benign, the patient should be treated with suppressive doses of L-thyroxine, and the biopsy should be repeated in 3 to 6 months.

What is the mechanism of thyroxine suppression?
The activity of the thyroid gland is regulated by the central nervous system and by the serum level of iodine. The hypothalamus secretes thyrotropin-releasing

hormone, which stimulates the anterior pituitary gland to release TSH (also known as thyrotropin). TSH stimulates the production and release of thyroid hormone and induces hyperplasia and vascularity of the thyroid gland. Secretion of TSH is inhibited by the negative feedback effect of the exogenous thyroid hormone. Oral L-thyroxine should therefore be given in doses sufficient to suppress TSH to barely detectable levels. This decrease in TSH may shrink the lesion.

How is thyroid hormone formed?
The principal function of the thyroid gland is to produce thyroid hormone, which regulates cellular metabolism. The production of thyroid hormone depends on dietary iodine, which is actively transported from the plasma into the thyroid, where it is oxidized and rapidly incorporated into a macromolecule, thyroglobulin. Tyrosine molecules are iodinated at one (monoiodotyrosine) or two (diiodotyrosine) sites, and these are subsequently coupled to form T_3 and T_4. Hydrolysis of thyroglobulin releases T_3 and T_4 into the circulation, but thyroglobulin is not released except in disease states (Figure 4.1). The active thyroid hormones attach to a plasma protein, thyroxine-binding globulin. In the

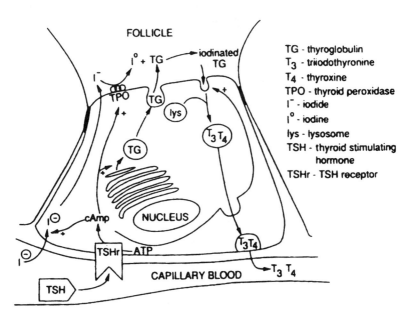

Figure 4.1.   Iodinated thyroglobulin stored as thyroid hormones in the follicle. (From Lawrence PF, Bell RM, Dayton MT, eds. Essentials of General Surgery. 2nd ed. Baltimore: Williams & Wilkins, 1992:294.)

plasma, the T_4-T_3 ratio ranges from 10:1 to 20:1. In the periphery, T_4 is converted to T_3, which enters the tissues quickly because of its lower affinity for protein and is three to four times as active as T_4. The half-life of T_4 (7 to 8 days) is longer than that of T_3 (3 days). The metabolic functions of thyroid hormone include increased calorigenesis, increased protein synthesis, and altered carbohydrate and lipid metabolism.

What are the indications for surgery in thyroid disease?
Surgical treatment of thyroid disease should be considered for the following conditions:

Malignancy
  • Carcinoma proved with FNA
  • A lesion suspicious for carcinoma on FNA
  • As prophylaxis for patients with familial thyroid cancer
Nonmalignant thyroid mass
  • Toxic multinodular goiter
  • Solitary toxic nodule
  • Graves' disease
Compression symptoms

Ms. Arnold's ultrasound examination reveals a solid nodule. A ^{123}I scan reveals a cold nodule, and FNA reveals papillary cells suggestive of carcinoma.

What are the pathologic types of thyroid cancers?
Four main types of thyroid cancers can be distinguished according to their pathology: papillary, follicular, medullary, and anaplastic. More than 90% of all thyroid cancers are papillary and follicular carcinomas.

Papillary carcinomas are well-differentiated lesions. More than 90% of thyroid carcinomas in patients with a history of irradiation are papillary. The peak incidence is in the third to fourth decades, and women are affected three times as often as men. Papillary carcinomas contain concentric layers of calcium called *psammoma bodies*. Papillary cancers are the slowest-growing thyroid tumors, and they spread through the lymphatic system. Lateral aberrant thyroid rest is a papillary cancer that has metastasized to a lymph node. The multicentricity rate is 80% on microscopic examination, but probably fewer than 5% have a clinical effect. Papillary metastases concentrate iodine and can be treated with radioiodine.

Follicular carcinomas are generally also well-differentiated tumors. They differ from papillary tumors in that they exhibit less multicentricity and are more likely to spread hematogenously to bone, lung, and liver. Follicular metastases concentrate iodine and can be treated with radioiodine.

Medullary carcinomas are less common tumors, comprising 3 to 10% of thyroid cancers. They are calcitonin-producing tumors that originate from the C cells; amyloid deposits in the stroma of the tumor are diagnostic. Bilateral multicentricity is commonly found in familial cases but is unusual in the sporadic variety. Medullary cancers occur in families as components of both multiple endocrine neoplasia (MEN) type II and the familial medullary carcinoma syndrome (see Chapter 23). MEN type IIA, or Sipple's syndrome, also includes pheochromocytomas and hyperparathyroidism. MEN type IIB is a less common form that includes mucosal neuromas, ganglioneuroma of the bowel, and a marfanoid appearance; hyperparathyroidism is rare. An elevated serum calcitonin level is diagnostic of medullary carcinoma and is also a useful screening tool for familial transmission. Evaluation of point mutations in the *Ret* protooncogene is part of the workup of these patients and their families (2).

Anaplastic carcinomas account for fewer than 5% of thyroid cancers and occur later in life than the other types. These cancers are characterized by extremely rapid and widespread growth. Patients present with a sometimes painful and enlarged thyroid gland. These tumors are highly aggressive and associated with very short life expectancy.

What is the treatment for a patient with a presentation such as Ms. Arnold's if the FNA indicates papillary carcinoma?
The lesion must be excised, but the extent of resection—thyroid lobectomy alone versus total or subtotal thyroidectomy (Figure 4.2)—has been debated (3, 4). Lobectomy is advocated because it minimizes the operative risks; multicentric disease rarely becomes a clinical problem; and thyroid cancers in general are not very aggressive. Extensive surgical ablation is promoted because it enhances postoperative scanning with ^{131}I for metastatic disease because no normal thyroid tissue (which concentrates iodine more vigorously than papillary or follicular metastases) remains in the neck; it facilitates follow-up with thyroglobulin levels; and it eliminates recurrence caused by multicentricity. A majority of endocrine surgeons favor total thyroidectomy for lesions larger than 2 to 3 cm.

After total thyroidectomy, L-thyroxine should be given for life in doses sufficient to suppress TSH secretion. Radioiodine is used to ablate any residual functional thyroid tissue in the neck after thyroidectomy and to destroy widespread metastases. Improved survival was demonstrated after treatment with total thyroidectomy, radioiodine ablation, and TSH suppression for life in a study of 1355 patients who were followed for 40 years (5, 6).

What is the treatment if the FNA shows atypical follicular cells?
The treatment decision in this instance is difficult. Although follicular carcinoma is not associated with multicentricity, the debate over the extent of operative

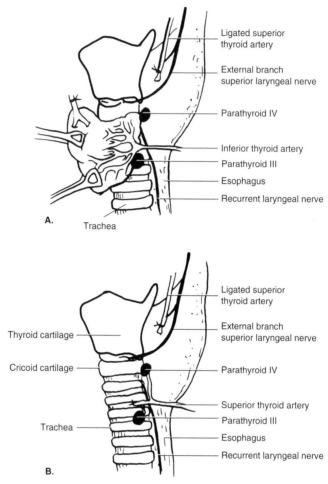

Figure 4.2. **A.** Anteromedial reflection of thyroid gland. **B.** Anatomy after total thyroidectomy. (Adapted from Doherty GM, Norton JA. Thyroid and parathyroid. In: Lawrence PF, ed. Essentials of General Surgery. 2nd ed. Baltimore: Williams & Wilkins, 1992:298.)

resection is similar to that for papillary carcinoma. Also, malignancy cannot be determined from intraoperative frozen sections (7), which adds to the uncertainty of the diagnosis. Advocates of total thyroidectomy for well-differentiated thyroid carcinoma recommend this procedure for lesions that cytology suggests are malignant and for lesions larger than 3 cm. An option for smaller lesions is lobectomy followed later by completion thyroidectomy if the permanent sections show malignancy. The surgeon and patient must balance the risk of a total thyroidectomy for possibly benign disease against the risk of further anesthesia and another procedure.

What are Hürthle cell carcinomas?
Hürthle cell carcinomas are aggressive variants of follicular cell origin. As with follicular carcinomas, capsular or vascular invasion by the tumor indicates malignancy, but some Hürthle cell tumors behave in a malignant fashion even without these pathologic features. Size appears to be an important criterion. As a general rule, lesions less than 3 cm in diameter behave benignly, whereas those larger than 4 cm behave as a malignancy (8).

How are medullary carcinomas treated?
Medullary carcinomas are aggressive lesions that are markedly multicentric and that commonly metastasize to the lymph nodes. Total thyroidectomy with a central node dissection should be performed for disease limited to the thyroid (9). A unilateral modified radical neck dissection is indicated only when metastatic disease is suspected because of elevated calcitonin levels and nodes that are either palpable or demonstrated by ultrasound studies to contain metastatic disease.

How are anaplastic carcinomas treated?
Anaplastic carcinomas are characterized by extremely rapid growth and a poor prognosis. Thyroidectomy does not improve the prognosis and is performed only to prevent airway compression. Chemotherapy and radiation therapy may offer some benefit as palliation (10).

Ms. Arnold is scheduled for neck exploration and thyroid resection for a papillary carcinoma.

What are the main steps in a thyroidectomy?
General endotracheal anesthesia is induced, and the head is placed in the extended position. A curvilinear transverse incision is made in the line of a natural skin crease over the cricoid cartilage. The incision is carried through the skin, subcutaneous tissue, platysma (innervated by the facial nerve), and the cervical fascia overlying the pretracheal muscles and anterior jugular veins. After the subplatysmal flaps are developed, the cervical fascia is divided in the midline. The strap muscles (sternohyoid and sternothyroid) are divided only for very large lesions. If the tumor infiltrates the sternothyroid muscle, the muscle should be resected en bloc with the thyroid (Figure 4.3).

What are the characteristics of the blood supply to the thyroid gland?
Abundant arterial blood is supplied to the thyroid by the superior thyroid arteries, which arise from the external carotid arteries, and by the inferior thyroid

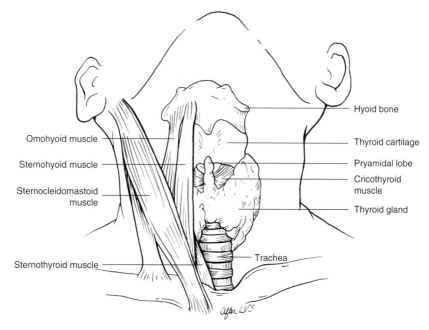

Figure 4.3.   Gross anatomy of the neck and thyroid gland. (Adapted with permission from Greenspan FS, ed. Basic and Clinical Endocrinology. 3rd ed. Norwalk, CT: Appleton & Lange, 1991:189.)

arteries, which arise from the thyrocervical trunks of the subclavian artery. There is no middle thyroid artery. Although the thyroid ima, an inferior artery, is mentioned in many texts, it is rarely found. The venous drainage consists of paired superior, inferior, and middle thyroid veins (Figure 4.2).

The patient undergoes total thyroidectomy for treatment of a papillary carcinoma.

What are the complications of thyroidectomy?
The most serious injury is to the recurrent laryngeal nerve.

How can that happen?
With an experienced thyroid surgeon and the use of magnification (loupes), this complication is infrequent. The nerve is most vulnerable at the level of the two upper tracheal rings, where the middle portion of the thyroid lobe is attached to the cricoid and tracheal cartilage by the suspensory ligament of Berry. The nerve is usually posterior to this ligament; however, in 25% of patients, it runs through this structure.

What happens if the recurrent laryngeal nerve is injured?
The recurrent laryngeal nerve is the motor nerve of all the muscles of the larynx except the cricothyroid. Therefore, injury results in an abductor laryngeal paralysis, and the affected vocal cord assumes a midline position. In most cases, nerve injury is an indirect result of adjacent dissection, and function returns within 3 to 6 months. Direct injury or severance of the nerve results in permanent damage. Unilateral injury causes various levels of hoarseness. Bilateral nerve injury may lead to airway obstruction and the need for a tracheostomy.

What other nerves may be injured during thyroidectomy?
Damage to the external branch of the superior laryngeal nerve during the mobilization of the superior pole of the thyroid is not as serious as injury of the recurrent laryngeal nerve. Injury to the external branch of the superior laryngeal nerve, which is the motor nerve of the inferior pharyngeal constrictor and cricothyroid muscles, is manifested by limitation of the force of projection of one's voice and lowering of the pitch. This function usually improves during the first 3 months after thyroidectomy.

What other complications may occur?
Hypoparathyroidism and hemorrhage.

What are the signs and symptoms of hypoparathyroidism, and how would you treat it?
With meticulous dissection, clinically significant hypoparathyroidism should be uncommon after thyroid resection. It is usually a temporary problem caused by minor injury to the blood supply during dissection around the parathyroid glands. The signs and symptoms of hypoparathyroidism occur within the first few days after surgery. The early symptoms are perioral numbness, tingling of the fingers, and intense anxiety. The threshold of muscular excitability is lowered, and involuntary spasms occur. The following are classic signs of hypoparathyroidism:

- *Chvostek's sign:* ipsilateral facial muscles contract when the facial nerve is tapped against the bone just anterior to the ear.
- *Trousseau's sign:* carpal spasm occurs after the brachial artery is occluded for 3 minutes with an inflated sphygmomanometer cuff.
- *Spontaneous carpopedal spasm:* hands and feet contract spontaneously.

Hypoparathyroidism may eventually progress to frank tetany. Laboratory indicators are a decreased serum calcium level with concomitantly increased serum phosphorus level and decreased or absent urinary calcium.

The calcium level should be measured postoperatively in any patient undergoing total thyroidectomy. It is probably unnecessary to perform this study when only one side has been explored. If the patient is symptomatic or if the calcium level falls to less than 7.5 to 8 mg/dL, oral calcium replacements should be given (500 mg of elemental calcium in the form of 1250 mg of calcium carbonate every 6 hours). Most postoperative hypoparathyroidism resolves over the first few days or weeks. If the hypocalcemia is unresponsive to oral calcium supplementation, oral vitamin D (calcitriol 0.25 μg daily) may be given.

Postoperative hypoparathyroidism can be prevented with the following intraoperative measures: (*a*) performing a gentle dissection and avoiding ligation of the inferior thyroid artery laterally (this can decrease blood flow to the parathyroid glands during a lobectomy or subtotal thyroidectomy) and (*b*) autotransplanting the parathyroid gland into the sternocleidomastoid muscles if the gland is clearly ischemic.

How is postoperative hemorrhage managed?
This potentially serious complication has become uncommon as surgical techniques have improved. Accumulation of blood or formation of a clot in the closed space around the trachea can lead to airway constriction. The treatment is to open the wound and evacuate the clot at the bedside and obtain hemostasis in the operating room. Tracheostomy is contraindicated if the clot is evacuated. If airway control is needed, the patient can be intubated orally.

After the thyroidectomy, Ms. Arnold's voice appears to be unchanged from the preoperative period, and she has no complications. She is discharged from the hospital.

What is the prognosis for the different types of thyroid cancers?
Several prognostic scoring systems have been developed for well-differentiated thyroid cancer. Two such systems are the AGES system (age of patient; grade, extent, and size of tumor) (11) and the AMES system (age, metastatic disease, and extent and size of tumor) (12). Papillary carcinoma has the most favorable prognosis, with approximately 95% survival at 10 and 20 years. The prognosis for follicular and medullary carcinomas is less favorable, with 80% of patients surviving at 10 years and 71% at 20 years (13). Anaplastic carcinomas have a poor prognosis: fewer than 10% of patients survive 1 year (14).

What is the recommended follow-up for the different types of carcinomas?
The follow-up for well-differentiated carcinomas consists of physical examination, thyroglobulin measurements, ultrasonography, chest radiography, and ^{131}I nuclear scanning. For patients with medullary carcinoma, the follow-up is similar, but it also includes calcitonin measurement and molecular analysis of the *Ret* protooncogene. This is important for family members for evaluation of familial carcinoma.

Ms. Arnold is prescribed L-thyroxine supplements. At the first post-operative clinic visit, her wound appears to be well healed, and she reports feeling well.

Barbara Morin has had a thyroid nodule for a few years and has been referred by her primary care physician. She has been told that the nodule is not cancer.

What are the common causes of thyroid nodules besides carcinoma?
Other causes are multinodular goiter, Hashimoto's disease (lymphocytic thyroiditis), and Graves' disease.

What does goiter mean, and what causes it?
Goiter is benign enlargement of the thyroid gland. The term is derived from the Latin *guttur,* which means throat. The pathogenesis of multinodular goiter in most cases is unknown; the involvement of growth factors is being investigated (15). TSH clearly plays a role in iodine deficiency states, but iodine deficiency is rare in the United States today.

What are the clinicopathologic manifestations of goiter, and what is the recommended therapy?
The thyroid gland may have nodules of variable size and number or be smooth and diffusely enlarged. Patients with goiter are usually asymptomatic, although they commonly complain of a neck mass or an increase in neck size, sometimes with pressure symptoms. On physical examination there may be a palpable mass that moves on swallowing. If the goiter extends retrosternally, the patient's face becomes suffused with blood when the arms are raised above the head because the goitrous mass obstructs venous return from the head (Pemberton's sign). Thyrotoxicosis can also develop in patients with a long-standing history of goiter (toxic multinodular goiter).

Multinodular goiter that produces no symptoms may not require treatment. If the goiter creates a cosmetic problem or pressure, initial treatment consists of supplemental thyroid hormone to suppress TSH secretion and its effects on the thyroid gland. Indications for surgery are pressure, cosmetic deformity, persistent growth of the goiter, and a suspect nodule.

What is Hashimoto's thyroiditis?
Hashimoto's thyroiditis is chronic lymphocytic thyroiditis, the most common form of chronic thyroiditis. It is an autoimmune disease in which antibodies to thyroglobulin are formed. The thyroid is often diffusely enlarged, pale, and firm. The presence of nodules may cause this condition to be confused with colloid goiter or carcinoma. Most patients are women, with a mean age of 50

years. Common complaints are neck enlargement and associated pain and tenderness. Most patients are euthyroid or hypothyroid, although some cases of
transient hyperthyroidism have been reported.

A high serum titer of thyroid antibodies is diagnostic of this disease. Needle aspiration and cytologic examination may be indicated to rule out carcinoma.

The treatment of Hashimoto's disease depends on severity. In some patients,
no therapy is indicated, whereas other patients require thyroid replacement
therapy to relieve hypothyroidism. Surgery is indicated for pressure, for suspected carcinoma, and for cosmetic reasons. After surgery, patients should take
chronic suppressive thyroid hormone.

What are the other types of thyroiditis and how do they differ from Hashimoto's disease?
These are the other types of thyroiditis:

Acute suppurative thyroiditis, the rarest form of thyroiditis, usually occurs
  after an acute upper respiratory tract infection. Clinical manifestations include sudden severe pain around the thyroid gland, dysphagia, fever, and
  chills. Treatment includes antibiotics and drainage of the abscess.
de Quervain's disease (subacute thyroiditis) is not thought to be autoimmune. Sudden onset of thyroid pain and swelling is a common presenting
  feature. The erythrocyte sedimentation rate is elevated. A brief course of
  steroids may relieve symptoms, and spontaneous recovery is common.
  Surgery is not indicated.
Riedel's struma (chronic thyroiditis) is a rare condition in which patients
  have profound hypothyroidism that is usually irreversible. The thyroid gland
  is so hard that an open biopsy must be performed to distinguish this lesion
  from thyroid carcinoma. Patients with chronic thyroiditis have lower titers
  of circulating autoantibodies than those with Hashimoto's disease. Thyroid
  hormone replacement therapy relieves the hypothyroidism but does not affect the disease.

*What is toxic multinodular goiter and how does it differ from Graves' disease or a soli-
tary toxic nodule?*
Patients with long-standing nontoxic multinodular goiter may develop hyperthyroidism because the nodules hyperfunction autonomously. This form of hyperthyroidism, known as Plummer's disease, is usually not as severe as Graves'
disease. Antithyroid drugs offer no long-term benefit because the disease is relatively resistant to these drugs. Similarly, radioiodine ablation is inefficient in
destroying hyperactive thyroid tissue, and recurrence is more common than
with Graves' disease because of the intrinsic autonomy of the thyroid tissue

(16, 17). Many patients have prominent thyroid masses and resulting compression; therefore, the preferred treatment for patients who are otherwise well is total or subtotal thyroidectomy after the patient has been made euthyroid with propylthiouracil or methimazole.

What is Graves' disease and how is it treated?
Graves' disease, or toxic diffuse goiter, is a systemic autoimmune disease caused by immunoglobulin-α (IgG) antibodies to the thyroid-stimulating hormone receptor. These antibodies bind the hormone receptor and stimulate the thyroid gland. Graves' disease affects women six to seven times as commonly as men. Both Graves' disease and Hashimoto's thyroiditis have a high familial incidence. The thyroid gland in these patients is symmetrically and diffusely enlarged. The cardinal signs of Graves' disease are thyroid enlargement, exophthalmos, tachycardia, and tremor. Common symptoms include heat intolerance and weight loss. Eye signs, mild in most patients, include (*a*) upper lid spasm with retraction, (*b*) external ophthalmoplegia, (*c*) exophthalmos with proptosis, (*d*) supraorbital and infraorbital edema, and (*e*) conjunctive congestion and edema.

Treatment is antithyroid drugs, radioactive iodine, or thyroid resection. Commonly used drugs include methimazole and propylthiouracil. These drugs block synthesis of thyroid hormone by inhibiting iodide organification and iodotyrosine coupling (Figure 4.1). In addition, propylthiouracil inhibits peripheral conversion of T_4 to T_3 by blocking the action of the $5'$ deiodinase enzyme. The normal metabolic rate is restored within 6 weeks of treatment. After drug withdrawal, hyperthyroidism recurs in 50 to 75% of patients. The advantages of radioactive iodine therapy are that remission occurs in 80 to 98% of patients, surgery with its potential for complications is avoided, and costs are reduced. Its disadvantages are that it takes longer to control the disease and the incidence of permanent hypothyroidism is high, up to 90% at 10 years. Radioiodine therapy is contraindicated in pregnant or lactating women.

When is surgical treatment indicated for Graves' disease?
Subtotal or total thyroidectomy is indicated in young adults with severe disease and large goiters, in patients who are refractory to medical therapy or whose symptoms recur after it, in patients who desire a rapid response, and in patients for whom radioiodine is contraindicated. The thyrotoxic state is corrected in more than 95% of patients. Total thyroidectomy has been advocated by some surgeons because (*a*) it is safe when performed by an experienced surgeon, (*b*) there is almost no recurrence of hyperthyroidism, and (*c*) the exophthalmos and other eye signs resolve more completely. Pretibial myxedema, which is seen in a few patients, also responds best to total surgical thyroid ablation (18).

What is the preoperative treatment?
Patients with active Graves' disease and those with toxic multinodular goiter require preoperative treatment to avoid thyroid storm (discussed next) and to shrink the thyroid gland. Antithyroid drugs establish a euthyroid state. Iodine is administered 8 to 10 days before surgery to decrease the vascularity of the thyroid gland. These large doses of iodine cause a dramatic but short-lived decrease in iodine organification (the Wolff-Chaikoff effect). Administering β-adrenergic blockers adds to the safety of this procedure. Propranolol decreases the pulse rate of patients with thyrotoxicosis. Many patients are treated preoperatively with a combination of propylthiouracil, iodine, and propranolol.

What is thyroid storm?
Thyroid storm is an acute adrenergic outburst that is augmented by the presence of thyroid hormone and that manifests clinically as hyperthermia, tachycardia, hypertension, and eventual hypotension and death. Thyroid storm was a frequent and life-threatening condition before preoperative control of thyrotoxicosis was possible. Today thyroid storm is rare, but it still occurs spontaneously in patients with unknown hyperthyroidism. Treatment is directed at inhibiting the production of thyroid hormone and at antagonizing its effects. Large doses of propranolol are beneficial in reducing the tachycardia. Intravenous iodine should be given in addition to steroids because of the danger of adrenal insufficiency. Oxygen and intravenous glucose should be given to treat the hypermetabolic state, and a hypothermia blanket may be used. This complication has a 10% mortality rate.

What is the management of a patient with a thyroid nodule who complains of heat intolerance and tremor?
Heat intolerance and tremor suggest that the patient may be thyrotoxic with an autonomous nodule. Under these circumstances, FNA should not be performed until thyroid function is studied. T_3, T_4, and TSH levels should be determined, and a thyroid scan should be performed. Although the nodule is the most likely source of hyperfunction, it is essential to rule out a cold nodule in an otherwise hyperfunctioning gland. Such a nodule is suspect for malignancy, whereas few hot nodules are malignant.

Ms. Morin's laboratory report indicates that she has elevated T_3 and T_4 levels and a low TSH level. A ^{99m}Tc scan shows a single hyperfunctioning nodule.

What is the recommended treatment?
There are two steps to management. The first is to achieve a euthyroid state with methimazole or propylthiouracil. After the patient is euthyroid, either a

thyroid lobectomy or radioiodine ablation can be performed. Generally, surgical resection is preferred because many nodules persist after radioiodine ablation (17). *See Algorithm 4.1 at the end of this chapter.*

PARATHYROID DISEASE

Mary Knowles is a 55-year-old woman with a long history of hypertension and recurrent nephrolithiasis who has had progressive fatigue and muscular weakness over the past 3 months. She is otherwise in good health and does not have weight loss, night sweats, or other constitutional complaints. She is taking clonidine for hypertension. The family history and physical examination are unremarkable, and she has no history of neck irradiation. She is afebrile and her vital signs are stable. The results of the blood chemistry screen are within normal limits except that the serum calcium level is 12.8 mg/dL and the serum phosphate level is 2.2 mg/dL.

What is the differential diagnosis for hypercalcemia in this patient?
The most common causes of hypercalcemia are primary hyperparathyroidism (HPT) and malignancy, which account for more than 90% of cases. Medications, most commonly thiazides; lithium, vitamin D, or vitamin A intoxication; and the milk-alkali syndrome (excessive intake of antacids, milk, or alkali) may cause hypercalcemia. Endogenous causes such as granulomatous disorders (sarcoidosis, berylliosis, tuberculosis, coccidioidomycosis, and histoplasmosis) and endocrine disorders (hyperthyroidism, hypothyroidism, adrenal insufficiency, and familial hypocalciuric hypercalcemia), immobilization, and Paget's disease may also lead to hypercalcemia (19, 20).

Which tests help confirm this diagnosis?
If exogenous causes are excluded, primary HPT is the most likely diagnosis because of the patient's history of symptomatic hypercalcemia in the absence of weight loss or other systemic symptoms that suggest neoplasm. Hypercalcemia should be confirmed first. In sick patients, it is important to correct serum calcium values for variations in serum albumin:

$$(Adjusted\ Ca^{2+}) = (Serum\ Ca^{2+}) + 0.8 \times [4 - (Serum\ albumin)]$$

However, in most patients it is unnecessary to measure the serum albumin. The level of ionized calcium can clarify any ambiguity. The serum phosphate level, which is less than 3 mg/dL in primary HPT, should also be determined. In a hypertensive patient, urinary catecholamine metabolites must be evaluated to rule out pheochromocytoma. Other helpful laboratory findings include a serum chloride level less than 102 mEq/L, serum chloride-phosphate ratio less than 33, elevated serum alkaline phosphatase, elevated urinary calcium, and elevated urinary cyclic adenosine monophosphate.

The next step is to obtain an intact parathyroid hormone (PTH) assay and a 24-hour urinary calcium measurement. An understanding of PTH physiology and the availability of the assay has made much of the extensive workup performed in the past unnecessary.

What is the function of PTH, and how does its measurement help diagnosis?
PTH is an 84–amino acid peptide secreted by the parathyroid glands. In the circulation, the intact hormone (half-life, less than 3 minutes) is rapidly cleaved into the active aminoterminal fragment containing amino acids 1 to 34 (short half-life) and an inactive carboxyterminal fragment (long half-life, about 20 hours) and cleared by the liver. Hormonal activity is exhibited by both the aminoterminal fragment and the intact hormone. Assays for the carboxyterminal, midregion, and aminoterminal fragments are available, but the assay for intact hormone (also known as the sandwich or two-site assay) is superior (21). This assay uses antibodies to PTH fragments 1 to 34 and 39 to 84. An elevated serum calcium level, together with increased intact PTH level and elevated 24-hour urinary calcium excretion, is diagnostic of primary HPT. The assay for intact PTH does not cross-react with parathyroid hormone–like peptide and thus effectively rules out malignancy as a cause of hypercalcemia.

Why is it important to measure 24-hour urinary calcium excretion?
It is important to measure urinary calcium excretion to rule out familial hypercalcemic hypocalciuria (FHH) (22). FHH is an autosomal dominant disease characterized by mildly elevated serum calcium, but unlike primary hyperparathyroidism, it is associated with decreased urinary calcium excretion. It is generally considered a disease not of the parathyroids but of renal calcium excretion. PTH levels may be low, normal, or high in FHH; when the value is high, an erroneous diagnosis of hyperparathyroidism may be suggested. The ratio of calcium clearance to creatinine clearance is less than 0.01.

What are the normal physiologic mechanisms for calcium and phosphate homeostasis?
PTH and vitamin D are the primary factors that regulate serum calcium and phosphate concentrations (23). PTH stimulates osteoclastic bone resorption, increases tubular reabsorption of calcium, retards renal tubular reabsorption of phosphate, and indirectly increases intestinal absorption of calcium by inducing renal hydroxylation of vitamin D. The action of PTH on the kidney occurs within seconds to minutes, whereas its effects on bone and gut take hours to days. PTH is synthesized in the chief cells of the parathyroid gland, and its release is controlled in a negative feedback loop by the calcium concentration.

Vitamin D is synthesized in the skin in response to sunlight and is also a dietary component. Two hydroxylations convert it to its active form. The first hydroxylation, in the liver, converts it to 25-hydroxyvitamin D. The second hydroxylation, which occurs in the kidney, produces the active form, 1,25-dihydroxyvitamin D; it is directly stimulated by PTH and low calcium or phosphate concentrations. This active form increases intestinal absorption of calcium and phosphate, promotes mineralization of bone by calcium and phosphate, and enhances PTH-mediated mobilization of calcium and phosphate from bone. Along with its primary effect of increasing serum calcium levels, 1,25-dihydroxyvitamin D inhibits PTH secretion (24). Increased serum calcium or phosphate levels inhibit the renal hydroxylating enzyme.

What is the role of calcitonin in serum calcium homeostasis?
Calcitonin plays an important role in the maintenance of skeletal mass during periods of calcium stress such as growth spurts, pregnancy, and lactation. The increased demands for calcium during these periods may cause calcium to be depleted from the bony skeleton by osteoclastic bone resorption. Calcitonin inhibits this effect (25).

What is the pathophysiology of hypercalcemia associated with malignancy?
Hypercalcemia secondary to an underlying malignancy occurs (*a*) through bone resorption by primary or metastatic tumor cells in direct contact with bone (breast cancer, multiple myeloma, and other hematologic cancers) or (*b*) through osteoclastic activity of a circulating humoral factor secreted by tumors such as renal, bladder, and ovarian cancers and squamous cell carcinoma of the lung. This factor, characterized in the late 1980s, is known as parathyroid hormone–related protein or peptide (PTHrP) (26). PTHrP has extensive homology with the N-terminal portion of PTH, which accounts for the similarity of its action in producing humoral hypercalcemia of malignancy (HHM). However, the C-terminals of PTH and PTHrP differ considerably, so the assay for intact PTH does not detect PTHrP. In the past, serum assays of C-terminal PTH were unreliable in differentiating primary hyperparathyroidism from HHM, necessitating an extensive workup. With the intact assay, patients with HHM are shown to have suppressed levels of PTH.

How is primary hyperparathyroidism differentiated from sarcoidosis and other causes of hypercalcemia?
Hypercalcemia in sarcoidosis is believed to result from increased production of vitamin D secondary to enhanced extrarenal production of 1,25-dihydroxyvitamin D in granulomata (27). Intact PTH levels are low in sarcoidosis as well as in other causes of hypercalcemia, such as Paget's disease, immobilization, excessive calcium intake, vitamin D intoxication, and thyrotoxicosis. Thiazides increase renal tubular absorption of calcium, and their use may be associated with increased levels of PTH. The diagnosis of primary hyperparathyroidism cannot therefore be made until thiazide treatment has been stopped and the patient has been restudied.

What is the relation between symptomatic disease and serum calcium levels in patients with hypercalcemia?
Symptoms of hypercalcemia are related to the degree and duration of the hypercalcemia. With regard to symptoms caused by hypercalcemia alone, patients with serum calcium levels less than 11.5 mg/dL are rarely symptomatic, whereas patients with levels between 11.5 and 13 mg/dL may or may not display symptoms. Severe hypercalcemia (calcium level higher than 13 mg/dL) is almost always associated with symptoms, and the risk of severe organ damage is significant.

Appropriate laboratory tests, including the PTH level, are performed on Ms. Knowles, and the diagnosis of primary hyperparathyroidism is confirmed.

What are the principal symptoms of primary hyperparathyroidism?
More than half of patients diagnosed with primary hyperparathyroidism after routine serum chemistry screening are asymptomatic, in comparison with 18% of patients before the introduction of routine screening in the 1970s. Symptoms include bone pain or fractures; nephrolithiasis; gastrointestinal distress such as peptic ulcer, pancreatitis, or constipation; lethargy or weakness; and delirium, depression, coma, or exacerbation of preexisting psychiatric disease.

What are typical radiologic findings in primary hyperparathyroidism?
Standard radiography of the middle and distal phalanges of the hand to show subperiosteal bone resorption and skull radiography to demonstrate the moth-eaten appearance of hyperparathyroidism are rarely done today because overt clinical bony disease is present in only about 10% of patients. Osteitis fibrosa cystica, which is characterized by resorption of bone, focal eroded areas, reactive fibrosis, cyst formation, and brown tumors, was once the major clinical manifestation of primary hyperparathyroidism but is now also uncommon. Bone densitometry, which is a much more sensitive indicator of bone disease such as osteoporosis, can guide decisions to operate on otherwise asymptomatic patients, especially women who are in or past menopause (28).

Ms. Knowles's radiologic workup is negative. She returns to the clinic for a discussion of possible surgery for primary hyperparathyroidism.

What are the indications for surgery in primary hyperparathyroidism?
Surgical intervention is indicated in all cases of symptomatic disease, except in patients for whom the operative risk is prohibitive. Indications include radiographic evidence of bone disease (including bone resorption, cysts, pathologic fractures, or osteoporosis demonstrated by bone densitometry), nephrolithiasis,

decreased renal function, gastrointestinal complications (peptic ulcer disease or pancreatitis), neuromuscular disease, and acute hypercalcemic symptoms.

Should asymptomatic patients undergo surgery?
Although it is a controversial recommendation, many groups advocate surgery for most cases of asymptomatic primary hyperparathyroidism. This course is recommended because (*a*) there are no defined criteria for early identification of patients whose disease will eventually become symptomatic and (*b*) patients strongly resist the prolonged and rather intensive follow-up required for nonoperative management. In addition, some authors believe that if an appropriate history has been obtained, only 10% of patients are found to be truly asymptomatic (29). Surgery can be delayed in asymptomatic patients who express interest in nonoperative management and are willing to undergo the prolonged, regular follow-up to evaluate progress of the disease. The most persuasive argument for recommending surgery in this group of patients is that the risks and cost of long-term nonoperative therapy exceed the cost and potential morbidity of parathyroidectomy. The incidence of complications (e.g., hypertension, nephrolithiasis, impaired renal function, nephrocalcinosis) arising from nonoperative disease within 5 years of follow-up is considerably higher than the 25% originally reported (30).

What are the embryologic and anatomic features of the parathyroid glands?
The upper parathyroid glands develop from the fourth branchial pouch and descend into the neck with the thyroid, remaining in close association with the upper portion of the thyroid lobes. Their blood supply is primarily from the superior thyroid artery. The lower parathyroid glands arise from the third branchial pouch along with the thymus, and they descend with the thymus, usually coming to rest in the neck but on occasion continuing into the mediastinum. This long migration in embryologic life appears to account for the variable location of these glands. In approximately 50% of persons, these glands are found on the lateral or posterior surface of the lower pole of the thyroid gland. The inferior thyroid artery supplies blood. Ordinarily, there are four parathyroid glands, but autopsy series have demonstrated five glands in 6% of cases and three glands in 13% of cases. The average total weight of the four parathyroid glands is 140 mg.

What are common ectopic locations of the parathyroid glands?
Parathyroid glands have been found as high as the carotid artery bifurcation and as low as the pericardium. The superior glands have the most constant position, behind the upper thyroid lobe or at the cricothyroid junction posteriorly in nearly 80% of cases. Most ectopic superior glands are within the surgical capsule of the upper pole of the thyroid. Roughly 1% of superior glands are in the retropharyngeal or retroesophageal region. Superior parathyroid adenomas

have a tendency to migrate from the normal position into the posterior superior mediastinum.

The inferior parathyroid glands are more widely distributed than the superior glands. The most common location for these glands is the anterolateral or posterolateral surface of the lower thyroid gland (in 40 to 50% of cases). The majority of ectopic glands are found within the thymus, either in the lower neck within the thymic tongue or inside the mediastinal thymus (in 1 to 2% of cases). Approximately 15% of inferior glands reportedly lie lateral to the thyrothymic tract and the lower thyroid pole, and an additional 5% are intrathyroidal. In rare instances, the lower parathyroid gland is high in the neck lateral to the upper thyroid lobes or in proximity to the carotid sheath because of early developmental arrest. These glands are typically associated with a thymic remnant (Figure 4.4).

What causes primary hyperparathyroidism, and what are its pathologic characteristics?
Single adenomas cause disease in approximately 80 to 85% of patients; 10 to 15% have multiglandular disease, either double adenomas or diffuse hyperplasia; and fewer than 1% have cancer. In most cases of primary hyperparathyroidism, the cause is unknown. A protooncogene and chromosomal mutations have been described in small subsets of patients, generally those who have inherited parathyroid abnormalities (31). As with hyperthyroidism, there is an association between irradiation of the head and neck and hyperparathyroidism. Patients who have been exposed to low-level radiation either for medical treatment or after a nuclear accident (e.g., the Chernobyl incident) are at increased risk.

What role do localization studies have in the preoperative assessment for parathyroid disease?
The localization techniques include scanning with 99mTc sestamibi or sestamibi alone. These agents are taken up rapidly by both the thyroid and the parathyroid glands but are washed out more quickly from the thyroid. Ultrasonography, computed tomography, magnetic resonance imaging, and selective venous sampling for PTH may also be used.

The need for preoperative localization studies has been questioned. Most surgeons believe that exploration of the neck by an experienced parathyroid surgeon (one who performs more than 12 parathyroid operations a year) can achieve a cure rate greater than 90%, which is better than the sensitivity of localization studies, and they therefore do not recommend preoperative localization (32). The arguments in favor of preoperative localization are that (*a*) a positive sestamibi scan in the neck virtually eliminates the possibility of an ectopic location for the parathyroid tissue and (*b*) the use of rapid intraoperative PTH assays (33) allows a limited exploration, which saves time and discomfort (34).

There is agreement, however, that preoperative localization studies should be performed in patients with persistent or recurrent hyperparathyroidism that has prompted reexploration. In these patients, an intensive effort should be made to localize the glands because of the high incidence of ectopic tumors and because the increased scarring and loss of tissue planes from previous surgery make extensive dissection difficult. With preoperative localization, unnecessary dissection can be avoided, complications can be reduced, and surgical results can be improved.

Ms. Knowles requires parathyroidectomy for treatment of her disease and gives her consent to proceed. At operation, both sides of the neck are examined through a transverse neck incision with use of loupe magnification. Exploration is carried out to identify all parathyroid glands before any resection is done. The right superior parathyroid gland is enlarged, but the remaining three glands appear normal.

What is the appropriate treatment in patients with such findings?
Enlargement of only one gland with the others being normal is an indication of adenoma, which must be removed. Evaluation of the other glands is controversial. Magnification allows confirmation of the normal glands and biopsy is not required (35). This reduces the rate of postoperative hypoparathyroidism. However, if the normalcy of the glands is in doubt, biopsy is essential. Sporadic cases, in which two glands are enlarged and the others appear normal, should be treated with removal of the enlarged glands and biopsy of the normal glands. Enlargement of four glands constitutes hyperplasia, and treatment consists of removing three glands and part of a fourth (subtotal parathyroidectomy); a well-vascularized remnant of roughly 50 mg of tissue should be retained. This remnant gland should be pared to size before all remaining glands are excised to ensure that the remnant is not ischemic.

How is the distinction between parathyroid adenoma and hyperplasia made intraoperatively?
This differentiation, which is made by the surgeon, requires bilateral exploration and identification of all parathyroid glands under magnification. An effective procedure is to resect abnormal glands on the basis of macroscopic criteria, such as any gland that weighs more than 70 mg, which are considered the upper normal limit. Histologic examination is generally unreliable for differentiating parathyroid adenoma from hyperplasia or abnormal from normal parathyroid tissue. Pathologic examination is important for identifying parathyroid tissue and distinguishing it from thyroid or lymph node.

How are parathyroid glands that are in unusual locations identified?
A helpful procedure to localize parathyroid glands during a neck exploration is to locate the junction of the inferior thyroid artery and the recurrent laryngeal

nerve. Most inferior parathyroid glands lie anterior and caudal to this point; most superior glands lie posterior and cephalad to it (Figure 4.4).

When glands are not found in the usual sites, attention must be directed to known ectopic sites. If a lower parathyroid gland is missing, the ipsilateral thymus should be surgically delivered into the field, removed, and examined for the missing gland. Failure to identify the missing gland in the thymus should prompt exploration of the ipsilateral carotid sheath. If this, too, is negative, thyroid lobectomy is indicated on the side of the missing gland. The rationale for this is that 2 to 5% of inferior parathyroid glands lie in the lower third of the ipsilateral thyroid lobe.

If an upper gland is missing, the retroesophageal, retrocarotid, carotid sheath, and posterior mediastinal regions should be explored. It is important that the upper pole of the thyroid be fully mobilized; division of the superior thyroid vessels must be included if necessary, because the upper parathyroids are fre-

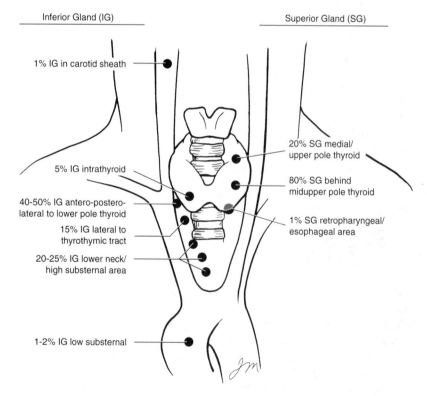

| Inferior Gland (IG) | Superior Gland (SG) |

1% IG in carotid sheath

5% IG intrathyroid

40-50% IG antero-postero-lateral to lower pole thyroid

15% IG lateral to thyrothymic tract

20-25% IG lower neck/ high substernal area

20% SG medial/ upper pole thyroid

80% SG behind midupper pole thyroid

1% SG retropharyngeal/ esophageal area

1-2% IG low substernal

Figure 4.4.   Possible locations and frequencies of the parathyroid gland.

quently tucked behind the superior pole. If fewer than two superior glands are identified at this point, a posterolateral thyroidotomy or a partial or total thyroid lobectomy is indicated (36, 37). Intraoperative ultrasonography may be used to determine whether an intrathyroidal nodule is a parathyroid gland.

What is the procedure if four normal glands are identified on exploration for primary hyperparathyroidism?
If four normal glands and no parathyroid tumor are found, the normal-appearing glands should be sampled for biopsy and confirmed to be normal parathyroid glands. Their positions should be marked with surgical clips. Although the supernumerary gland is usually in the mediastinum, all possible ectopic sites should be explored. If a tumor still remains unidentified, it is unlikely to be in the neck, and the neck should be closed.

Why is mediastinal exploration not the initial neck exploration if no abnormal parathyroid glands have been found in the neck?
There are several reasons to delay mediastinal exploration in this situation: (*a*) the neck dissection may have interrupted the blood supply of an ectopic parathyroid adenoma, rendering the patient normocalcemic; (*b*) a correctly performed neck exploration that shows negative results raises concern about the diagnosis and indicates the need for additional studies; (*c*) the actual site of an ectopic gland may not have been determined, and localization studies may be needed to distinguish between a parathyroid gland high in the neck and a mediastinal gland; and (*d*) if the lesion is in the thorax, careful planning and use of minimally invasive technology may avoid a formal median sternotomy.

What is the incidence of normocalcemia after surgery for primary hyperparathyroidism?
The incidence of normocalcemia after an initial neck exploration performed by an experienced parathyroid surgeon is greater than 95%.

What are the major complications of surgery?
Major complications include hypoparathyroidism, recurrent laryngeal nerve injury, and persistent or recurrent hyperparathyroidism. Postoperative hemorrhage is rare (see earlier section).

Ms. Knowles's single enlarged gland, an adenoma, is removed. Her immediate postoperative period is unremarkable. During morning rounds the next day, Ms. Knowles complains of numbness around her mouth and is found to have a positive Chvostek's sign.

What are Chvostek's and Trousseau's signs?
Chvostek's sign, an indicator of hypocalcemia, is a contraction of the facial muscles in response to tapping the facial nerve trunk in front of the ear. This

sign results from the increased neuromuscular irritability induced by hypocalcemia. Chvostek's sign may be found in up to 10% of the normal population.

Another useful sign of hypocalcemia is Trousseau's sign, in which carpal spasm, an indication of latent tetany, is induced by occluding the brachial artery for 3 minutes with a blood pressure cuff. Trousseau's sign is caused by increased tetanic activity resulting from ischemia in patients with hypocalcemia.

What are the symptoms of hypocalcemia, and when are they likely to occur?
Circumoral numbness, apprehension with or without dyspnea, weakness, headaches, extremity paresthesia (tingling of the fingertips), muscle cramps, laryngeal stridor, and convulsions may occur in hypocalcemia. The drop in calcium level is variable. Although the lowest serum calcium levels are usually seen 24 to 48 hours after surgery, symptomatic hypocalcemia is fairly common within the first 12 to 18 hours.

What are the most common causes of hypocalcemia after surgery for parathyroid disease?
Hypocalcemia after surgery is usually caused by hungry bone syndrome, or hypoparathyroidism resulting from operative trauma or underactivity of the suppressed remaining glands; it has a reported incidence of 13 to 30%. Other causes include hypomagnesemia, which may exaggerate hypocalcemia through impairment of PTH secretion and action on target tissues, and alkalosis, which can produce tetany even in the presence of a normal total blood calcium level by lowering the ionized calcium level.

What is hungry bone syndrome and how is it treated?
Hungry bone syndrome develops after parathyroidectomy as a result of extensive remineralization of the skeleton. It should be suspected in patients with known osteopenia on bone densitometry, in women who are in or past menopause, and in patients with long-standing disease (38). Postoperatively, as normal parathyroid function resumes, the calcium level should fall, and the phosphate level should increase. Hungry bone syndrome should be suspected when the phosphate level fails to increase or falls even further. In addition, calcium levels in hungry bone syndrome tend to decrease fast and dramatically. Calcium and phosphate levels should be monitored closely beginning the evening of surgery, and calcium replacement should be given as oral calcium supplements (500 mg of elemental calcium in the form of 1250 mg of calcium carbonate every 6 hours). Intravenous calcium and vitamin D (given orally as calcitriol 0.25 μg daily) are not commonly required. Since most patients are discharged the day after surgery, outpatient follow-up must include close monitoring of calcium levels. In patients at risk, calcium replacement should be begun immediately after the operation without a wait for a decline in serum calcium levels.

What are other possible causes of hypoparathyroidism in the postoperative period?
Hypoparathyroidism can be caused by direct operative trauma, removal of all parathyroid tissue, transient vascular compromise of the remaining parathyroid tissue, or reduced secretion of PTH from atrophic parathyroid tissue (a result of long-term hypercalcemic suppression).

What is the treatment for hypoparathyroidism?
Hypoparathyroidism is treated if there are symptoms or signs of neuromuscular irritability (positive Chvostek's or Trousseau's signs) together with hypocalcemia; hypocalcemia alone is not treated unless the calcium level decreases to less than 8 mg/dL. The treatment is similar to that for hungry bone syndrome.

How is the recurrent laryngeal nerve injured?
The recurrent laryngeal nerve is injured as the result of excessive trauma to the nerve during exposure, inclusion of the nerve in a ligature, or inadvertent sectioning of the nerve. The damage may be unilateral or bilateral and temporary or permanent.

What are the physical and laryngoscopic findings of unilateral injury to the recurrent laryngeal nerve, and how is it treated?
Physical examination reveals paralysis of one vocal cord from nerve injury, resulting in huskiness of the voice with varying degrees of hoarseness. On laryngoscopic examination, the vocal cord appears in a median or paramedian position because of abductor laryngeal paralysis. Hoarseness unassociated with laryngoscopic abnormalities is most likely caused by vocal cord edema from intubation and is usually adequately treated by humidifying inspired air.

In unilateral injury, cord paralysis results in narrowing of the glottic aperture, which is not sufficient to cause airway obstruction unless concurrent glottic edema is present. If the injury is related to dissection and the nerve is intact, function usually returns within 3 to 6 months. Typically, asymptomatic unilateral cord paralysis does not require treatment.

Ms. Knowles is found to have postoperative hypocalcemia, which is treated with oral calcium. With the increase of her serum calcium level, her perioral symptoms resolve. She is discharged home in satisfactory condition and scheduled for follow-up in the clinic a week later.

Do other features of hyperparathyroidism, such as kidney stones, high blood pressure, and neuromuscular symptoms, persist after surgery?
After surgery and normalization of urinary calcium excretion, formation of urinary calculi ceases in 91% of patients; however, deterioration of renal func-

tion and hypertension may persist. Psychiatric disturbances and neuromuscular problems caused by primary hyperparathyroidism are usually reversed. Parathyroidectomy does not reverse the diffuse osteopenia, but the rate of skeletal deterioration should be slowed or halted. Patients with osteopenia should receive calcium replacements for life.

What is the role of medical therapy in primary hyperparathyroidism?
Although surgery is the mainstay of treatment in primary hyperparathyroidism, medical therapy is used in cases of life-threatening hypercalcemia (acute primary hyperparathyroidism) and in patients for whom surgery is unacceptably risky.

Management of acute primary hyperparathyroidism. Acute life-threatening hypercalcemia is a rare manifestation of hyperparathyroidism. Typical features include serum calcium levels higher than 14 mg/dL and central nervous system disorders (confusion, disorientation, coma), gastrointestinal problems (abdominal pain, anorexia, nausea, weight loss), and neuromuscular dysfunction (fatigue, muscle weakness). The precipitating cause is usually volume depletion or stress. Two thirds of these patients have diagnostic features of hyperparathyroidism (history of hypercalcemia, presence of nephrolithiasis or nephrocalcinosis, radiographically demonstrated bone disease) (39). Emergency treatment consists of volume repletion with intravenous saline followed by furosemide to promote a sodium, hence calcium, diuresis. Mithramycin, through its inhibition of osteoclastic activity, can often prevent further accelerated bone resorption. The large amounts of potassium and magnesium lost during hyperparathyroid crisis must be replaced. Parathyroidectomy is typically performed after the patient has improved and the diagnosis is confirmed; however, urgent operative intervention is advocated by many surgeons in the absence of a prompt response to medical therapy by the patient (39).

Management of patients for whom surgery is unacceptably risky. The medical treatment of chronic hypercalcemia caused by primary hyperparathyroidism is much less effective than parathyroidectomy. Management includes walking to decrease mobilization of calcium from bone and judicious use of diuretics, as these may worsen a negative calcium balance. Other agents that inhibit or counteract the actions of parathyroid hormone on bone or intestine include oral phosphate, estrogens for postmenopausal women, and bisphosphonates, which impair the function of osteoclasts. These treatments are sometimes used for patients with mild asymptomatic hypercalcemia and those with persistent or recurrent disease. To date, there is no effective long-term medical management of primary hyperparathyroidism. A new class of agents that affect the extracellular calcium-sensing receptor function is being studied (40).

What preoperative findings suggest parathyroid carcinoma?
Parathyroid carcinomas are rare (incidence less than 0.5%), but any of these preoperative findings suggest that diagnosis: severe hypercalcemia (greater than 13 mg/dL), a markedly elevated PTH level (above 1000 pg/mL), a palpable cervical mass in a hypercalcemic patient (adenomas are almost never palpable), hypercalcemia associated with an unexplained unilateral vocal cord paralysis, or hyperparathyroidism recurring several months after an apparently successful parathyroidectomy.

What findings at surgery confirm this diagnosis?
The tumors are hard and surrounded by dense fibrous tissue, giving them a whitish appearance that is in marked contrast to the reddish-brown color of hyperactive glands in benign disease. A histologic diagnosis of parathyroid carcinoma is difficult, especially from a frozen section. The only findings diagnostic of malignancy are invasion of surrounding structures and lymph node metastases.

How does a diagnosis of malignancy alter surgical management?
En bloc resection should be performed, with care being taken to maintain capsular integrity. Cure rates have been reported in more than 50% of patients with this technique. Penetration of the tumor capsule disseminates cancer cells and is likely to result in local implantation in the operative site. Radical neck dissection should be performed only if clinically involved lymph nodes are present. Excision of recurrent or metastatic disease is only palliative and is usually indicated for control of severe hypercalcemia.

What are the most likely diagnoses in a young woman who has persistent asymptomatic hypercalcemia a year after subtotal parathyroidectomy and who has a family history of hypercalcemia?
After a diagnosis of FHH has been ruled out by repeat urine studies, the diagnosis of familial hyperparathyroidism and MEN syndromes should be considered. Familial hyperparathyroidism is a rare disorder that appears to be autosomal dominant with incomplete penetrance (41). Unlike the MEN syndromes, this is a single disease without associated abnormalities. The clinical and laboratory presentations are identical to those of nonfamilial primary hyperparathyroidism. The incidence of multiglandular disease with chief cell hyperplasia is high.

What is the incidence of hyperparathyroidism in the MEN syndromes?
Hyperparathyroidism is a significant element of the MEN-I and MEN-IIA syndromes, both of which are autosomal dominant disorders. The MEN-I syndrome consists of hyperparathyroidism in 90 to 97% of those affected, pancreatic tumors in 30 to 80%, and pituitary tumors in 15 to 50%. The MEN-IIA syndrome

consists of pheochromocytomas (commonly bilateral) or bilateral adrenal medullary hyperplasia in 50%, hyperparathyroidism in 10 to 25%, and medullary carcinoma of the thyroid or C-cell hyperplasia in 100%. Hyperparathyroidism is rare in the MEN-IIB syndrome, which consists of medullary carcinoma, pheochromocytomas, marfanoid habitus, neuromas of the tongue or conjunctiva, and ganglioneuromas of the plexuses of Meissner and Auerbach. The hyperparathyroidism in these syndromes is typically caused by chief cell hyperplasia (42, 43).

What are the appropriate screening tests for family members?
Initial screening for MEN-I should include measurement of serum calcium, whereas screening for MEN-II entails basal and stimulated calcitonin assays. Screening for MEN-II is particularly important because it allows diagnosis of medullary carcinoma at an early stage, when it is still curable.

How does a diagnosis of MEN syndrome affect treatment?
For treatment of the parathyroid component of these syndromes, a diagnosis of MEN-I should alert the surgeon to perform an adequate parathyroid resection when hyperplasia is present, because of the increased risk (as high as 33%) of recurrent disease postoperatively. Some surgeons continue to perform subtotal parathyroidectomy in these patients; others recommend total parathyroidectomy with autotransplantation of the parathyroid remnant into the forearm. If graft-dependent hypercalcemia occurs, the transplanted tissue can be resected easily. In patients with MEN-IIA, attention should first be directed to treatment of pheochromocytoma or adrenal hyperplasia and then to thyroidectomy. All four parathyroid glands should be identified and samples taken for biopsy, with subsequent resection of enlarged glands only. When this principle is followed, recurrent disease is rare.

What leads to an unsuccessful initial parathyroid resection?
Some 5 to 10% of patients undergoing parathyroid explorations subsequently require reexploration for persistent hyperparathyroidism. The factors implicated include inexperience of the surgeon leading to inadequate exploration of the neck and superior mediastinum, abnormal parathyroid gland location, and underestimation of multiglandular disease.

What is the preoperative evaluation in patients being considered for parathyroid reoperation?
The preoperative evaluation should include reconfirmation of the biochemical diagnosis of hyperparathyroidism, exclusion of FHH and MEN as possible diagnoses, careful review of previous operative notes and pathologic specimens, and localization studies.

How are abnormal glands localized in patients with recurrent or persistent hyperparathyroidism?
Noninvasive studies include computed tomography, ultrasonography, ^{99m}Tc sestamibi scintigraphy, and magnetic resonance imaging. Although computed tomography and magnetic resonance imaging are best for imaging the mediastinum, ultrasonography is sensitive to lesions in the neck and is much cheaper. If noninvasive imaging is inadequate, invasive studies, such as intraarterial digital subtraction angiography, conventional selective angiography, parathyroid venous sampling, and intraoperative ultrasonography are conducted. These procedures have allowed localization in up to 95% of cases.

Are there alternatives to surgical reexploration in patients with recurrent or persistent hyperparathyroidism in whom a mediastinal adenoma has been localized by angiography?
An alternative to surgical reexploration is angiographic ablation of the adenoma with ionic contrast material. Ablation is feasible in approximately 70% of patients with mediastinal adenomas. Even if it is unsuccessful, this procedure does not preclude surgical resection (44).

What is the operative strategy for parathyroid reoperation?
Disease will be found on neck reexploration in 60 to 70% of patients. Thus, the neck is usually explored first at reoperation unless a mediastinal adenoma has been found preoperatively. In the latter instance, either a partial or a complete sternotomy is performed, and attention is first directed to the thymus and then to posterior dissection of the mediastinum. The same surgical procedures recommended for a thorough neck exploration at initial operation apply on reexploration with regard to locating ectopic adenomas or parathyroid tissue in the neck. When hyperparathyroidism recurs in patients who were thought to have had adequate resection after initial neck exploration, the parathyroid disease should be treated as hyperplasia; subtotal parathyroidectomy or total parathyroidectomy with autotransplantation should be performed. During reexploration of patients in whom only biopsy-proven normal glands were detected at initial operation, identification and removal of the abnormal gland without further attempts to identify normal glands is usually successful.

What is secondary hyperparathyroidism?
Secondary hyperparathyroidism, or reactive hyperparathyroidism of renal disease, a compensatory response to lowered serum calcium levels by the parathyroid glands, is the result of progressive loss of nephrons. Several interrelated factors promote it. Renal disease suppresses the addition of the second hydroxyl group to form active 1,25-dihydroxyvitamin D; it also leads to decreased phosphate excretion and hyperphosphatemia. As a result, calcium absorption from the gut is decreased and ionized calcium levels are lowered, which enhances pro-

duction of PTH. This in turn leads to hyperplasia of parathyroid chief cells. The hypocalcemia is also fueled by a skeletal resistance to the action of PTH (45).

What are the major clinical manifestations of this disorder?
Clinical manifestations include bone pain and tenderness, especially in the pelvic girdle; pathologic fractures; proximal muscle weakness; severe pruritus; gastrointestinal problems, including peptic ulcer disease, nausea, and vomiting; painful extraskeletal calcifications, especially in periarticular sites; and ischemic necrosis of various tissues caused by progressive vascular calcification (46).

What is the recommended treatment?
The initial goals of therapy are to prevent parathyroid hyperplasia and secondary hyperparathyroidism by controlling hyperphosphatemia and negative calcium balance. Hyperphosphatemia is treated by lowering phosphate intake and administering aluminum hydroxide or carbonate to minimize intestinal absorption of phosphorus. Calcium levels are enhanced by oral calcium supplements and calcitriol and by dialysis with solutions containing high concentrations of ionized calcium (3 to 3.5 mEq/L).

What are the indications for parathyroidectomy in secondary hyperparathyroidism?
Indications for parathyroidectomy include hypercalcemia, either spontaneous or appearing during treatment with small doses of vitamin D; progressive increase in serum PTH to more than 20 times normal levels; bone pain; skeletal complications; pruritus; and soft tissue calcifications. For maximum benefit, parathyroidectomy should be performed before renal osteodystrophy leads to extensive bone involvement. Four hyperplastic glands are usually found at surgery, and a total parathyroidectomy with autotransplantation of parathyroid tissue is recommended (47). However, some surgeons recommend total parathyroidectomy without transplantation, relying on the presence and function of additional parathyroid rests and oral calcium supplementation to control calcium levels (48).

What is the significance of aluminum intoxication in patients with chronic renal failure, and how is it treated?
Aluminum accumulation in patients with chronic renal failure impedes bone mineralization, with resultant osteomalacia, which may occur with bone pain, fractures, and proximal muscle weakness. This condition is easily confused with renal osteodystrophy from secondary hyperparathyroidism and should be ruled out before surgery. Desferrioxamine, an aluminum chelator, is used to treat aluminum intoxication.

What are the effects of renal transplantation on secondary hyperparathyroidism?
Hypercalcemia and the skeletal effects of secondary hyperparathyroidism may be diminished or even cured by renal transplantation.

What is tertiary hyperparathyroidism, and how is it treated?
Tertiary hyperparathyroidism is secondary hyperparathyroidism in which PTH secretion has become autonomous. Hypertrophied parathyroid tissue continues to secrete increased quantities of PTH despite hypercalcemia. The diagnosis is established by an elevated serum calcium level in a previously hypocalcemic patient with chronic renal failure and secondary hyperparathyroidism. The most pertinent example is persistent hyperparathyroidism after successful renal transplantation.

Management should be conservative, and adequate time must be allowed for PTH levels to return to normal. Parathyroidectomy should be reserved for pa-

Management Algorithm for Palpable Thyroid Nodule

Algorithm 4.1. (Adapted from Doherty GM, Norton JA. Thyroid and parathyroid. In: Lawrence PF, ed. Essentials of General Surgery. 2nd ed. Baltimore: Williams & Wilkins, 1992:299.)

Management Algorithm for Primary Hyperparathyroidism

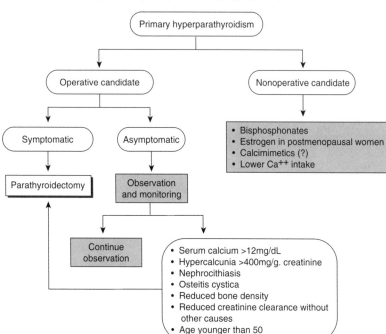

Algorithm 4.2.

tients with symptomatic disease and for those in whom severe asymptomatic hypercalcemia (serum calcium level higher than 12.5 mg/dL) persists for more than a year after the transplant (49).

REFERENCES

1. Frank R, Vander Velde TL, Doherty GM. Management of nodular thyroid disease and thyroid cancer associated with neck irradiation. Probl Gen Surg 1997;14:27–33.
2. Gagel RF, Goepfert H, Callender DL, et al. Changing concepts in the pathogenesis and management of thyroid carcinoma. CA Cancer J Clin 1996;46:261–283.
3. Cady B. Arguments against total thyroidectomy. Probl Gen Surg 1997;14:44–51.
4. Clark OH, Levin K, Zeng QH, et al. Thyroid cancer: the case for total thyroidectomy. Eur J Cancer 1988;24:305–313.
5. Mazzaferri EL, Jhiang SM. Long term impact of initial surgical and medical therapy on papillary and follicular thyroid cancer. Am J Med 1994;97:418–428.
6. Schlumberger MJ. Papillary and follicular thyroid carcinoma. N Engl J Med 1998; 338:297–306.
7. Chen H, Nicol TL, Udelsman R. Follicular lesions of the thyroid: does frozen section alter operative management? Ann Surg 1995;222:101–106.

8. Chen H, Nicol TL, Zeiger MA, et al. Hürthle cell neoplasms of the thyroid: are there factors predictive of malignancy? Ann Surg 1998;27:542–546.

9. Soybel DI, Wells SA. Medullary thyroid carcinoma. In: Cady B, Rossi R, eds. Surgery of the Thyroid Glands. 3rd ed. Philadelphia: Saunders, 1991:152–178.

10. Clark OH, Duh QY. Thyroid cancer. In: Greer MA, ed. The Thyroid Gland. New York: Raven, 1990:537–572.

11. Hay ID, Grant CS, Taylor WF, et al. Ipsilateral lobectomy versus bilateral lobar resection in papillary thyroid carcinoma: a retrospective analysis of surgical outcome using a novel prognostic system. Surgery 1987;102:1088–1095.

12. Cady B, Rossi R. An expanded view of risk-group definition in differentiated thyroid carcinoma. Surgery 1988;104:947–953.

13. Grant CS, Hay ID. Staging and prognosis in differentiated thyroid carcinoma. Probl Gen Surg 1997;14:34–43.

14. Lee HK, Graham ML. Anaplastic thyroid cancer: diagnosis, prognosis and treatment. Probl Gen Surg 1997;14:124–131.

15. Studer H, Gerber H. Non-toxic goiter. In: Greer MA, ed. The Thyroid Gland. New York: Raven, 1990:391–404.

16. Orgiazzi JJ, Mornex R. In: Greer MA, ed. The Thyroid Gland. New York: Raven, 1990:405–495.

17. Soh EY, Duh QY. Diagnosis and management of hot nodules (Plummer's disease). Probl Gen Surg 1997;14:165–173.

18. Winsa B, Rastad J, Larrson E, et al. Total thyroidectomy in therapy-resistant Graves' disease. Surgery 1994;116:1068–1075.

19. Bilezikian JP. Etiologies and therapy of hypercalcemia. Endocrinol Metab Clin North Am 1989;18:389–413.

20. Chan FKW, Koberle LMC, Thys-Jacobs S, Bilezikian JP. Differential diagnosis, causes, and management of hypercalcemia. Curr Probl Surg 1997;34:456–461.

21. Nussbaum SR, Potts JT. Advances in immunoassays for parathyroid hormone: clinical applications to skeletal disorders of bone and mineral metabolism. In: Bilezikian JP, Marcus R, Levine MA, eds. The Parathyroids. New York: Raven Press, 1994:157–169.

22. Heath H III. Familial benign (hypocalciuric) hypercalcemia: a troublesome mimic of mild primary hyperparathyroidism. Endocrinol Metab Clin North Am 1989;18:723–740.

23. Brown EM. Homeostatic mechanisms regulating extracellular and intracellular calcium metabolism. In: Bilezikian JP, Marcus R, Levine MA, eds. The Parathyroids. New York: Raven Press, 1994:15–54.

24. Mallette LE. Regulation of blood calcium in humans. Endocrinol Metab Clin North Am 1989;18:601–610.

25. Brunt LM, Halverson JD. The endocrine system. In: O'Leary JP, Capote LR, eds. The Physiologic Basis of Surgery. 2nd ed. Baltimore: Williams & Wilkins, 1996:388.

26. Broadus AE, Mangin M, Ikeda K, et al. Humoral hypercalcemia of cancer: identification of a novel parathyroid hormone-like peptide. N Engl J Med 1988;319:556.

27. Chan FKW, Koberle LMC, Thys-Jacobs S, Bilezikian JP. Differential diagnosis, causes, and management of hypercalcemia. Curr Probl Surg 1997;34:489–492.

28. Silverberg SJ, Gartenberg F, Jacobs TP, et al. Longitudinal measurements of bone density and biochemical indices in untreated primary hyperparathyroidism. J Clin Endocrinol Metab 1995;80:723–728.

29. Thomas JM, Cranston D, Knox AJ. Hyperparathyroidism: patterns of presentation, symptoms and response to operation. Ann R Coll Surg Engl 1985;67:79–82.

30. Mowschenson PM, Silen W. Developments in hyperparathyroidism. Curr Opin Oncol 1990;2:95–100.

31. Chan FKW, Koberle LMC, Thys-Jacobs S, Bilezikian JP. Differential diagnosis, causes, and management of hypercalcemia. Curr Probl Surg 1997;34:462–464.

32. Kaplan EL, Yoshiro T, Salti G. Primary hyperparathyroidism in the 1990's. Ann Surg 1992;215:300–317.

33. Irvin GL, Prudhomme DL, Deriso GT. A new, practical intraoperative parathyroid hormone assay. Am J Surg 1994;219:574–581.

34. Sfakianakis GN, Irvin GL, Foss WM, et al. Efficient parathyroidectomy guided by SPECT-MIBI and hormonal measurements. J Nucl Med 1996;37:798–804.

35. Oertli D, Richter M, Kraenzlin M, et al. Parathyroidectomy in primary hyperparathyroidism: preoperative localization and routine biopsy of unaltered glands are not necessary. Surgery 1995;117:392–396.

36. Levin KE. The reasons for failure in parathyroid operations. Arch Surg 1989;124:911–915.

37. Rossi RL, Cady B. Surgery of the parathyroid glands. In: Cady B, Rossi RL, eds. Surgery of the Thyroid and Parathyroid Glands. 3rd ed. Philadelphia: Saunders, 1991:283–294.

38. Brasier AR, Nussbaum SR. Hungry bone syndrome: clinical and biochemical predictors of its occurrence after parathyroid surgery. Am J Med 1988;84:654–660.

39. Fitzpatrick LA, Bilezikian JP. Acute primary hyperparathyroidism. Am J Med 1987;82:275–282.

40. Chan FKW, Koberle LMC, Thys-Jacobs S, Bilezikian JP. Differential diagnosis, causes, and management of hypercalcemia. Curr Probl Surg 1997;34:477.

41. Goldsmith RE, Sizemore GW, Chen I, et al. Familial hyperparathyroidism: description of a large kindred with physiologic observations and a review of the literature. Ann Intern Med 1976;84:36–43.

42. Metz DC, Jensen RT, Bale AE, et al. Multiple endocrine neoplasia type I. In: Bilezikian JP, Marcus R, Levine MA, eds. The Parathyroids. New York: Raven Press, 1994:591–646.

43. Gagel R. Multiple endocrine neoplasia type II. In: Bilezikian JP, Marcus R, Levine MA, eds. The Parathyroids. New York: Raven Press, 1994:681–698.

44. Miller DL, Doppmann JL, Chang R. Angiographic ablation of parathyroid adenomas: lessons from a 10-year experience. Radiology 1987;165:601–607.

45. Martin KJ, Slatopolsky E. The parathyroids in renal disease. In: Bilezikian JP, Marcus R, Levine MA, eds. The Parathyroids. New York: Raven Press, 1994:711–745.

46. Sitges-Serra A, Caralps-Riera A. Hyperparathyroidism associated with renal disease. Surg Clin North Am 1987;67:359–377.

47. Romanus ME, Farndon R, Wells SA. Transplantation of the parathyroid glands. In: Johnston IDA, Thompson NW, eds. Endocrine surgery. Stoneham MA: Butterworth, 1983:25–40.

48. Kaye M, D'Amour P, Henderson J. Elective total parathyroidectomy without autotransplant in end-stage renal disease. Kidney Int 1989;35:1390–1399.

49. D'Alessandro AM, et al. Tertiary hyperparathyroidism after renal transplantation: operative indications. Surgery 1989;106:1049–1056.

Gastroesophageal Reflux Disease

Prashant K. Narain and Eric J. DeMaria

Andrew Grant is a 45-year-old man who has a 3-year history of heart-burn that is particularly bothersome at night when he is in bed. The heartburn worsens when he bends over; antacids provide relief. Occasionally he wakes up at night coughing and choking.

Mr. Grant's medical history is significant for hypertension and bronchial asthma, for which he takes calcium channel blockers and albuterol by inhaler, respectively. He smokes a pack of cigarettes and drinks 10 cups of coffee daily. He also admits to significant intermittent consumption of alcohol.

The physical examination reveals no problems; Mr. Grant is well developed and well nourished, his vital signs are within normal limits, and examination shows his chest, cardiovascular system, and abdomen to be normal. The rectal examination is normal and the stool is guaiac negative. The physician makes a provisional diagnosis of gastroesophageal reflux disease (GERD) on the basis of the history.

What is the prevalence of GERD in the United States?
Approximately 40 million persons in the United States have GERD. Although about 38% of the population has heartburn, only those with severe symptoms (approximately 10% of this group) seek the advice of their physician (1).

What are the clinical features of GERD?
The typical symptoms of GERD are heartburn and regurgitation. However, the absence of these symptoms does not exclude GERD. Conversely, only about a third of patients with typical symptoms have endoscopic evidence of GERD.

Atypical symptoms of GERD include substernal chest pain (approximately 50% of patients with noncardiac chest pain have reflux disease), hoarseness caused by reflux laryngitis, hiccups, asthma, ear pain, loss of dental enamel, night sweats, heartburn during intercourse (reflux dyspareunia), and dysphagia secondary to stricture.

What is the pathophysiology of GERD?
Gastroesophageal reflux to a certain extent is a normal continual phenomenon. Prolonged contact of the esophageal mucosa with gastric juice leads to pathologic conditions such as esophagitis and subsequently to stricture and metaplasia (Barrett's esophagus). Innate mechanisms protect the esophagus from abnormal reflux (2), and when these fail, signs and symptoms of GERD appear. These protective mechanisms can be described as esophageal, gastric, and duodenal.

1. Esophageal factors
   Lower esophageal sphincter (LES) mechanism. Dysfunction of the LES is the most important esophageal factor in the pathophysiology of reflux. Once the high-pressure zone of the lower esophageal sphincter is lost, reflux of gastric contents occurs. Many factors affect the LES and can precipitate reflux symptoms. The anatomic factors that are believed to contribute to the LES are mentioned later in this chapter.
   Peristalsis. Another important factor is esophageal peristalsis. Primary peristalsis results from a swallowing reflex that propels the bolus of food down the esophagus and lowers the LES to allow the bolus passage into the stomach. Secondary peristaltic waves are initiated in the esophagus. These so-called stripping waves clear any refluxed material from the esophagus into the stomach.
   Salivary bicarbonate. Swallowed salivary bicarbonate neutralizes gastric acid in the esophagus and thus protects the esophageal lining.
   Esophageal mucosa. The esophageal mucosa has inherent defense mechanisms against the noxious gastric secretions. Bicarbonate in the unstirred water layer adjacent to the mucosa protects the mucosa from H^+ and pepsin. This mechanism is believed to play only a minor role in humans. Other protective mechanisms of the esophageal mucosa are intercellular tight junctions, epithelial transport (Na^+-H^+ exchange), epithelial buffers, and the lipid bilayer of the stratum corneum (3). Along with these factors, an adequate esophageal blood supply helps in cell replication, regeneration, repair, and adequate nutrition of the epithelium.
2. Gastric factors
   Gastric distention. Gastric distention reduces the LES pressure and promotes reflux. Patients with Zollinger-Ellison syndrome are prone to reflux disease because of the increased gastric volume secondary to gastric hypersecretion.
   Increased intraabdominal pressure. Obese patients and pregnant women have increased intraabdominal pressure, which raises the pressure gradient across the LES, causing reflux of gastric contents.

3. Duodenal factors

Alkaline reflux. The alkaline reflux of biliary and pancreatic juices can injure the esophagus (4), a well-documented occurrence after resection of the LES following total gastrectomy.

At present, there is no evidence that *Helicobacter pylori* plays any significant role in reflux disease.

What investigations aid in the diagnosis of GERD?
The initial diagnosis is based largely on the history. Several tests can help in diagnosis and management of the disease:

1. Tests for mucosal injury
   Esophagogastroduodenoscopy (EGD). EGD is usually the first test to be performed. It is useful for the detection of mucosal injury and for the surveillance of Barrett's metaplasia. Endoscopic appearance can be misleading, as biopsy of a "normal" mucosa may reveal florid inflammatory changes. Histology helps make the diagnosis of esophagitis and Barrett's metaplasia.
   Barium esophagram. Reflux may be demonstrated with a barium esophagram even in normal persons. Reflux becomes pathologic when it is excessive, frequent, and associated with symptoms and signs of reflux disease. A barium esophagram reveals mucosal abnormalities, strictures, motility dysfunction, and a short esophagus. This allows surgery to be customized to the patient's needs.
2. Tests for abnormal reflux
   The 24-hour pH monitor. One of the most specific and sensitive tests for GERD, pH monitoring quantifies the actual periods when acid is in contact with the esophageal mucosa. It allows the correlation of these exposures with the subjective feeling of heartburn. A normal 24-hour pH study virtually rules out reflux disease. Some new probes (e.g., Bilitec) also monitor any biliary contents in the esophagus.
   Barium study. A barium study of the upper gastrointestinal (GI) tract can demonstrate reflux and the presence of hiatal hernia. Reflux itself is not considered pathologic because some degree of reflux is normal, as mentioned earlier. A barium study may also show evidence of mucosal injury, abnormalities of esophageal motility, and gastroparesis.
3. Test for gastric emptying
   Gastroesophageal scintiscan. Delayed gastric emptying can be detected with this scan, in which a ^{99}Tc sulfur colloid–labeled diet is used. About 5% of patients with reflux disease have poor gastric emptying. If these patients undergo antireflux surgery, the steep increase in intragastric

pressure postoperatively can cause wrap disruption or gastric perforation. To prevent these complications, a pyloroplasty may be added to the fundoplication.

4. Test for esophageal motility

   Esophageal manometry. This test is helpful in individualizing the surgery. The LES pressure in patients with reflux disease is usually 6 mm Hg or less. Most patients therefore require a 360° wrap. A partial wrap is indicated if the LES pressure is high or if the esophageal motility is poor. Patients with a high LES pressure may still have abnormal reflux, and patients with a low LES pressure may have a normal esophagus.

5. Other test

   Bernstein's test of acid perfusion in the distal esophagus to elicit esophageal sensitivity has mostly historical value.

What are the recommended changes to Mr. Grant's lifestyle?
The first step in the treatment of reflux disease is a change in lifestyle.

Diet. A diet low in fat, mint, chocolates, coffee, and alcohol improves the LES pressure and reduces reflux. Obese patients who lose weight by dieting may have less heartburn as the result of both better diet and decreased intra-abdominal pressure.

Sleeping position and time. Patients are advised to raise the head end of the bed and sleep on their left side. Gravity helps to clear the esophagus of the gastric refluxate and decrease the symptoms of reflux. Patients are also advised to delay going to bed until 3 to 4 hours after the last meal to allow the stomach to empty.

Smoking. Smoking worsens reflux disease by decreasing the LES pressure and increasing the time taken for esophageal clearance.

Medications. Medications that decrease the LES (e.g., calcium channel blockers in the case of Mr. Grant) should be changed. Medications that worsen reflux are listed in Table 5.1.

Other factors. Tight clothes and exercise can aggravate the symptoms of reflux. Although stress does not directly cause GERD, it makes the patient more sensitive to the symptoms of reflux and has therefore been historically associated with GERD.

Mr. Grant tries conservative measures for a few months, but his symptoms do not improve.

Which single test is appropriate at this stage?
Upper GI endoscopy (EGD) is the initial test usually recommended for diagnosing the extent and severity of the disease. EGD also allows for concurrent biopsy and dilation (5).

Table 5.1. FACTORS THAT AFFECT LES PRESSURE

Factors that increase LES pressure
Diet: Protein, coffee
Drugs: Cisapride, metoclopramide, bethanecol, norepinephrine, phenylephrine
Hormones: Gastrin, bombesin, motilin, substance P, L-encephalin
Other: Antireflux surgery, gastric alkalization
Factors that decrease LES pressure
Diet and lifestyle: Fatty diet, old age, exercise, chocolate, mint, alcohol, cigarettes
Drugs: Atropine, epinephrine, theophylline, nitroglycerin, prostaglandin F_2, oral
   contraceptives, diazepam, dopamine, meperidine, calcium channel blockers,
   barbiturates, prostaglandins E_1 and E_2
Hormones: Secretin, cholecystokinin, glucagon, somatostatin, neuropeptide Y,
   vasoactive intestinal peptide, and calcitonin gene–related peptide
Medical conditions: Diabetes, pregnancy, hiatal hernia, gastric acidification,
   hypothyroidism, amyloidosis, gastrectomy, placement of nasogastric tube

EGD on Mr. Grant reveals inflammation in the lower portion of the esophagus and a small sliding hiatal hernia. No other abnormalities are noted. A biopsy is performed on the distal esophagus.

What are the histologic features of GERD?
Some 94% of the patients with significant GERD have histologic abnormalities; in 40 to 65% of patients, abnormalities are visible during endoscopy. The histologic features that correlate with reflux are the subject of considerable debate. Findings, even in carefully controlled experiments on animals, are inconsistent. These features are common in GERD:

1. Segmented leukocytes (neutrophils and eosinophils) infiltrating the mucosa
2. Balloon cells: enlarged, round squamous cells with a pale-staining cytoplasm and a degenerative nucleus caused by the pathologic swelling of the cell
3. Epithelial hyperplasia (basal cell zone thickness of the mucosa)
4. Papillomatosis (elongated papillae of lamina propria extending to within a few epithelial cell layers of the mucosal surface)
5. Erosions (denudation of the superficial layers of the mucosa)
6. Ulcers (full-thickness destruction of the mucosa and muscularis mucosae)
7. Distention and congestion of the microvasculature in the papilla of the lamina propria
8. Barrett's esophagus

What is a hiatal hernia, and what is its association with GERD?
Hiatal hernia is herniation of the stomach through the esophageal hiatus. There are three types of hiatal hernia:

Sliding hernia. The phrenoesophageal membrane becomes lax; the LES is pulled up in the thorax along with a portion of the stomach.
Paraesophageal hernia. The stomach herniates into the thorax, but the LES remains in its intraabdominal location.
Mixed hernia. The hiatal hernia is a combination of the sliding and paraesophageal types.

GERD and hiatal hernia are common conditions that may coexist in a patient. No evidence supports a cause-and-effect theory. Hiatal hernia can exacerbate reflux disease by two mechanisms. With the sliding hernia, the LES gets pulled up in the thorax; the LES pressure is thereby reduced and reflux increases. A hiatal hernia may also trap the gastric secretions that have refluxed into the esophagus and hinder their clearance, prolonging exposure to acid juices and worsening the esophageal injury.

Where is the esophagogastric junction?
The precise location of the esophagogastric junction is a matter of controversy. There are three opinions:

1. It is the junction of the squamous and columnar epithelium (Z line, or ora serrata). This is not accepted by many because the last few centimeters of the esophagus may be normally lined with columnar epithelium.
2. It is the junction of the esophageal circular muscle layer and the oblique muscle fibers of the stomach known as the collar of Helvetius.
3. It is the site at which the tubular esophagus joins the gastric pouch.

What is the normal resting pressure of the LES? What anatomic features contribute to the sphincter mechanism?
The LES is more a physiologic than an anatomic entity. It is the name given to the distal 1 to 5 cm of the esophagus that acts as a high-pressure zone. The resting pressure of the LES is normally 10 to 20 mm Hg. In GERD the resting pressure is usually less than 6 mm Hg.

Various anatomic factors may contribute to the sphincter mechanism of the LES:

1. Reflection of the phrenoesophageal membrane from the muscular margins of the diaphragmatic hiatus to the esophagus. This tethers the LES in the intraabdominal position.
2. Intraabdominal position of the LES. The transmission of positive intraabdominal pressure to the distal esophagus increases the LES pressure above the negative pressure of the intrathoracic esophagus.
3. The right crus of the diaphragm encircles the esophagus and on contraction may act as a pinchcock, closing the esophagus.

4. The acute angle of insertion of the esophagus into the stomach (angle of His) helps prevent reflux.
5. The oblique sling fibers of the muscle layer of the stomach at the gastro-esophageal (GE) junction.
6. The rosettelike configuration of the gastric mucosa at the GE junction helps prevent reflux.

What factors affect LES pressure?
The factors that affect LES pressure are listed in Table 5.1.

How is GERD managed medically?
GERD is a chronic disease, and most patients' symptoms can be controlled with medications. The objectives of treatment are relief of symptoms, avoidance of complications, healing of esophagitis, and ideally, healing of any mucosal metaplasia. However, the natural history of the disease does not change with medications, and symptoms recur after therapy is stopped. The following therapies may be used:

Lifestyle changes. These have been discussed in a previous section.
Antacid therapy. Antacids may provide short-term systematic relief, but they are ineffective for long-term therapy of GERD. Ingestion of large quantities of calcium-containing antacids may result in serum electrolyte abnormalities, such as the milk-alkali syndrome.
H_2 receptor blockers. When changes in lifestyle and antacid therapy are ineffective, H_2 receptor blockers are used. The commonly used ones are ranitidine (Zantac), cimetidine (Tagamet), nizatidine (Axid), and famotidine (Pepcid); famotidine is the most potent.
Proton pump inhibitors (H^+-K^+ ATPase inhibitors). These drugs are much more powerful than H_2 blockers. One dose of inhibitor reduces gastric acid secretion by 90% in a normal person. When H_2 blockers fail, omeprazole (Prilosec) is the drug most commonly used. Other proton pump inhibitors are lansoprazole (Prevacid) and pantoprazole.
Prokinetic agents. Other medications, such as prokinetic agents and sucralfate, may be added as adjunctive therapy to control GERD symptoms. Sucralfate provides a protective lining for the mucosa in an acid environment. It is used in the treatment of peptic ulcer disease and to prevent stress gastritis; however, its role in GERD is small. Cisapride (Propulsid) is the most common prokinetic agent used. Others include metoclopramide (Reglan), domperidone (Motilium), bethanechol (Urecholine), and erythromycin.

The drugs may be combined for synergistic effect. When standard doses are ineffective, higher doses of these medications may be used. It is fairly common for patients with severe reflux symptoms to be treated with twice the normal doses of omeprazole, cisapride, and sucralfate.

What are the side effects of H_2 blockers and H^+-K^+ ATPase inhibitors?
H_2 blockers are fairly safe. Common side effects include diarrhea, headache, fatigue, muscular pains, drowsiness, and constipation. Cimetidine and to a lesser extent ranitidine reversibly bind to oxidases of the cytochrome P450 system and inhibit hepatic metabolism of drugs such as phenytoin, warfarin, and theophylline, which raises the serum level of these medications. Other effects may include gynecomastia resulting from elevated serum prolactin levels and a reduction in procainamide secretion by the renal tubules, leading to higher serum levels.

Proton pump inhibitors are similarly well tolerated; common GI side effects are dyspepsia, nausea, vomiting, flatulence, and diarrhea. Headaches are less common, as is inhibition of P450 system of liver enzymes and attendant drug interactions. Reduction of acid secretion causes hypergastrinemia, bacterial overgrowth, and nitrosamine production, all of which may lead to gastric malignancy. Long-term administration of high doses of omeprazole to rats causes gastric carcinoid tumors; however, this has not been observed in humans.

Mr. Grant is prescribed a 3-month course of high-dose omeprazole and cisapride. However, his symptoms persist after therapy, and he still wakes up with a choking sensation at night and has coughing spells. He now complains of dysphagia with solid food. Endoscopy is repeated; it reveals esophagitis and a stricture in the lower esophagus; the latter problem is corrected successfully by endoscopic dilation.

What are the different types of esophageal dilators and what are their respective advantages and disadvantages?
Three types of esophageal dilators are commonly used:

Mercury-filled rubber bougie. Examples are the Hurst (round tip) and Maloney (tapered tip) types. These are easy to use but require repeated blind passages. The operator has a good feel for the resistance. These dilators are not useful in very tight or irregular strictures.

Guided, fixed-size dilator. Examples are Eder Puestow metal olives and Celestin, Savary Gilliard, Buess, and Keymed advanced dilators. They are passed over a guide wire, and because of their relative stiffness, they can negotiate tight and irregular strictures. The disadvantages include pharyngeal and dental injury; also, the operator does not have a good feel for resistance.

Balloon dilator. Various types of balloon dilators can traverse irregular strictures. They have the advantage of not causing any shearing damage because the force applied is radial, but the balloons are fragile and easily displaced.

Surgery is recommended to Mr. Grant at this stage.

What are the indications for surgery in GERD?
The indications for surgery are as follows:

- Failed medical therapy with persistent esophagitis and/or persistent symptoms
- Complications of GERD, such as Barrett's esophagus, stricture refractory to medical treatment, or bleeding from refractory esophagitis
- Healthy young patient who prefers surgery to lifelong medication
- Extraesophageal symptoms from reflux that are refractory to medical treatment

What are some antireflux procedures?
Antireflux procedures can be divided into these groups (6):

Partial fundoplication
- Belsey Mark IV (thoracic approach, anterior 270° wrap, crural repair)
- Toupet (abdominal approach, posterior 270° wrap, crural repair)
- D'or (abdominal approach, anterior 270° wrap, crural repair)
- Hill (abdominal approach, posterior wrap, anchor GE junction to the median arcuate ligament)

Total fundoplication
- Floppy Nissen (abdominal approach, 360° wrap, crural repair)
- Rosetti Nissen (same as floppy Nissen but no division of short gastric arteries)

Antireflux prosthesis
- Angelchik prosthesis (discredited because of problems of slippage, perforation, and stricture)

Experimental procedures
- Endoscopic injection of collagen in LES
- Endoscopic injection of sodium morrhuate into gastric cardia
- Narbona sling procedure (abdominal approach, mobilization of hepatic ligamentum teres, and formation of a sling around the gastroesophageal junction onto the anterior stomach)

Common laparoscopic procedures used for reflux disease are the floppy Nissen and Toupet fundoplications.

What are the goals of surgery for reflux disease?
The primary goal of surgery is to reestablish the competency of the LES. These are the technical goals:

1. To place an adequate length (1.5 to 2 cm) of the distal esophagus in the positive pressure environment of the abdomen

2. To maintain or restore overall LES pressure to twice the resting gastric pressure (e.g., 12 mm Hg for a gastric pressure of 6 mm Hg)
3. To avoid too competent an LES by use of a 60-F bougie in the esophagus prior to wrap placement and use of a wrap no longer than 1.5 cm
4. To perform crural repair

A floppy Nissen procedure is performed laparoscopically on Mr. Grant. He is discharged home the day after surgery. Initially, he notices some dysphagia and inability to belch, but these problems improve with time. Heartburn and regurgitation decrease, and he does not have choking spells at night.

What are some complications of antireflux surgery?
The mortality from antireflux surgery is approximately 1%, and the morbidity after surgery approaches 10%.

Specific complications of antireflux surgery can be operative or postoperative. Operative complications specific to reflux surgery include splenic trauma leading to splenectomy and its attendant problems, perforated esophagus, and inadvertent vagotomy. The usual postoperative complications specific to reflux surgery are gas bloat syndrome, inability to vomit or belch, and dysphagia.

General complications of any surgery include atelectasis, pleural effusion, bleeding, wound infection, deep venous thrombosis, and pulmonary embolism.

Most of these complications specific to antireflux surgery are self-limited and diminish with time. Good results are evident in more than 90% of patients 10 years after a Nissen procedure (7).

What are some technical reasons for a failed surgical repair?
The following are some common reasons for surgical failure:

1. Partial or complete breakdown of the repair
2. Placement of the wrap around the stomach instead of around the esophagus
3. Overtight wrap (fails to mobilize the short gastric vessels) or overlong wrap
4. Herniation of the wrap into the chest
5. Necrosis or fistula in the lower esophagus
6. Inadvertent division of the vagus nerve

What are the complications of GERD?
Severe GERD can cause erosions, ulcerations, stricture, and metaplasia. The difference between an erosion and an ulcer is that an erosion is only a mucosal

injury, whereas an ulcer is deeper. Ulcers can bleed, perforate, or cause strictures. Metaplasia (Barrett's esophagus) can lead to dysplasia and malignancy.

Other complications attributed to GERD are laryngitis, hoarseness, cough, bronchitis, asthma, pneumonitis, and hemoptysis. Apnea and sudden infant death syndrome have been associated with reflux disease in children.

What is the stepwise progression for diagnosis and management of GERD?
An algorithm for management is presented at the end of this chapter.

What is Barrett's esophagus and why is it important? What are the usual histologic features?
Barrett's esophagus was first described in 1950 by Sir Norman Barrett of England. His initial hypothesis that this was a congenital condition with columnar cells lining the distal esophagus has largely been discarded. It is now considered to be acquired from long-standing reflux disease. Repeated and prolonged peptic acid and alkaline reflux damage the esophageal mucosa, which undergoes repair and regeneration. Barrett's esophagus is essentially a metaplasia of the damaged squamous epithelium of the esophagus to the columnar type, which has a propensity for dysplasia and neoplasia. Approximately 10% of patients with severe GERD have Barrett's disease (1), and 0.5 to 10% of patients with Barrett's esophagus eventually develop carcinoma. Even patients with easily controlled symptoms of reflux disease may have severe dysplasia accompanying Barrett's esophagus. Patients with Barrett's disease have a risk of malignancy that is 40 times as high as in the general population. This translates into a sevenfold lifelong risk of developing adenocarcinoma. The risk is the same as that of a 55-year old smoker developing lung cancer (8). The histologic features of Barrett's disease are usually subdivided into three distinct patterns:

1. **Specialized, or intestinal, type,** the most common variety, is characterized by villous architecture, mucous glands, and goblet cells, features that are normally seen in the small bowel.
2. **Junctional type** has mucosa resembling the cardia of the stomach.
3. **Fundic type,** in which the mucosa resembles the gastric fundus, with parietal and chief cells, is the type associated with malignancy. Coexistence of different types is usual.

How is Barrett's disease treated, and what are the results of surgery?
The treatment of Barrett's disease is controversial. An algorithm for management is presented at the end of this chapter. It is not clear whether nonoperative treatment prevents dysplasia or reduces the degree of dysplasia that may already be present. Similarly, although some literature suggests that surgery may cure a few

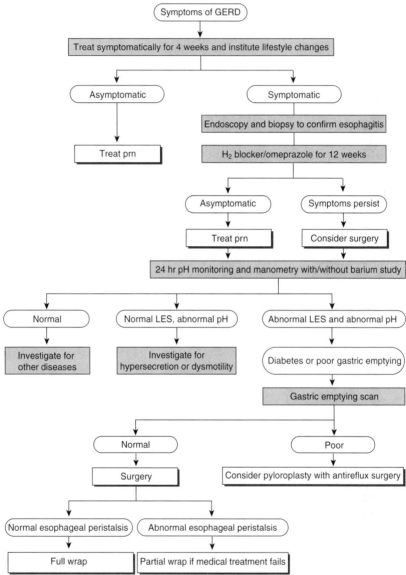

Algorithm 5.1.

Management Algorithm for Barrett's Esophagitis

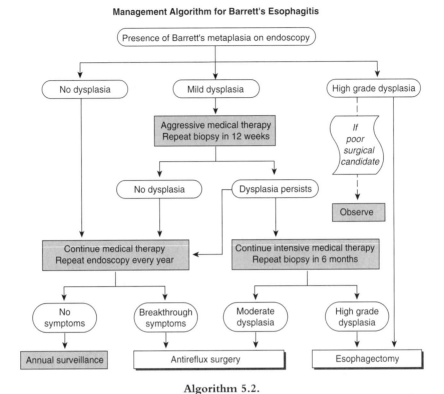

Algorithm 5.2.

patients with dysplastic Barrett's disease, the consensus is that antireflux surgery does not cure the condition, although it may delay or prevent the development of dysplasia.

How are esophageal motility disorders classified?
Esophageal motility disorders can be primary or secondary.

Primary disorders include achalasia, diffuse and segmental esophageal spasm, nutcracker esophagus, hypertensive lower esophageal sphincter, and other nonspecific disorders.

Secondary disorders, which include systemic sclerosis, polymyositis, dermatomyositis, systemic lupus erythematosus, and mixed connective tissue disease, chronic idiopathic intestinal pseudo-obstruction, neuromuscular disorders, endocrine disorders, and metastatic disorders, are secondary to collagen disorders.

REFERENCES

1. Nebel OT, Fornes MF, Castell DO. Symptomatic gastro-esophageal reflux: incidence and precipitating factors. Am J Dig Dis 1976;21:953–956.
2. Cohen S. The pathogenesis of gastro-esophageal reflux disease: A challenge in clinical physiology. Ann Intern Med 1992;117:1051–1052.
3. Orlando RC. Esophageal epithelial defenses against acid injury. Am J Gastroenterol 1994;89:S48–S52.
4. Lillemoe KD, Johnson LF, Harmon JW. Alkaline esophagitis: a comparison of the ability of components of gastroduodenal contents to injure the rabbit esophagus. Gastroenterology 1983;85:621–628.
5. Weinberg DS, Kadish SL. The diagnosis and management of gastroesophageal reflux disease. Med Clin North Am 1996;80:411–429.
6. Peters JH, DeMeester TR. Minimally Invasive Surgery of the Foregut. St. Louis: Quality Medical Publishing, 1994.
7. DeMeester TR, Bonavina L, Albertucci M. Nissen fundoplication for gastro-esophageal reflux disease: evaluation of primary repair in 100 consecutive patients. Ann Surg 1986; 204:9–20.
8. Dent J, Bremner CG, Collen MJ, et al. Barrett's Esophagus: Working Party Reports of the Ninth World Congress of Gastroenterology. Melbourne: Blackwell Scientific, 1990: 17–26.

Esophageal Cancer

Richard Maley and Cornelius M. Dyke

Richard Smith is a 51-year-old white man who was in good health until 8 weeks ago, when he began having progressive dysphagia, especially with solids. A review of symptoms is remarkable only for heartburn, which was controlled with omeprazole (Prilosec) for many years. He has not been vomiting, nor does he have odynophagia, weight loss, or pulmonary symptoms. He has hypertension and diabetes mellitus, and his medications are fosinopril (Monopril), omeprazole, and insulin. He has had no previous surgery. He is a former smoker (50-pack-year history) and a social drinker.

Mr. Smith's vital signs are normal, and a head and neck examination reveals no oral lesions, adenopathy, or carotid bruits. His chest is clear to auscultation, and the cardiovascular examination is normal. No mass or organomegaly is detected during the abdominal examination. The rectal examination does not identify a mass and is negative for occult blood. The neurologic examination is unremarkable.

What is the differential diagnosis of Mr. Smith's dysphagia?
In general, difficulty in swallowing can be caused by central nervous system lesions, motility disorders of the esophagus, or obstructive disorders of the esophagus. Mr. Smith does not have neurologic problems. However, he does have a history of reflux, so peptic stricture of the esophagus is a possibility. Benign and malignant obstructive lesions are also possibilities.

Which screening tests are recommended for initial evaluation of dysphagia?
Many causes of dysphagia (e.g., esophagitis, esophageal cancer) result in chronic anemia, which may be detected with a complete blood count. The chest radiograph may show pulmonary metastases, aspiration pneumonitis, a large thoracic aneurysm, a dilated esophagus, or a large periesophageal hernia. The barium contrast examination should be the first evaluation of a patient with dysphagia. In

cases of dysphagia caused by obstruction, it accurately defines the cause and the anatomy. Anatomic definition is essential before esophagoscopy.

Mr. Smith's primary care physician orders a complete blood count, chest radiograph, and barium contrast examination. Mr. Smith's hemoglobin level is 14 g/dL (normal range is 12 to 15 g/dL); his chest radiograph is normal; and his barium swallow examination shows distal esophageal irregular narrowing, consistent with esophageal cancer.

Mr. Smith is referred to a thoracic surgeon because of the barium swallow results. The thoracic surgeon performs esophagoscopy and performs a biopsy of a 6-cm irregular exophytic mass 32 to 38 cm from the incisors in the distal esophagus. The biopsy specimen is positive for adenocarcinoma. A computed tomography (CT) scan of the chest and abdomen demonstrates no metastases.

What important assessments are made during esophagoscopy?
Endoscopists locate tumors in the esophagus by measuring the distance of the tumor from the incisor teeth. With this method, the esophagus begins 15 cm from the incisors and terminates at the gastroesophageal (GE) junction (38 to 45 cm). A tumor mass should always be sampled for biopsy, and the pathology findings should be confirmed before treatment is begun. Because the stomach is the most frequently used conduit for replacement of the esophagus after resection, the endoscopist must examine the stomach carefully for any disease. The endoscope can be turned back on itself once in the stomach for a careful examination of the GE junction to confirm that the tumor does not extend into the stomach.

How are esophageal cancers classified anatomically?
The esophagus (23 to 30 cm long) can be divided into four parts:

1. Cervical esophagus: C6 to T2 (cricoid cartilage to suprasternal notch)
2. Thoracic esophagus, upper third: T2 to T5 (suprasternal notch to carina)
3. Thoracic esophagus, middle third: T5 to T8 (carina to inferior pulmonary vein)
4. Thoracic esophagus, lower third: T8 to T12 (inferior pulmonary vein to GE junction)

Mr. Smith's cancer is a distal third thoracic esophageal adenocarcinoma.

Should the airway of patients with esophageal cancer be examined?
Mr. Smith does not need a bronchoscopic examination because he has no symptoms related to the airway and because his tumor is in the distal third of the thoracic esophagus. Patients who have pulmonary symptoms (cough, hemoptysis,

pneumonia) should undergo bronchoscopy at the time of esophagoscopy. Tumor in the cervical esophagus or upper third of the thoracic esophagus can invade the trachea and larynx; tumor in the middle third of the thoracic esophagus can invade the carina. Patients whose tumor can locally invade the airway should undergo bronchoscopy even if they have no symptoms.

Should tests other than CT of the chest and abdomen be performed to detect metastases?
In most cases this is not necessary. For specific complaints (e.g., headache or bone pain), CT of the brain and a nuclear bone scan may be obtained. The CT of the chest and abdomen may demonstrate liver, lung, and lymph node metastasis, which as a rule cause no symptoms until disease is extensive. However, the relative inaccessibility of the esophagus has limited accurate tumor staging, and new techniques are being developed. These include endoscopic ultrasonography (1), positron emission tomography, and minimally invasive surgical staging. Endoscopic ultrasonography is critically important for clinical staging and should be performed wherever possible.

What is the most common malignant tumor of the esophagus?
In 1980, squamous cell carcinoma accounted for more than 90% of malignant esophageal tumors, with adenocarcinoma constituting 7% of the malignancies. By 1987, adenocarcinoma accounted for 34% of esophageal tumors, and the incidence of adenocarcinoma now approaches 50% (2). The reasons for these changes are unclear.

What are the risk factors for esophageal cancer?
The main risk factors for developing esophageal squamous cell carcinoma are tobacco use, alcohol use, and nutritional deficiencies. Lesser risk factors for squamous cell carcinoma are male sex, black race, achalasia, Plummer-Vinson syndrome, scleroderma, lye stricture, and nitrosamine ingestion. China and Iran have a particularly high incidence of squamous cell cancers. The risk factors for adenocarcinoma are less well defined; they include esophageal reflux disease, Barrett's esophagus, and being a white man.

What are the treatment options and cure rates for esophageal cancer?
Surgery, radiation therapy, and chemotherapy have been used either alone or in combinations to treat esophageal carcinoma. Radiation therapy alone in high doses (40 to 50 Gy) carries a 5-year survival rate of 5 to 10% (3). Surgery alone results in a 5-year survival of 20% (4). This percentage is higher for patients operated for cure and significantly lower for patients operated for palliation. The addition of preoperative radiation to surgery confers no survival benefit, very likely because surgery and radiation are both forms of local treatment, and patients are most likely to die of disseminated disease. Cisplatin-based combination chemotherapy has yielded response rates ranging from 25 to 35% in

metastatic esophageal carcinoma and rates of 50 to 75% for local or regional disease. Trials of combinations of chemotherapy with surgery or radiation, now under way, have shown promise (5).

How is esophageal cancer staged, and what is the survival rate for each stage?
Esophageal cancer is staged with the tumor, node, and metastasis (TNM) system described by the American Joint Committee for Cancer Staging (Tables 6.1 and 6.2). Survival for esophageal cancer is broken down by the stage of disease. The 5-year survival reported by Roth et al. (6) is as follows: stage 1, 61%; stage II, 25 to 40%; stage III, 16%; and stage IV, less than 5%.

Mr. Smith's CT scan does not show evidence of metastasis, so he does not have stage IV tumor. He undergoes endoscopic ultrasonography and is found to have tumor through the esophageal wall (T_3) and periesophageal lymph node involvement (N_1). Therefore, he has a stage III tumor with an expected 5-year survival of 16%.

What is the best treatment for Mr. Smith?
Mr. Smith's thoracic surgeon recommends a multimodal treatment plan consisting of two courses of fluorouracil and cisplatin and 40 Gy of radiation therapy followed by surgery. In a prospective, randomized trial comparing surgery alone with combined chemotherapy, radiation therapy, and surgery, 3-year survival for surgery alone was 6% compared with 32% for combination therapy (5).

Mr. Smith proceeds with the multimodal treatment plan. After he receives chemotherapy and radiation therapy, he returns to the thoracic surgeon.

Table 6.1. TUMOR, NODE, METASTASIS CLASSIFICATION OF ESOPHAGEAL CANCER

Tumor (T)
  T_0, no evidence of tumor
  T_1, tumor invasion of the lamina propria or submucosa
  T_2, tumor invasion of the muscularis propria
  T_3, tumor invasion of adventia
  T_4, tumor invasion of adjacent structures
Nodal (N)
  N_0, no lymph node metastasis
  N_1, regional lymph node metastasis
Metastasis (M)
  M_0, no evidence of distant metastasis
  M_1, distant metastasis

Table 6.2.   STAGING OF ESOPHAGEAL CANCER

Stage	Tumor (T)	Node (N)	Metastasis (M)
I	T_1	N_0	M_0
IIa	T_2	N_0	M_0
	T_3	N_0	M_0
IIb	T_1	N_1	M_0
	T_2	N_1	M_0
III	T_3	N_1	M_0
	T_4	Any N	M_0
IV	Any T	Any N	M_1

What are the surgical options for adenocarcinoma of the distal esophagus?
A tumor of the esophagus must be removed so that proximal and distal margins are negative as evaluated in frozen sections. This usually requires removal of a large portion of the esophagus because the tumor spreads in the submucosa. In most cases the stomach is mobilized and advanced cephalad to replace the resected esophagus. The blood supply of the stomach used as an esophageal replacement is based on the first gastroepigastric artery. The stomach can easily reach the neck without causing tension. The two most commonly performed procedures are Iver-Lewis esophagectomy (laparotomy, right thoracotomy, and anastomosis in the right chest) (7) and transhiatal esophagectomy (laparotomy and cervical incisions with a blunt esophagectomy and an anastomosis in the neck) (8).

What are possible complications of esophagectomy?
In addition to the usual complications after any major surgery, complications specific to esophagectomy are anastomotic leak, anastomotic stricture, and reflux. In general, the risk of anastomotic leak from a cervical anastomosis is higher (19% plus or minus 15%) than that reported for an intrathoracic anastomosis (11% plus or minus 6%). However, mortality from a cervical anastomotic leak was 20% plus or minus 11% compared with 69% plus or minus 16% for an intrathoracic leak (9). The more cephalad the anastomosis, the less the reflux symptoms. Anastomotic stricture is most common with a cervical anastomosis. These may be satisfactorily managed with dilation.

What are alternative conduits if the stomach cannot be used because of tumor involvement or previous surgery?
The colon and less commonly the jejunum have been used for conduits. Some thoracic surgeons routinely obtain barium enemas before surgery and have the patient undergo a mechanical colon preparation the day before surgery in case

these sites have to be used. The left or right colon may be used, depending on the surgeon's preference, although the smaller caliber of the left colon may confer some advantage.

Which additional surgical procedures are performed because of esophagectomy?
Because esophagectomy entails removal of both vagus nerves, pyloroplasty or pyloromyotomy is performed. A feeding jejunostomy is also performed in case postoperative nutritional problems arise.

Mr. Smith has a transhiatal esophagectomy, pyloromyotomy, and feeding jejunostomy. His postoperative course is uncomplicated and a barium swallow examination on postoperative day 5 is normal. He is discharged home on postoperative day 6, eating soft food and receiving nutritional supplements via the jejunostomy tube.

Can surgery be performed in all patients with esophageal cancer?
Patients with tumor involvement of only the esophagus, of the esophagus and regional nodes (Mr. Smith's case), or even with minimal metastatic disease such as a single liver nodule are best treated with resection and reconstruction. However, several conditions preclude resection and reconstruction:

Advanced age or coexistent severe medical conditions
Extensive metastatic disease
Esophageal cancer that is technically unresectable because of invasion of structures such as the aorta
Malignant esophagorespiratory fistula

In these situations, the thoracic surgeon must palliate the patient's symptoms, which most often are severe progressive dysphagia, chronic blood loss from the tumor surface, and, in the case of an airway fistula, continual aspiration of ingested food, saliva, and refluxed gastric contents.

How is dysphagia palliated?
Radiation therapy, surgical bypass, dilation and stent placement, and laser therapy have all been used.

Is external beam radiation satisfactory for the palliation of dysphagia?
This treatment frequently causes tumor shrinkage, but palliation is only modest because the tumor is replaced by a stricture, so dysphagia persists. Adenocarcinoma tends to respond less well to external beam radiation than does squamous cell carcinoma. Radiation to the upper two-thirds of the esophagus is tolerated better than radiation to the lower third because irradiation of the GE junction and celiac axis causes significant nausea and vomiting.

What is brachytherapy?
Brachytherapy is the use of intracavitary radioactive materials to treat tumors. Intracavitary radiation is the standard treatment for early carcinoma of the cervix and the body of the uterus. The radioactive agents used are ^{137}Cs, ^{60}Co, and ^{129}Ir. In 1985, Flores et al. (10) used endoesophageal radiation to treat esophageal cancer. Its use is still investigational.

What is the most common route of surgical bypass, and what is the most common esophageal substitute?
There are four possible anatomic bypass routes: posterior mediastinal; anterior mediastinal and retrosternal; subcutaneous over the sternum and antesternal; and intrapleural. The most common is the retrosternal route, and the most common conduit is the stomach. The subcutaneous route is usually used in patients with no retrosternal space—for example, patients who have had cardiac surgery. In a recent large series, a hospital mortality rate of 11% was reported; 90% of the survivors could tolerate an unrestricted diet (11). For patients in whom the risk of surgery is acceptable but who are not candidates for resection, surgical bypass can offer durable lifelong palliation.

A variety of minimally invasive techniques can palliate esophageal cancer. Pneumatic dilation of tumors at any level can be done through the flexible upper endoscope. This procedure, if performed alone, results in rapid restenosis, but expandable metal stents can help maintain the lumen of the esophagus. If a malignant esophagorespiratory fistula is present, a covered stent can be used. A covered stent does not grip the tissue as well as an uncovered stent and may therefore migrate distally because of ongoing esophageal peristalsis. Hence, an uncovered stent is preferred if there is no fistula. Endoscopic esophageal laser therapy, first described in 1982, can control bleeding and rapidly restore the patency of the esophageal lumen to allow oral nutrition (11). Complications include bleeding, perforation, and fistula, but the rate is low.

What is photodynamic therapy and how does it work?
Photodynamic therapy is an experimental treatment in which a photosensitizing chemical that is activated by light selectively destroys neoplastic tissue. Three components are needed to cause cell death: a sensitizer, light, and oxygen. The sensitizer is a porphyrin-based compound that is injected intravenously. This chemical is initially taken up by all cells in the body but is released more rapidly by normal cells than by cancerous cells over the next 48 hours. After 48 hours, the tumor is exposed to light, most commonly a red light produced by an argon pump dye laser. In esophageal cancer, the light is delivered through the esophagoscope down a fiberoptic cable. The tip of the fiber delivers a cylindrical field of light perpendicular to the axis of the fiber and thus makes treatment along the side walls of the esophagus easy and rapid. In the

Management Algorithm for Esophageal Cancer

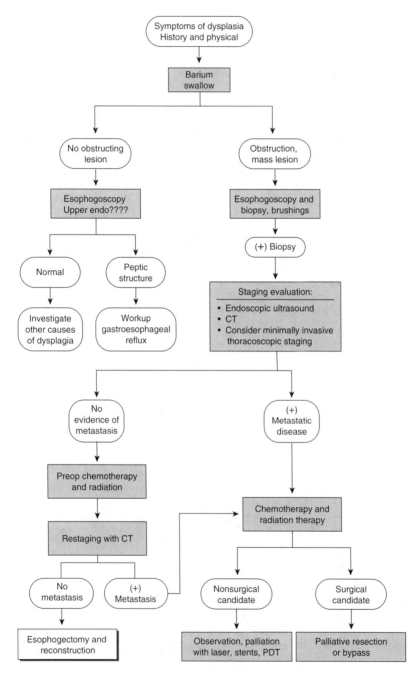

Algorithm 6.1.

presence of oxygen, the light-activated sensitizer triggers formation of singlet oxygen and other oxygen-free radicals, which damage the tumor vasculature and lead to tumor ischemia and necrosis (12).

What is the main complication of photodynamic therapy?
The sensitizer remains in skin macrophages in declining concentrations for about 30 to 45 days. Patients must avoid direct and reflected sunlight during this period and wear protective clothing if they go outdoors. Exposure to sunlight can lead to first- or second-degree burns. Tumor regrowth is the main shortcoming of both laser ablation therapy and photodynamic therapy.

What is Barrett's esophagus?
Barrett's esophagus, or columnar-lined esophagus (CLE) is caused by severe, long-standing reflux of gastric contents into the esophagus. Repeated injury-repair processes cause a metaplastic condition in which the normal squamous epithelium is replaced by glandular epithelium. This condition is present in 10% of patients with symptomatic gastroesophageal reflux disease, as revealed in endoscopic biopsy specimens.

Why is CLE an important clinical finding?
CLE can ulcerate, cause a stricture, and possibly degenerate into adenocarcinoma. The estimated risk of developing adenocarcinoma of the esophagus in patients with CLE is 30 to 40 times that of the general population (13). CLE is treated by treating gastroesophageal reflux disease and screening for dysplasia. Biopsy samples from patients with CLE show a range of disease including no dysplasia, low-grade dysplasia, high-grade dysplasia, and carcinoma in situ. In general, patients with CLE should undergo esophagoscopy and biopsy every year, with the interval reduced to every 6 months if low-grade dysplasia is present. Esophagectomy is required for carcinoma and in the opinion of some surgeons, for high-grade dysplasia also. In one study, carcinoma was present in 40 to 50% of esophagectomy specimens removed for high-grade dysplasia. The majority of these carcinomas were intramucosal and had a high likelihood of cure (14).

REFERENCES

1. Botet JF, Lightdale CJ, Zauber AG, et al. Preoperative staging of esophageal cancer: comparison of endoscopic US and dynamic CT. Radiology 1991;181:419.
2. Blot WJ, Devesa SS, Kneller RW, Fraumeni JF. Rising incidence of adenocarcinoma of the esophagus and gastric cardia. JAMA 1991;265:1287.
3. Newaishy GA, Read GA, Duncan W. Results of radical radiotherapy of the squamous carcinoma of the esophagus. Clin Radiol 1982;33:347.
4. Ellis FH Jr. Treatment of carcinoma of the esophagus or cardia. Mayo Clin Proc 1989;64:945.
5. Walsh TN, Noonan N, Hollywood D, et al. A comparison of multimodal therapy and surgery for esophageal adenocarcinoma. N Engl J Med 1996;335:462–467.

6. Roth JA, Ruckdeschel JC, Weisenburger TH, eds. Thoracic Oncology. Philadelphia: Saunders, 1989.
7. Skinner DB. En bloc resection for neoplasms of the esophagus and cardia. J Thorac Cardiovasc Surg 1983;85:59.
8. Orringer NM. Transhiatal esophagectomy without thoracotomy for carcinoma of the thoracic esophagus. Ann Surg 1984;200:282.
9. Muller JM, Erasmi H, Stelzner M, et al. Surgical therapy of oesophageal carcinoma. Br J Surg 1990;77:845.
10. Flores AD, Nelem B, Evans KG, et al. Impact of new radiotherapy modalities on the surgical management of carcinoma of the esophagus and cardia. Int J Radiat Oncol Biol Phys 1989;17:937.
11. Fleischer D, Kessler F, Bage O. Endoscopic Nd:YAG laser therapy for carcinoma of the esophagus: a new palliative approach. Am J Surg 1982;143:280.
12. Pass HI. Photodynamic therapy in oncology: mechanisms and clinical use. J Natl Cancer Inst 1993;85:6.
13. Spechler SJ, Robbins AA, Rubins HB, et al. Adenocarcinoma and Barrett's esophagus: an overrated risk? Gastroenterology 1984;87:927.
14. Rice TW, Falk GW, Achkar E, Petras RE. Surgical management of high-grade dysplasia in Barrett's esophagus. Am J Gastroenterol 1993;88:1832.

Peptic Ulcer Disease

David Page

Robbie Steele is a 49-year-old insurance agent with epigastric pain. For approximately 6 months, Mr. Steele has had vague abdominal distress after meals and at night, and he now uses antacids on a regular basis. However, the antacids are no longer effective. Although he admits to one instance of blood in his stool and occasional nausea, he denies repeated melena, change in bowel habits, or weight loss. He smokes a pack of cigarettes a day, uses aspirin sparingly, and drinks socially. The remainder of his history is negative.

What other important information should be obtained?
The following information should be elicited:

• When antacid use was started
• Use of other over-the-counter antacids or histamine receptor antagonists
• Any vomiting of blood
• Diminished ability to eat a whole meal
• Heartburn

Mr. Steele has used antacids for 1 to 2 years for epigastric pain as well as for heartburn. He vomited blood once 6 months ago, but his appetite has not been impaired. His weight dropped 10 pounds during the past year. Mr. Steele has an average build with normal vital signs, and other than being nervous, he is not in acute distress. The findings of the head, neck, and chest examinations are normal. The abdominal examination reveals epigastric tenderness with deep palpation. There is no guarding or rebound tenderness, and bowel sounds are present. No mass or groin hernia is present. Findings of rectal examination and hemoccult tests are negative.

What is the first step in assessing a new patient with symptoms such as Mr. Steele's?
The clinician must determine how sick the patient is. Factors that must be

considered include severity of pain and associated symptoms, hemodynamic status, and any indications for immediate surgery. The need for urgent workup for acute symptoms must be determined, and a plan for resuscitation, if needed, must be made.

What is the differential diagnosis for epigastric pain?
Diagnoses include but are not limited to peptic ulcer disease, gastritis, pancreatitis, pancreatic cancer, biliary tract disease, abdominal aortic aneurysm, early appendicitis, gastroenteritis, and ischemic heart disease.

Why is acute myocardial infarction included in the differential diagnosis of epigastric pain?
Pain from the inferior wall of the left ventricle may be referred to the epigastrium and can be associated with nausea, vomiting, and diaphoresis.

Mr. Steele's laboratory tests show the following: hemoglobin level, 14.2 g/dL; hematocrit, 41%; white blood cell count, 12,800/mL; normal blood urea nitrogen, creatinine, amylase, and lipase levels. Liver function is normal. An electrocardiogram shows normal sinus rhythm at 82/minute with no acute changes.

What is the most likely diagnosis according to the laboratory results?
The normal electrocardiogram eliminates acute myocardial infarction. Normal liver function studies suggest there is probably no acute biliary tract disease, although an ultrasound examination is needed if cholecystitis is suspected. Normal amylase and lipase levels rule out pancreatitis and along with a normal hemoglobin reduce the likelihood of pancreatic carcinoma. Gastritis, gastroenteritis, and early appendicitis are unlikely but possible according to his history and presentation. The absence of a palpable pulsatile mass on initial examination reduces the possibility of abdominal aortic aneurysm. Peptic ulcer disease is the most likely diagnosis.

How is peptic ulcer disease confirmed?
Upper endoscopy (esophagogastroduodenoscopy) is the next step for confirming the diagnosis and defining the extent of the disease. Not only can ulcers be seen but this test also helps rule out other diagnoses such as reflux esophagitis, Barrett's esophagus, and gastritis. All gastric ulcers must be sampled for biopsy (four-quadrant specimens must be obtained); and if the ulcers appear suspect for malignancy, gastric washings must be obtained for cytologic examination. Gastric ulcers that have not healed as determined by endoscopy after several weeks of treatment must also be aggressively assessed with repeat biopsies. Although cancer of the duodenum is unusual, biopsy of anomalous, nonhealing duodenal ulcers is necessary. Experience in Japan has demonstrated that early diagnosis and treatment of gastric ulcer improves survival (1).

What is the incidence of peptic ulcer disease?
Approximately 5 million Americans have peptic ulcer disease (2). Ulcers occur most commonly in men aged 45 to 55, although they also occur in the elderly and occasionally in children and adolescents.

What causes peptic ulcer disease?
Historically, excess gastric acid was believed to cause peptic ulcer disease. Now, however, it is estimated that 90% of duodenal ulcers and 80% of gastric ulcers are associated with *Helicobacter pylori,* the putative causative agent (3). This organism is found in the gastric mucous layer or on the gastric mucosa. Other factors associated with peptic ulcers are cigarette smoking, high alcohol intake, nonsteroidal antiinflammatory drug use, and a stressful lifestyle. Excess gastric acid production continues to accompany peptic ulceration.

Mucosal injury of the stomach (gastric ulceration or stress gastritis) is associated with specific stressors such as major body surface burns (Curling's ulcer), multiple organ failure, multiple trauma, and head injuries (Cushing's ulcer) (4).

What is H. pylori *and how is* H. pylori *infection diagnosed?*
H. pylori is a spiral flagellated organism found worldwide. In countries such as China, in which *H. pylori* infects more than half the population during early childhood, the rate of gastric cancer, which is also associated with this organism, is high. *H. pylori* infection is linked to both duodenal and gastric ulcers and to the lymphoid type of mucosal lymphoma. Approximately two-thirds of the world population is infected with *H. pylori*. In the United States the organism is most often seen in African-Americans, Hispanics, the elderly, and the poor (5). Three tests diagnose *H. pylori* infection: rapid urease test, serologic antibody measurement, and urea breath test.

What is the treatment for peptic ulcer disease?
Uncomplicated peptic ulcer disease is treated medically with any of a number of agents. Surgical intervention is reserved for recalcitrant cases that progress to complications such as bleeding, obstruction, perforation, and intractability. Before the role of *H. pylori* in peptic ulcer disease was discovered, primary treatment centered on histamine receptor antagonists such as cimetidine, ranitidine, and famotidine. Omeprazole, a parietal cell proton pump blocker, has proved to be a more potent agent for acid suppression but is not used for long-term treatment. Sucralfate, an aluminum salt of sulfated sucrose that binds to the ulcer base and promotes healing, is used to treat acute duodenal ulcers. Pain resolution with sucralfate is less prompt than with H_2 blockers.

The standard treatment of peptic ulcer disease focuses on treatment of *H. pylori* infection with any of several drug combinations. The most common regimen is a 14-day course of triple treatment, which consists of bismuth, metronidazole, and either tetracycline or amoxicillin. Other choices include regimens combining (*a*) omeprazole and clarithromycin; (*b*) ranitidine, bismuth citrate, and clarithromycin; and (*c*) lansoprazole and either amoxicillin alone or amoxicillin with clarithromycin (6–8). The choice of treatment is up to the individual physician.

What are the goals of peptic ulcer treatment and how is therapy assessed?
The goals of treatment are to provide rapid relief of symptoms; promote permanent healing of the ulcer (avoid recurrence); reduce ulcer-related complications; and control treatment costs (9). After treatment, the eradication of *H. pylori* must be confirmed by either endoscopic biopsy or a urea breath test. If the results are negative, no further medical treatment is needed.

How successful is treatment with triple or alternative therapy for H. pylori?
The rates of recurrence of gastric and duodenal ulcers are 4% and 6%, respectively, after successful eradication of *H. pylori,* compared with 59% and 67%, respectively, if the organism persists (10).

Mr. Steele completes a course of triple therapy consisting of bismuth, metronidazole, and ampicillin, and his symptoms resolve. He returns to his investment job with his usual enthusiasm and resumes smoking. About 2 months later, he goes to the emergency department because of gnawing epigastric pain. Endoscopy, performed within the next 2 weeks, reveals a recurrent duodenal ulcer. He is reluctant to undergo further medical treatment and requests a more permanent alternative.

What are the alternatives to medical treatment for gastric ulcer disease?
Laparoscopic (minimally invasive) surgery has had a great influence on the surgical management of peptic ulcers (11). Enthusiasm for surgical therapy has been renewed because of shorter hospital stays, acceptable recurrence rates after proximal gastric vagotomy, and probable overall reductions in cost as compared with long-term pharmacologic management. Surgical treatment is mandatory if medical therapy fails and symptoms become intractable or if gastric outlet obstruction, significant bleeding, or perforation occurs. However, a patient should undergo more than one course of conservative, nonsurgical treatment before a surgeon is consulted.

Mr. Steele ignores his doctor's advice to undergo another course of medical treatment and refuses surgery. About 4 months later he arrives in the emergency room vomiting bright red blood. His blood

pressure is 80/60 mm Hg, his pulse is 110 beats per minute, and he is diaphoretic.

What is the first step in managing a patient in a condition such as Mr. Steele's?
Mr. Steele is in hemorrhagic shock and must be resuscitated immediately. Normal saline or lactated Ringers solution must be administered via one or two large-bore intravenous lines, and blood must be drawn for typing, cross-matching, and routine laboratory tests. A Foley catheter and a nasogastric tube must also be inserted and the fluid balance monitored. Preparations must be made for emergency upper endoscopy.

What is the differential diagnosis for upper gastrointestinal hemorrhage?
Possible diagnoses include but are not limited to reflux esophagitis, esophageal cancer, esophageal varices, gastritis, gastric cancer, foreign body trauma to the esophagus or stomach, Dieulafoy's ulcer, gastric and duodenal ulcers, and swallowed blood from an upper aerodigestive lesion.

What endoscopic findings suggest ongoing bleeding or rebleeding from a peptic ulcer?
Endoscopic assessment of upper gastrointestinal bleeding identifies patients at high risk for rebleeding, who may require prolonged hospitalization and repeat assessment. Patients who have ulcers with a clean base or with small, flat blood spots do not require endoscopic treatment and may be sent home with appropriate medications (12, 13). Those with active arterial bleeding or with a visible nonhemorrhaging vessel should be treated endoscopically with a heat probe or, rarely, injection therapy. If bleeding is recurrent, a second endoscopic treatment may be attempted as long as it does not delay any necessary surgery.

An emergency upper endoscopic examination of Mr. Steele reveals a pyloric channel ulcer that has a clot at the base. The endoscopist elects not to disturb the clot and terminates the procedure.

What are the indications for surgical treatment of bleeding peptic ulcers?
Emergency surgery for hemorrhage must be performed for the following three conditions:

1. The patient continues to hemorrhage and remain in shock despite maximum resuscitation; surgery is usually contemplated if the patient does not respond to administration of 6 to 8 units of blood.
2. The patient stops bleeding clinically and rebleeds as proven endoscopically; if a patient rebleeds massively, surgery is indicated without repeat endoscopy.
3. The patient bleeds slowly but persistently and requires 2 or 3 units of blood per day for several consecutive days.

What is the recommended surgical procedure for a hemorrhagic ulcer?
Three standard procedures may be considered in this setting:

Oversewing of the bleeding ulcer with highly selective (proximal gastric) vagotomy may be performed open or laparoscopically. In the urgent setting with massive bleeding, the open approach is expedient and stops the hemorrhage more quickly. The recurrence rate is 10 to 15%, but few postoperative complications occur.

Oversewing of bleeding ulcer with truncal vagotomy and pyloroplasty, probably the most often used procedure, is performed open. Complete division of the vagus nerve requires a drainage procedure, such as pyloroplasty, to overcome gastric stasis.

Oversewing of ulcer with antrectomy (hemigastrectomy) and truncal vagotomy has the lowest recurrence rate (2 to 3%) but is associated with more postoperative complications than the other procedures.

What are other indications for surgery in peptic ulcer disease?
In addition to massive bleeding, other indications for surgery in patients with peptic ulcer disease are perforation, obstruction, and intractability. Evaluations of the cost of peptic ulcer disease suggest that earlier surgery may be a less expensive alternative to lifelong pharmacologic therapy (10).

What is the recommended surgical procedure in a patient with a perforated ulcer?
The definitive operative options for a perforated peptic ulcer are similar to those for bleeding. In an emergency, the surgeon uses an omental patch (called a Graham patch) to close the perforation rather than oversewing as with a bleeding point. The rigidity of the surrounding tissue makes oversewing a perforation risky or impossible.

How is gastric outlet obstruction (acquired pyloric obstruction) treated?
Both nonsurgical and surgical procedures are effective, depending on the degree of scarring and stenosis. Balloon dilation via endoscopy, which is preferred for a small obstruction, may be repeated as needed. For pyloric stenosis that is not remediable by dilation, operative intervention is needed.

Which operation is indicated for gastric outlet obstruction secondary to peptic ulcer disease?
Either truncal vagotomy with pyloroplasty or antrectomy with truncal vagotomy is useful for patients with symptoms of gastric outlet obstruction. After gastric resection, reconstruction of the stomach may be with either a Billroth I (gastroduodenostomy) or a Billroth II (gastrojejunostomy) anastomosis (Figure 7.1). Truncal vagotomy with gastroenterostomy or a Roux-en-Y anastomosis is a less desirable option.

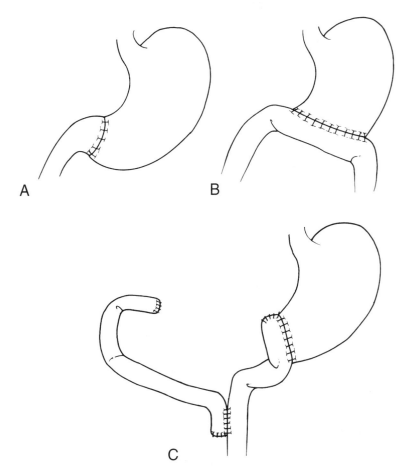

Figure 7.1. **A.** Billroth I (gastroduodenostomy) anastomosis. **B.** Billroth II (gastroje-junostomy) anastomosis. **C.** Billroth II with Roux-en-Y anastomosis.

Which surgical procedures are used for intractability?
The same procedures as for gastric obstruction are used. Laparoscopic proximal (parietal cell) gastric vagotomy is least invasive; open gastric resection with trun-cal vagotomy is most aggressive and has the highest complication rate. However, results with laparoscopic surgery should be assessed and compared with the time-tested open procedures before laparoscopic surgery is accepted as the standard (11).

Over time, Mr. Steele takes his medication less consistently, and his ulcer symptoms worsen. Eventually he develops intractable pain and some gastric outlet obstruction. He is counseled about options and agrees to undergo elective antrectomy and truncal vagotomy.

What are the short-term complications and long-term problems of gastric resection and vagotomy?
Postgastrectomy complications may be related to anatomic changes (absence of pyloric meter), influence of vagotomy, and several nutritional factors. Although many patients have these symptoms to varying degrees immediately after peptic ulcer surgery, only 1 to 2% have debilitating symptoms. Short-term problems include the following:

Early and late dumping syndromes are thought to result from the absence of the pylorus and the presentation of a high osmolar fluid load to the small bowel in a bolus. This causes epigastric pain, nausea, light-headedness, and possi-

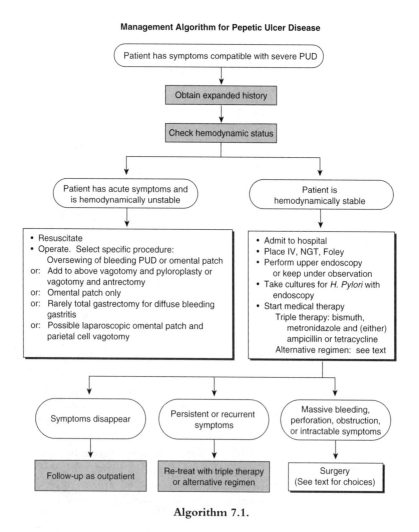

Management Algorithm for Pepetic Ulcer Disease

Patient has symptoms compatible with severe PUD

Obtain expanded history

Check hemodynamic status

Patient has acute symptoms and is hemodynamically unstable

Patient is hemodynamically stable

• Resuscitate
• Operate. Select specific procedure:
   Oversewing of bleeding PUD or omental patch
or: Add to above vagotomy and pyloroplasty or vagotomy and antrectomy
or: Omental patch only
or: Rarely total gastrectomy for diffuse bleeding gastritis
or: Possible laparoscopic omental patch and parietal cell vagotomy

• Admit to hospital
• Place IV, NGT, Foley
• Perform upper endoscopy or keep under observation
• Take cultures for *H. Pylori* with endoscopy
• Start medical therapy
   Triple therapy: bismuth, metronidazole and (either) ampicillin or tetracycline
   Alternative regimen: see text

Symptoms disappear

Persistent or recurrent symptoms

Massive bleeding, perforation, obstruction, or intractable symptoms

Follow-up as outpatient

Re-treat with triple therapy or alternative regimen

Surgery (See text for choices)

Algorithm 7.1.

bly syncope. Early dumping symptoms occur within minutes of eating; similar distress characterizes late dumping, which occurs an hour or more after a meal and which may be associated with reactive hypoglycemia.

Alkaline reflux gastritis occurs when alkaline bile is refluxed into the stomach in the absence of a pyloric barrier and patients have postprandial epigastric discomfort, nausea, and occasionally vomiting. These persons have endoscopic evidence of bile in the stomach, as well as biopsy-proven gastritis. Treatment includes H_2-receptor antagonists, changes in diet, and bile-binding drugs. A Roux-en-Y gastrojejunostomy is the surgical treatment for recalcitrant cases.

Postvagotomy diarrhea occurs in a small proportion of patients undergoing truncal vagotomy. Its prevention is one of the primary rationales for parietal cell vagotomy.

Nutritional deficiencies include iron-deficiency anemia, vitamin B_{12} anemia (loss of intrinsic factor), and protein-calorie deficits.

Cancer in the gastric remnant may occur 15 to 20 years after surgery. Long-term endoscopic follow-up is important (4).

REFERENCES

1. Fielding JWL. Gastric cancer: different diseases. Br J Surg 1989;76:1227.
2. Vakil, N, Fennerty B. The economics of eradicating *Helicobacter pylori* infection in duodenal ulcer disease. Am J Med 1996;100:60S–63S.
3. NIH Consensus Development. *Helicobacter pylori* in peptic ulcer disease. JAMA 1994; 272:65–69.
4. Mulholland MW. Stomach and duodenum. In: Greenfield LJ, et al, eds. Surgery: Scientific Principles and Practice. Philadelphia: JB Lippincott, 1993:661–702.
5. Hunt RH. Eradication of *Helicobacter pylori* infection. Am J Med 1996;100:42S–51S (review).
6. Hunt RH. Peptic ulcer disease: defining the treatment strategies in the era of *Helicobacter pylori*. Am J Gastroenterol 1992;92(4 Suppl):36S–43S.
7. Walsh JH, Peterson WL. The treatment of *Helicobacter pylori* infection in the management of peptic ulcer disease. N Engl J Med 1995;333:984–991.
8. Howden CW. Optimizing the pharmacology of acid control in the acid-related disorders. Am J Gastroenterol 1997;92(4 Suppl):17S–21S.
9. Hunt RH et al. Optimizing acid suppression for treatment of acid-related diseases. Dig Dis Sci 1995;40(2 Suppl):24S–49S.
10. Hopkins RJ, Girardi LS, Turney EA. Relation between *Helicobacter pylori* eradication and reduced duodenal and gastric ulcer recurrence: a review. Gastroenterology 1996; 110:1244–1252.
11. Casas AT, Gadacz TR. Laparoscopic management of peptic ulcer disease. Surg Clin North Am 1996;76:515–522.
12. Villanueva C, Balanzo J. A practical guide to the management of bleeding ulcers. Drugs 1997;53:389–403.
13. Jiranek GC, Kozarek RA. A cost-effective approach to the patient with peptic ulcer bleeding. Surg Clin North Am 1996;76:83–103.

Gastric Cancer

D. Scott Lind

Henry Jones is a 65-year-old man who has been having anorexia, postprandial fullness, and vague epigastric discomfort for the past 6 months. He has lost 20 pounds over this period but does not have dysphagia or vomiting. A peptic ulcer was diagnosed 4 months ago, and he was treated with an H_2 blocker, but his symptoms, anorexia, postprandial fullness, and vague epigastric discomfort, are now persistent. His medical history is unremarkable with the exception of hypertension that is well controlled by a thiazide diuretic. Mr. Jones's physical examination is also unremarkable, other than mild midepigastric tenderness to deep palpation. Rectal examination reveals no masses, but his stool is positive for occult blood. Laboratory examination reveals a hemoglobin of 9.2 g/dL, which indicates mild anemia. Levels of serum transaminases and alkaline phosphatase are within normal limits, and his albumin level is normal.

What are some early symptoms of gastric cancer?
Some of the initial symptoms of gastric cancer include weight loss, abdominal pain, nausea, and anorexia. These symptoms are nonspecific and are often overlooked by both the patient and the physician and as a result, the disease is often advanced when it is diagnosed. Proximal gastric cancer (i.e., cancer of the gastrointestinal junction) causes dysphagia, and distal gastric cancer (i.e., prepyloric cancer) results in gastric outlet obstruction, but both symptoms are common with advanced cancers. Gastrointestinal hemorrhage resulting from gastric cancer is usually occult; rarely is it severe enough to result in gross hematemesis (1).

What is an acceptable initial diagnostic step for this patient?
Empiric therapy with H_2 blockers for presumed ulcerative disease is probably inappropriate considering Mr. Jones's age and symptoms. An acceptable initial diagnostic test is an upper gastrointestinal radiographic study. This study has an overall accuracy of about 90%; however, normal results should not preclude further evaluation of the patient's symptoms (2). An alternative initial study is

flexible fiberoptic endoscopy (esophagogastroduodenoscopy). Endoscopy and contrast studies of the upper gastrointestinal tract are complementary in their diagnostic capabilities. In other words, endoscopy may provide information that was missed by upper gastrointestinal radiography and vice versa. If the surgeon does not perform endoscopy as part of his or her practice, upper gastrointestinal radiography provides a road map for any surgery that is contemplated. The advantage of endoscopy as a diagnostic test is that it permits biopsy of lesions that are visualized.

An upper gastrointestinal radiographic study reveals a 4-cm ulcer on the greater curve of the distal stomach.

What is the next step in the continuing evaluation of this patient?
Endoscopy is the next step for diagnostic workup for gastric cancer. Endoscopy allows the physician to obtain a tissue sample for histologic diagnosis (e.g., to distinguish between benign and malignant ulcers) and to define the extent of the lesion. Because a single endoscopic biopsy sample has not much diagnostic value, the endoscopist should take six or more samples from various parts of the ulcer (e.g., the base, slope, and rim). Histologic analyses of these biopsy specimens must be combined with brush cytology to increase diagnostic accuracy (3). Occasionally, endoscopy fails to detect a gastric malignancy. In addition, false-negative results are obtained with endoscopic biopsies from patients with gastric lymphoma because this malignancy is submucosal (4).

Pathology studies on the endoscopic brushings and biopsy specimens from Mr. Jones reveal poorly differentiated adenocarcinoma.

What are the histologic types of gastric malignancies, and what is the relative incidence of each type?
Approximately 95% of malignant neoplasms of the stomach are adenocarcinomas. The most common sarcoma of the gastrointestinal tract is leiomyosarcoma of the stomach, which accounts for 1 to 4% of malignant gastric tumors. Primary gastric lymphoma constitutes 1 to 5% of all gastric neoplasms and is the most common extranodal lymphoma. Adenosquamous, squamous, and carcinoid neoplasms occur in the stomach, but these account for less than 1% of gastric malignancies (5).

What is linitis plastica?
Linitis plastica means leather bottle. It is a morphologic variant of gastric adenocarcinoma characterized by a diffusely infiltrating tumor that incites a desmoplastic response, which results in a rigid, nondistendible stomach with no intraluminal mass. Patients with linitis plastica have a dismal prognosis.

What additional tests can help determine the extent of the disease?
In addition to a chest radiograph to detect pulmonary metastases, radiologic studies may include computed tomography (CT) of the abdomen. CT yields information about possible liver metastases, invasion of adjacent organs, and lymph node involvement. However, CT is relatively insensitive to peritoneal carcinomatosis, nor can it reliably establish unresectability of a tumor (6). Recently, endoscopic ultrasonography (EUS) has been used to assess the depth of penetration of the lesion and lymph node enlargement. EUS can accurately identify all the gastric layers (i.e., mucosa, submucosa, muscularis, subserosa, and serosa), and its findings correlate well with operative and pathologic findings (7). Although a precise role for EUS remains to be defined, it may allow more accurate preoperative staging and thus help identify patients who may benefit from neoadjuvant (preoperative) therapy. Unfortunately, with both CT and EUS, it is difficult to distinguish between inflammatory changes and tumor.

What is the anatomic distribution of adenocarcinoma of the stomach and its pattern of spread?
Approximately half of all gastric cancers arise in the gastric antrum, and about one-fourth arise in the body of the stomach. Recently, there has been an increase in cancer of the proximal stomach and gastroesophageal junction, particularly in young white men. However, the incidence of distal cancers has decreased (8). A thorough understanding of the patterns of spread of the disease is necessary to plan rational therapy for gastric cancer. The patterns of extension of gastric carcinoma are as follows:

1. Direct spread within the wall of the stomach, either proximally to involve the esophagus or less commonly, distally to involve the pylorus and duodenum
2. Direct extension to involve contiguous organs, such as the spleen, pancreas, colon, and left lobe of the liver
3. Peritoneal dissemination as a result of serosal penetration by the tumor
4. Lymphatic spread to involve local or distant lymph nodes
5. Bloodborne metastases, particularly to the liver

Virchow's node, Irish's node, Sister Mary Joseph's node, Krukenberg's tumor, and Blumer's shelf are all eponyms that may be associated with gastric cancer. How is each defined?

Virchow's node is a palpable left supraclavicular node that is often associated with an advanced gastrointestinal malignancy.
Irish's node denotes a palpable left axillary node.
Sister Mary Joseph's node is a palpable periumbilical node.
Krukenberg's tumor is a malignant tumor of the ovary that arises from a gas-

trointestinal malignancy because of either peritoneal or hematogenous metastases.

Blumer's shelf is an extraluminal mass that is palpable during a rectal or pelvic examination; it is the result of peritoneal metastases from a gastrointestinal malignancy.

Is the incidence of gastric cancer increasing or decreasing worldwide?
Over the past 50 years, the incidence of gastric cancer has declined dramatically in the United States. In 1930, gastric cancer was the most frequent cancer in adults, with an incidence of 38 in 100,000. The incidence decreased to 8 in 100,000 in 1980 and then leveled off in the mid-1980s. With approximately 25,000 new cases being reported per year and with about 15,000 deaths per year, gastric cancer remains a significant national health problem (9). In addition, gastric cancer is an enormous health problem worldwide. The incidence of gastric cancer in countries such as Japan and Chile is 10 times as high as that of the United States. In Japan, gastric cancer screening programs have greatly improved the detection of early lesions. In Western countries, screening for gastric cancer in the general population is probably not cost-effective with existing technology (10). However, some groups of patients in the United States are at high risk for gastric cancer and may benefit from screening.

What are some risk factors for gastric cancer?

1. **Gastric polyps** occur in two histologic types: hyperplastic and adenomatous. Hyperplastic polyps are not considered premalignant; however, patients with adenomatous polyps of the stomach are at increased risk for gastric cancer. The incidence of malignancy in patients with adenomatous gastric polyps correlates with the size and number of the polyps (11).
2. **Chronic atrophic gastritis and intestinal metaplasia** are both associated with an increased risk of gastric cancer. In fact, some physicians have proposed a pathway of disease progression from chronic atrophic gastritis (with intestinal metaplasia as a maladaptive response) to dysplasia and finally invasive carcinoma (12).
3. **Pernicious anemia** is not precisely defined as a risk factor for gastric cancer, but the risk is established. Patients may benefit from periodic endoscopic surveillance.
4. **Ménétrier's disease, or giant hyperplasia of the gastric mucosal folds** is a rare protein-losing enteropathy associated with a slightly increased incidence of gastric cancer.
5. **Gastric stump, or gastric remnant, carcinoma** arises in the part of the stomach that remains after a previous gastric resection. Whether the frequency of carcinoma is increased in the gastric remnant remains controversial. If such an association does exist, one proposed theory is that the high

pH in the gastric remnant permits the overgrowth of bacteria that convert dietary nitrates and nitrites into carcinogenic compounds. In addition, bile reflux may also promote gastric cancer. These cancers develop many years after gastric resection, and therefore some physicians advocate endoscopic screening of patients beginning 10 to 20 years after surgery. However, existing data do not justify endoscopic screening of asymptomatic patients (13). On the other hand, symptomatic patients who have undergone a gastric resection merit intensive investigation, including endoscopy.

6. **Benign gastric ulcer** is associated with cancer probably in fewer than 1% of cases (14). Nevertheless, nonhealing gastric ulcers should raise suspicion of malignancy because such ulcers are probably malignant from the outset.

7. *Helicobacter pylori* **infection** has been strongly implicated in adenocarcinoma of the stomach in recent studies because almost all patients with gastric cancer are infected with this gram-negative bacillus. It is postulated that *H. pylori* leads to chronic gastritis that slowly progresses to cancer. In addition, certain strains of *H. pylori* may be more carcinogenic than others (14). Whether adequate antibiotic treatment of *H. pylori* reduces the risk of gastric adenocarcinoma remains to be determined. There is also an association between *H. pylori* and low-grade B-cell lymphoma of the stomach. These tumors have been called mucosal-associated lymphoid tumors (MAL-Tomas). These lesions usually regress with eradication of *H. pylori*, and patients have a good prognosis (15). Although the oncogenic potential of viruses has long been known, the association between *H. pylori* and gastric malignancy suggests that bacteria may also play a role in cancer.

What are some of the molecular mechanisms of gastric cancer?
Our understanding of the molecular biology of gastric cancer is still in its infancy, but some important advances have been made (16). Several abnormalities in oncogenes, tumor suppressor genes, and growth factor expression have been identified in gastric cancer. The tumor suppressor gene p53 on the short arm of chromosome 17 plays a key role in regulating the cell cycle. Advanced gastric cancers have a higher rate of p53 tumor suppressor gene mutations than do early gastric cancers, suggesting that p53 expression may have prognostic significance. Overexpression of the *ras* protein p21 has also been found in gastric cancer. In addition, the bcl-2 protooncogene, which plays a critical role in programmed cell death (apoptosis), is associated with gastric cancer. Abnormalities of several growth factors and growth factor receptors have also been found in gastric cancer, including fibroblast growth factor, transforming growth factor, and epidermal growth factor receptor. Overexpression of epidermal growth factor receptor is associated with aneuploidy, proliferation, and lymph node involvement in gastric cancer. Understanding the molecular basis of gastric cancer will lead to more effective methods of primary prevention, secondary prevention (early diagnosis), and treatment.

What is early gastric cancer?
Early gastric cancer is confined to the mucosa and submucosa and does not penetrate the muscularis. Patients have an excellent prognosis when treated with
adequate surgery, with more than 90% of patients surviving 5 years. As a result
of aggressive endoscopic screening, early gastric cancer makes up a larger percentage of gastric cancer in Japan than it does in the United States. In part, this
accounts for the better survival of patients with gastric cancer in Japan (17).

**Mr. Jones undergoes EUS, which reveals that the lesion has pene-
trated the serosa; however, no nodal enlargement is detected. CT
fails to delineate any adenopathy or contiguous organ involvement,
and his liver appears to be free of metastases. His chest radiograph
is unremarkable.**

Does laparoscopy have a role in the management of gastric cancer?
Because imaging studies are somewhat insensitive for detecting peritoneal
spread of the cancer, laparoscopy has been used increasingly to stage gastric cancer patients with greater accuracy. Laparoscopy may identify occult peritoneal
metastasis and avoid unnecessary laparotomy in patients with advanced disease.
In addition, a jejunostomy tube can be placed under laparoscopic guidance to
provide enteral support for the patient during neoadjuvant chemoradiation
(18). Further improvements in laparoscopic instruments will probably broaden
the role for laparoscopy in the management of gastric cancer.

What is neoadjuvant therapy and what is its role in the management of gastric cancer?
Neoadjuvant therapy is the use of chemotherapy and/or radiation therapy before surgery. The response rates achieved with neoadjuvant therapy for esophageal cancer, combined with the disappointing results with postoperative adjuvant therapy for gastric cancer, have stimulated investigators to evaluate
preoperative chemotherapy and/or radiation therapy for gastric cancer (19).
Possible advantages of delivering chemotherapy or radiation therapy preoperatively include the following:

1. Surgery produces scarring and ischemia, and there is greater blood flow to
   the tumor before surgery. This preoperative improved blood flow facilitates
   the delivery of chemotherapeutic agents and improves the effectiveness of
   radiation therapy.
2. Resection may stimulate the growth of remaining tumor cells and cause the
   proliferation of tumor cell clones that are resistant to chemotherapy and radiation therapy.
3. Postoperative complications may delay the initiation of adjuvant therapy
   and thereby limit its effectiveness.
4. Because most patients with gastric cancer present with advanced disease,

either locally or regionally, preoperative chemotherapy or radiation therapy may downstage unresectable tumors to resectable lesions.

5. Neoadjuvant therapy serves as an in vivo assay of the tumor's sensitivity to chemotherapy or radiation therapy and therefore more readily predicts which patients will benefit from these therapies after surgery.

What are some disadvantages of neoadjuvant therapy for gastric cancer?
Disadvantages of neoadjuvant therapy for gastric cancer include the following:

1. Chemotherapy or radiation therapy may show toxicity.
2. If neoadjuvant therapy is ineffective, the delay of definitive surgical therapy may result in tumor growth.
3. Increased surgical morbidity and mortality are associated with preoperative chemotherapy or radiation therapy.

Recent clinical trials have demonstrated that chemotherapy or radiation therapy can produce response rates and may convert unresectable tumors to resectable tumors (19). Whether these response rates translate into disease-free or improved overall survival has not been proved. Furthermore, caution must be used when interpreting data from neoadjuvant trials because of variation in techniques used for pretherapy staging (e.g., CT, laparoscopy, or laparotomy), lack of standardized surgical techniques and histopathologic evaluation, and relatively short median duration of follow-up. Neoadjuvant treatment cannot now be routinely recommended other than during a clinical trial. Further data from well-designed prospective, randomized trials are needed.

What is the treatment of choice for Mr. Jones in the absence of any neoadjuvant protocol?
Resection offers the best chance for cure, and surgery (resection or bypass) can provide effective palliation.

What preoperative preparation should Mr. Jones receive?
Routine preoperative blood work should be performed, an electrocardiogram should be obtained, and the patient should be adequately hydrated. In addition, attention must be directed to full bowel preparation and nutritional support.

Bowel preparation. Although CT may not detect adjacent organ involvement, gastric cancer can invade either the colon or the transverse mesocolon (i.e., the blood supply to the transverse colon) directly, necessitating partial colectomy at the time of gastrectomy. Bowel preparation reduces the septic complications of colon surgery and allows the surgeon to perform a primary colonic anastomosis rather than a colostomy. An oral purgative given the day before the operation is a standard mechanical procedure for preparing the bowel. In addition, the patient is administered nonabsorbable oral antibiotics (i.e., erythromycin base and neomycin) on the day before the operation. Also, because the achlorhydria often associated with gastric malignancy predisposes to bacterial overgrowth in the stomach, some surgeons advocate preoperative gastric lavage with antibiotics (delivered through a nasogastric tube) to reduce the likelihood of postoperative infectious complications (20).

Nutritional support. In patients such as Mr. Jones, who have significant weight loss and low serum albumin levels, some surgeons may advocate intensive preoperative nutritional support via a nasoenteral feeding tube or with total parenteral nutrition provided through a central venous catheter. However, in the absence of profound malnutrition or the need for a prolonged preoperative evaluation, advocacy for preoperative total parenteral nutrition is limited, and this approach may simply prolong the hospital course and predispose the patient to infection of the central venous catheter.

After a detailed description of the operative procedure and its risks and benefits, Mr. Jones gives informed consent. During exploratory celiotomy, bimanual palpation reveals that the liver is grossly free of tumor and that peritoneal implants and palpable intraabdominal adenopathy are absent. The tumor itself is in the antrum, on the greater curvature of the stomach, and it grossly penetrates the serosa.

How is the appropriate surgical procedure for patients with gastric cancer selected?
The surgical approach (i.e., transabdominal incision, abdominal incision and right thoracotomy, or left thoracoabdominal incision) and extent of gastric resection for gastric cancer depend primarily on the location of the lesion.

Proximal gastric cancer is probably best treated by radical total gastrectomy. This procedure entails en bloc removal of the omentum, the stomach, and the first portion of the duodenum. Microscopic spread of proximal gastric cancer frequently occurs beyond the gross extent of the tumor and may involve a significant portion of the distal esophagus. Although radical total gastrectomy can be performed solely via the transabdominal route, the surgeon may have to enter the chest to obtain a sufficient esophageal margin. One option is to use a right subcostal incision that extends across the midline with extension through the eighth intercostal space into the left side of the chest (21). The disadvantage of this approach is that if a high esophageal transection is required, the beating heart and aortic arch severely limit the exposure and make the anastomosis technically demanding. An alternative approach is to perform a celiotomy and a separate right thoracotomy, the so-called Ivor-Lewis technique (22). This affords excellent exposure for an esophageal anastomosis. The extent of lymph node dissection with radical total gastrectomy is controversial, and this issue is addressed later. Radical proximal gastrectomy, in which part of the distal stomach is left intact and anastomosed to the esophagus, results in severe alkaline (bile) reflux gastritis and should be avoided.

Distal gastric cancer is best treated by radical distal subtotal gastrectomy. This procedure consists of en bloc removal of the omentum, 80 to 85% of the stomach, and the first portion of the duodenum. The lymph node dissection is the same as for a radical total gastrectomy.

Who performed the first successful gastrectomy?
Theodore Billroth carried out the first successful gastrectomy on January 29, 1881, for an obstructing adenocarcinoma of the pylorus. Unfortunately, the patient died of recurrent disease about 14 months later (23).

To what extent should lymphadenectomy be performed for gastric cancer?
The extent of lymphadenectomy necessary for gastric cancer is controversial in the United States. In Japan, an aggressive approach has been adopted, and extended lymphadenectomy during gastric resection has been championed. The routes of lymphatic spread have been precisely mapped, and extended lymphadenectomy is performed to remove not only all lymph nodes at risk but also nodes that are one level beyond those predicted to contain microscopic disease. The Japanese staging system for nodal disease is as follows (24):

N_1: Perigastric nodes along the greater and lesser curve of stomach within 3 cm of the primary tumor
N_2: Nodes around the blood vessels supplying the stomach (common hepatic, splenic, left gastric arteries)
N_3: Nodes in the hepatoduodenal ligament, retropancreatic area, or celiac plexus and near the superior mesenteric artery
N_4: Nodes in the para–aortic area

Gastric resections are categorized according to the radicalism (R–value) of the dissection. An R–0 gastrectomy has incomplete dissection of the N_1 (perigastric nodes), and an R–1 resection entails en bloc dissection of the N_1 nodes. R–2, R–3, and R–4 resections denote complete dissection of the nodes at the corresponding levels (i.e., N_2, N_3, and N_4 nodes, respectively). In the absence of randomized controlled clinical trials, most American surgeons have been reluctant to perform extended lymphadenectomy for gastric cancer.

What variations of the blood supply to the stomach should surgeons be aware of?
The stomach has a rich blood supply. The lesser curvature of the stomach is supplied by the left gastric artery, which arises from the celiac axis, and by the right gastric artery, which arises from the hepatic artery; it in turn branches off the celiac axis. The greater curvature is supplied by the right gastroepiploic

artery, a branch of the gastroduodenal artery, and by the left gastroepiploic artery, a branch of the splenic artery. In addition, the splenic artery sends numerous short branches, the vasa brevia, or short gastric arteries, to the upper portion of the greater curve. There is an anatomic variation in the blood supply that the surgeon must know about when performing a gastrectomy. Occasionally the left hepatic artery arises from the left gastric artery, and if the surgeon is not aware of this aberrant vessel, ligation of the left gastric artery can result in ischemia of the left lobe of the liver.

Does radical total or subtotal gastrectomy require splenectomy?
The lymphatic tissue along the splenic vessels is a route of spread of gastric cancer and theoretically should be included in any potentially curative en bloc resection. Nevertheless, retrospective data suggest that prophylactic splenectomy offers no benefit and may increase morbidity and mortality (25). However, direct adherence of a gastric tumor to the distal pancreas or spleen must not preclude en bloc resection of these organs.

How is gastrointestinal continuity restored after resection of the tumor?
After radical total gastrectomy, reconstruction is usually accomplished by a Roux-en-Y esophagojejunostomy. The small bowel is transected at a convenient point distal to the ligament of Treitz. The distal limb of the small intestine is then anastomosed to the esophagus by connecting the end of the esophagus to the side of the jejunum.

The esophagojejunostomy can be hand sewn, but because of limited exposure in this area, an end-to-end anastomosis stapler may facilitate construction of the anastomosis. To restore gastrointestinal continuity, the transected end of the proximal small bowel is anastomosed to the side of the Roux limb. To minimize bile reflux, this anastomosis is constructed 45 to 60 cm from the esophagojejunostomy. If a radical subtotal gastrectomy has been carried out, a Billroth II anastomosis (gastrojejunostomy) may be performed. A Billroth I anastomosis (gastroduodenostomy), which is often performed for reconstruction after gastric resection for benign disease, is avoided because there is concern that recurrence at the line of duodenal transection will lead to obstruction of the anastomosis.

A number of reconstructive techniques attempt to provide some reservoir capacity after gastrectomy. The Hunt-Lawrence double-lumen jejunal pouch is an example, but whether jejunal reservoir procedures offer any advantage over the simpler, standard Roux-en-Y esophagojejunostomy remains controversial (26).

At exploration, Mr. Jones undergoes a radical gastrectomy and Roux-en-Y esophagojejunostomy. The pathology results show poorly differentiated adenocarcinoma that extends through all the layers of the

stomach to the serosa, with 3 of 20 lymph nodes positive for cancer. The margins of the resection are free of tumor.

Which early complication unique to radical gastrectomy must be avoided?
Other than bleeding and infection, perhaps the most feared complication of radical gastrectomy is a leak at the esophagojejunostomy site. Clinically, this may manifest as fever, abdominal tenderness, and leukocytosis. An anastomotic leak in the chest can be catastrophic and requires prompt recognition, immediate drainage, and institution of parenteral hyperalimentation. In spite of aggressive therapy, the mortality from an anastomotic leak remains high (27).

How soon after surgery can feedings by mouth be reinstituted?
Opinions vary on the postoperative management of patients who have undergone a radical gastrectomy. Some surgeons obtain an oral contrast radiograph, usually on postoperative day 5 or 6, and if no leak is demonstrated, the nasoenteral feeding tube is removed and oral intake begun. Other surgeons defer the radiographic studies and use clinical criteria alone (i.e., no signs of a leak and return of bowel function) to determine when oral feeding can be resumed.

What postgastrectomy dietary measures prevent dumping syndrome?
Any operation that bypasses, ablates, or alters the pyloroantral pump mechanism of the stomach can lead to the so-called dumping syndrome. (See Selected Topics at the end of this chapter.) Several dietary measures can obviate this problem. The postgastrectomy diet generally consists of six small daily meals that are high in protein and low in carbohydrate. In addition, fluid intake with meals should be restricted. Generally, dumping is not common after a Roux-en-Y reconstruction, and in fact, delayed emptying of the Roux-en-Y limb, also known as the Roux-en-Y stasis syndrome, may occur if the limb is made too long (28).

What is the most common staging system for gastric cancer in the United States, and what stage is Mr. Jones's tumor?
A precise staging system is required for any malignancy for accurate comparison of various treatments. The most common staging system used in the United States is the American Joint Committee for Cancer (AJCC) tumor, node, metastases (TNM) system (Tables 8.1 and 8.2) (29). A more sophisticated system is used in Japan but has not been adopted in the United States. Mr. Jones's stage is $T_3N_1M_0$, or stage IIIA.

What is the long-term prognosis for patients with gastric carcinoma?
The overall 5-year survival for adenocarcinoma of the stomach in the United States is only 5 to 15%. In the absence of lymph node involvement with tumor, the 5-year survival is 30 to 40%; with lymph node involvement, survival

Table 8.1.   TUMOR, NODE, METASTASIS SYTEM FOR CLARIFYING GASTRIC CANCER

Primary Tumor (T)
T_0: no primary tumor evident
T_{is}: carcinoma in situ
T_1: tumor invading lamina propria
T_2: tumor invading muscularis propria
T_3: tumor penetrating serosa
T_4: tumor invading adjacent structures

Lymph Node (N)
N_0: no regional lymph node metastasis
N_1: metastasis in perigastric nodes ($<$3 cm from tumor)
N_2: metastasis in perigastric nodes ($>$3 cm from tumor)

Distant Metastasis (M)
M_0: no distant metastasis
M_1: distant metastasis

Table 8.2.   STAGING OF GASTRIC CANCER

Tumor, Node, Metastases Classification	Tumor Stage
$T_{is} N_0 M_0$	0
$T_1 N_0 M_0$	IA
$T_1 N_1 M_0$	IB
$T_2 N_0 M_0$	
$T_1 N_2 M_0$	II
$T_2 N_1 M_0$	
$T_3 N_0 M_0$	
$T_2 N_2 M_0$	IIIA
$T_3 N_2 M_0$	
$T_4 N_0 M_0$	
$T_3 N_2 M_0$	IIIB
$T_4 N_1 M_0$	
$T_4 N_2 M_0$	IV
Any T, any N, M_1	

is reduced to 15 to 20% (2). The survival rates for gastric cancer are superior in Japan. That may be the result of numerous factors, including the following:

1. Inherent biologic differences between gastric cancer in Japan and the United States

2. Mass screening for and earlier detection of gastric cancer in Japan
3. Better staging of gastric cancer in Japan owing to aggressive nodal dissection and intensive histopathologic examination
4. Technical superiority of Japanese surgeons with gastric cancer because of their enormous experience
5. The Japanese body habitus (i.e., less body fat), which facilitates a more radical dissection

What is the role of postoperative adjuvant therapy in the treatment of this patient?
Most studies in the United States do not demonstrate any clear advantage to adjuvant chemotherapy. In a prospective randomized trial, the Gastrointestinal Tumor Study Group (30) reported an improvement in survival in patients receiving 5-fluorouracil and semustine after curative resection. However, these results were not substantiated by two other prospective randomized multicenter trials conducted by the Eastern Cooperative Oncology Group (31) and the Veterans Administration Surgical Oncology Group (32). Japanese surgeons have been much more aggressive with chemotherapy, often initiating therapy in the operating room or immediately afterward. In addition, they have reported some success with hyperthermic intraperitoneal chemotherapy with mitomycin C (33). The rationale for the use of intraperitoneal chemotherapy is the high incidence of peritoneal recurrences, particularly with transmural tumors, as in Mr. Jones's case. Also, higher drug levels can be reached in the peritoneal cavity with less systemic toxicity. Hyperthermia enhances the effectiveness of intraperitoneal chemotherapy. These results are preliminary and should be evaluated in the context of a controlled study; therefore, the routine use of adjuvant chemotherapy for gastric cancer has not been proved beneficial.

Is there any role for adjuvant radiation therapy in the treatment of this patient?
Gastric cancer has historically been considered a relatively radioresistant tumor. The dose of radiation that is required is often limited by the toxicity to the surrounding tissues. Radiation therapy delivered after curative resection has no proven benefit. In an attempt to lessen toxicity, some centers have tried delivering radiation therapy in the operating room. This technique requires specialized equipment and therefore is limited to a few major centers. External beam radiation therapy is given as a palliative measure, predominantly for locally unresectable tumors or for recurrent cancer.

What follow-up care should be provided to patients who have undergone a curative resection for gastric cancer?
There are no rigid guidelines for follow-up, but patients should be monitored closely for the first 3 years, because most recurrences fall within this period. Initially, patients should be seen monthly and questioned about dysphagia, abdominal pain, weight loss, and blood in the stools. In addition, physical exam-

ination should focus on the appearance of any abdominal tenderness, masses, or ascites, and a digital rectal examination should be performed to check for occult blood. Laboratory studies may include hemoglobin determinations and liver function tests. Although it has low yield, a chest radiograph may be obtained yearly. Some physicians perform a barium swallow study or endoscopy postoperatively to obtain baseline results and at arbitrary intervals thereafter. The opposing view is that postoperative tests that screen for recurrent disease neither are cost-effective nor improve survival and that it is therefore more prudent simply to investigate symptomatic patients with barium swallow studies or esophagoscopy. A consequence of gastrectomy is that the patients lack intrinsic factor and therefore require periodic vitamin B_{12} injections to prevent megaloblastic anemia.

A year after surgery, Mr. Jones develops dysphagia associated with a 20-pound weight loss. A barium swallow study and esophagoscopy confirm a recurrence of tumor (proved by biopsy) at the anastomosis. CT reveals a 4- to 5-cm mass in the area of the esophagojejunostomy and suggests considerable adenopathy around the celiac axis, but the liver appears to be free of tumor. A chest radiograph is also clear. Mr. Jones is still very active, but he can swallow only liquids.

What is the pattern of recurrence of gastric cancer after a presumably curative resection?
Although many patients eventually develop distant disease, local regional disease recurs alone or as a component of treatment failure in as many as 80% of patients after apparently curative resection (34). Local regional recurrence is tumor at the site of anastomosis, in the bed of resection, or in adjacent lymph nodes. The reported magnitude of local regional recurrence depends on how it is detected: by nonoperative means, during reoperation, or at autopsy. The stage of the initial tumor influences the incidence of local regional recurrence; lesions that extend through the wall and lesions with lymph node involvement have the highest incidence. Local regional recurrences are associated with a poor prognosis and are rarely resectable.

What are some options for treatment after recurrence of tumor?
Although resection of recurrent gastric cancer is rarely curative, selected patients may benefit from surgical palliation. The goal in the case of patients such as Mr. Jones is to offer palliation to control the dysphagia with the least harm to quality of life. These are the options for palliation of Mr. Jones's symptoms:

1. Surgical exploration with re-resection or surgical bypass (i.e., palliative esophagojejunostomy)
2. Endoscopic pneumatic dilation or laser ablation and placement of an expandable metallic endoprosthesis (35)

3. Palliative chemotherapy or radiation therapy
4. Some combination of these therapies (e.g., endoscopic dilation and stent placement combined with intraluminal brachytherapy and systemic chemotherapy)

Mr. Jones is treated with endoscopic pneumatic dilation and stent placement, which is well tolerated and which palliates his dysphagia. Eventually, however, he develops metastases and dies 3 months after the detection of his recurrent cancer.

SELECTED TOPICS

POSTGASTRECTOMY SYNDROMES

The postgastrectomy syndromes are a collection of disorders that are the sequelae of ablation or bypass of the pylorus and of truncal vagotomy. Fortunately, these disorders are relatively uncommon and, when they do occur, can be managed successfully without surgery. However, remedial operations may be required in patients who remain refractory to conservative measures.

Dumping Syndrome

Dumping syndrome consists of vasomotor and gastrointestinal symptoms that follow a meal; it is often divided into an early and a late component. The vasomotor component consists of diaphoresis, weakness, dizziness, and palpitations; the gastrointestinal symptoms consist of nausea, abdominal fullness, pain, cramping, and diarrhea. Early dumping becomes manifest within the first 30 minutes after ingestion of a meal and is thought to result from the rapid passage of hyperosmolar chyme into the small bowel. The resulting fluid shifts cause a rapid decrease in circulating plasma volume and are partially responsible for the vasomotor symptoms. In addition, some hormones (serotonin, bradykinin, and enteroglucagon) may play a role (36). Most patients can be managed with dietary measures (i.e., small, frequent low-carbohydrate, high-protein meals, with restriction of fluid intake with meals). Pectin (a gel-forming starch), serotonin antagonists, and somatostatin analogs have also been used to treat dumping syndrome (37). Operative intervention is rarely required; the best results are obtained with reversed jejunal segments and Roux-en-Y diversion (38).

Late dumping, which is less common, characteristically occurs 2 to 4 hours after meals, with vasomotor symptoms predominating. Late dumping is thought to result from insulin hyperresponsiveness to a carbohydrate load, and profound hypoglycemia ensues. Pectin can also ameliorate some of the symptoms associated with late dumping. Pectin can normalize the glucose tolerance curve.

Management Algorithm for Gastric Cancer

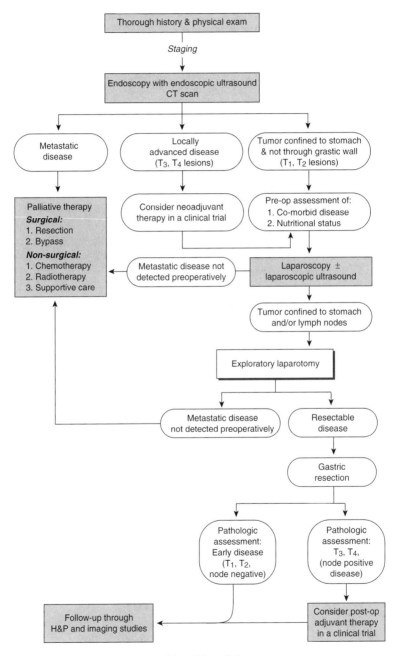

Algorithm 8.1.

Alkaline Reflux Gastritis

Alkaline reflux gastritis is associated with epigastric pain and sometimes with bilious vomiting. It is attributed to reflux of bile into the gastric pouch or esophagus. Endoscopy reveals erythematous, bile-stained mucosa. However, the severity of the gastritis seen endoscopically does not correlate well with the extent of symptoms (39). Some physicians favor the measurement of the degree of enterogastric reflux by using technetium-labeled sulfur colloid (40). Medical therapy involves administration of bile salt–binding agents, such as cholestyramine and metoclopramide, to facilitate gastric emptying. Nonoperative measures for genuine alkaline reflux gastritis frequently fail. The procedure of choice for operative repair is the creation of a 45- to 60-cm Roux-en-Y limb (40).

Afferent Loop Syndrome

Afferent loop syndrome is manifested by postprandial epigastric fullness and pain that is relieved by bilious vomiting. It is caused by intermittent obstruction of the afferent limb of the gastrojejunostomy after eating. Pancreaticobiliary secretions distend the afferent loop, causing pain. With time, the pressure in the limb builds up and is finally released in the form of projectile bilious vomiting. Endoscopy and radionuclide scans aid in diagnosis. Afferent loop syndrome is often the consequence of an excessively long afferent limb. The treatment is operative, including a variety of procedures such as conversion of the gastrojejunostomy to a Billroth I anastomosis (gastroduodenostomy) or creation of a Roux-en-Y limb or a distal enteroenterostomy.

Postvagotomy Diarrhea

Postvagotomy diarrhea is an increase in stool frequency that occurs after truncal vagotomy. This diarrhea subsides in most patients, but in a few patients it persists and can be disabling. Although the cause of the diarrhea is not fully understood, cholestyramine has therapeutic value. Remedial surgery is necessary in a few cases; it consists of interposition of a 10-cm reversed jejunal loop to slow intestinal transit (41).

REFERENCES

1. Sawyers JL. Gastric carcinoma. Curr Prob Surg 1995;32:101–178.
2. Laufer I, Mullens J, Hamilton J. The diagnostic accuracy of barium studies of the stomach and duodenum: correlation with endoscopy. Radiology 1975;115:569–573.
3. Graham D, Schwartz J, Cain G. Prospective evaluation of biopsy number in the diagnosis of esophageal and gastric carcinoma. Gastroenterology 1982;82:228–231.
4. Schwartz R, Conners JM, Schmidt M. Diagnosis and management of stage IE and stage IIE gastric lymphoma. Am J Surg 1993;165:561–565.
5. Brenes F, Correa P. Pathology of gastric cancer. Surg Oncol Clin North Am 1993;2: 347–370.

6. Ajani JA, Mansfield PA, Ota DM. Potentially resectable gastric carcinoma: current approaches to staging and preoperative therapy. World J Surg 1995;19:216–220.

7. Pollack BJ, Chak A, Sivak MV. Endoscopic ultrasonography. Semin Oncol 1996;23: 336–346.

8. Inamdar N, Levin B. Epidemiology and causes of gastric cancer. Surg Oncol Clin North Am 1993;2:333–345.

9. Parker SL, Tongs T, Bolden S, Wingo PA. Cancer statistics. CA Cancer J Clin 1996; 46:5–27.

10. Hisamichi S. Screening for gastric cancer. World J Surg 1989;13:31–37.

11. Hughes RW Jr. Diagnosis and treatment of gastric polyps. Gastroenterol Endocrinol Clin North Am 1992;2:457–467.

12. Thompson GB, Van Heerden JA, Sarr MG. Adenocarcinoma of the stomach: are we making progress? Lancet 1993;342:713–718.

13. Offerhaus GJA, Tersmette AC, Giadiello et al. Evaluation of endoscopy for early detection of gastric stump cancer. Lancet 1992;340:33–35.

14. Nightingale TE, Gruber J. *Helicobacter* and human cancer. J Natl Cancer Inst 1994;86: 1505–1509.

15. Wotherspoon AC, Doglioni C, Diss TC, et al. Regression of primary low-grade B-cell gastric lymphoma of mucosa-associated lymphoid tissue type after eradication of *Helicobacter pylori*. Lancet 1993;342:575–577.

16. Wright PA, Williams GT. Molecular biology and gastric carcinoma. Gut 1993;34: 145–147.

17. Farley DR, Donohue JH. Early gastric cancer. Surg Clin North Am 1992;72:401–421.

18. Hemming AW, Nagy AG, Scudamore CH, Edelmann K. Laparoscopic staging of intra-abdominal malignancy. Surg Endosc 1995;9:325–328.

19. Kelsen DP. Adjuvant and neoadjuvant therapy for gastric cancer. Semin Oncol 1996; 23:379–389.

20. Zinner MJ, Mcfadden DW. Surgery for recurrent peptic ulcer disease. In: Fry DE, ed. Reoperative Surgery of the Abdomen. New York: Marcel Decker, 1986:531.

21. McNeer G, Vandenberg H, Donn F. A critical evaluation of subtotal gastrectomy for the cure of cancer of the stomach. Ann Surg 1951;134:2.

22. Brennan MF, Karpeh MS. Surgery for gastric cancer: the American view. Semin Oncol 1996;23:352–359.

23. Pack GT. Cancer of the stomach. Am J Gastroenterol 1965;44:18–25.

24. Adachi Y, Oshiro T, Okuyama T, et al. A simple classification of lymph node level in gastric carcinoma. Am J Surg 1995;169:382–385.

25. Brady MS, Rogatko A, Dent LL, Shiu MH. Effect of splenectomy on morbidity and survival following curative gastrectomy for carcinoma. Arch Surg 1991;126:359–364.

26. Troidl H, Kushe J, Vestweber K. Pouch versus esophagojejunostomy after total gastrectomy: a randomized clinical trial. World J Surg 1989;11:699–704.

27. Urschel JD. Esophagogastrostomy anastomotic leaks complicating esophagectomy: a review. Am J Surg 1995;169:634–640.

28. Fromm D. Complications of gastric surgery. New York: Wiley, 1977:35–49.

29. Beahrs OH, Henson DE, Hutter RVP, Kennedy BJ. Manual for Staging of Cancer. 4th ed. Philadelphia: Lippincott, 1992.

30. Gastrointestinal Tumor Study Group (GITSG). Controlled trial of adjuvant chemotherapy following curative resection for gastric cancer. Cancer 1982;49:1116–1122.

31. Higgins GA, Amadeo JH, Smith DE. Efficacy of prolonged intermittent therapy with combined 5-FU and methyl-CCNU following resection for gastric carcinoma. Cancer 1983;52:1105–1112.

32. Engstrom PF, Lavin PT, Douglass HO, Brunner KW. Postoperative adjuvant 5-fluorouracil plus methyl-CCNU therapy for gastric cancer patients (Eastern Cooperative Oncology Group). Cancer 1985;55:1868–1873.

33. Macdonald JS, Schnall SF. Adjuvant treatment of gastric cancer. World J Surg 1995;19: 221–225.

34. Minsky BD. The role of radiation therapy in gastric cancer. Semin Oncol 1996;23: 390–396.

35. Topazian M, Ring E, Grendell J. Palliation of obstructing gastric cancer with steel mesh, self-expanding endoprostheses. N Engl J Med 1992;38:58–60.

36. Sawyers JL. Management of postgastrectomy syndromes. Am J Surg 1990;159:8–14.

37. Jenkins DJA, Gassull MA, Leeds AR. Effect of dietary fiber on complications of gastric surgery: prevention of postprandial hypoglycemia by pectin. Gastroenterology 1977;73: 215–217.

38. Miranda R, Steffes B, O'Leary JP, Woodward ER. Surgical treatment of the postgastrectomy dumping syndrome. Am J Surg 1980;139:40–43.

39. Ritchie WP Jr. Alkaline reflux gastritis: an objective assessment of its diagnosis and treatment. Ann Surg 1980;192:288–298.

40. Herrington JL, Sawyers JL. Surgical management of reflux gastritis. Ann Surg 1974; 180:526–537.

41. Sawyers JL, Herrington JL. Antiperistaltic jejunal segments for control of dumping syndrome and postvagotomy diarrhea. Surgery 1971;69:263–267.

Small Bowel Obstruction

K. Francis Lee

George Chapman is a 42-year-old man who presents to the emergency department complaining of a 3-day history of crampy abdominal pain, nausea, and vomiting. Prior to the onset, he has had occasional abdominal colic that was relieved by intermittent bowel movement. However, for the past 3 days he has not had a bowel movement, and his abdominal pain has become diffuse and crampy, relieved only by emesis. He states that his vomitus is somewhat foul-smelling and dark green. His last meal was 3 days ago, and he has been having difficulty tolerating even liquids for the past 12 hours. His medical history is significant for exploratory surgery following a stab wound to the abdomen 5 years ago.

What is the differential diagnosis?
The patient's history of crampy abdominal pain relieved by emesis and a previous abdominal surgery suggests that this patient has small-bowel obstruction (SBO) until proven otherwise. Other possibilities include adynamic ileus, large-bowel obstruction, volvulus, gastroenteritis, pancreatitis, and mesenteric vascular occlusion.

What are the most common causes of SBO?
In adults, *postoperative adhesion* is the most common cause of SBO, producing up to two-thirds of cases (26 to 64%); next are *incarcerated hernia* (6 to 21%) and *neoplasms*. Inflammatory bowel disease, diverticulitis, gallstone ileus, and bezoars are other less common causes (1).

What are the three most salient features of SBO on history, and why is it important to recognize them?
A history of abdominal pain, obstipation, and emesis typify SBO. More frequently than not the diagnosis must be made by history alone, because the physical examination and laboratory tests are not diagnostic. A delay in diagnosing SBO can lead to catastrophe.

On physical examination, Mr. Chapman's vital signs are found to be as follows: blood pressure, 140/92 mm Hg; heart rate, 100 beats per minute; respirations, 18 per minute; temperature, 98.2°F. Cardiopulmonary findings are within normal limits. His abdomen is noteworthy for a well-healed midline scar from the xiphoid process to the pubic bone, moderate distension, and somewhat hyperactive bowel sounds. Except for some discomfort upon palpation, there is no significant tenderness or abnormal mass. The rectal examination is normal and heme negative.

Why is testing for blood important?
Heme-positive stool may be an early indication of ischemic bowel. The mucosal layer of the bowel wall is most susceptible to ischemia and may bleed before full-thickness bowel injury occurs. Also, in elderly patients, one should keep in mind cancer as a possible cause of bowel obstruction.

What is the significance of the quality of the bowel sounds?
In the early period of obstruction, peristalsis is increased, and hyperactive bowel sounds can be heard as the intestines attempt to overcome the obstruction. As the bowel distends, reflex inhibition of bowel motility results in a quiet abdomen (2). The quality of the bowel sounds does not help in differentiating between a partial and a complete obstruction.

What are the most common physical findings associated with SBO?
The most common physical abnormalities found in a patient with SBO are those associated with dehydration (e.g., low-grade fever, dry skin turgor or mucosa, tachycardia). Other than distension, the abdominal examination is most commonly *equivocal* (i.e., moderate subjective discomfort upon palpation without a bona fide tenderness or rebound).

Why does SBO not usually produce significant abdominal tenderness? What is the distinction between abdominal pain and tenderness? How is this related to the pathophysiology of SBO?
Abdominal pain is a subjective experience reported by the patient during review of history. Abdominal tenderness is an objective physical finding obtained during examination of the patient. It is absolutely critical to understand the pathophysiology of SBO to formulate the correct therapeutic approach. Whether the obstruction is caused by postoperative adhesions, hernia, or neoplasm, the result is either (*a*) simple distal intestinal obstruction with proximal distension and no vascular compromise, or (*b*) strangulation of bowel or closed-loop intestinal obstruction, with or without significant vascular compromise due to the twisting of the mesentery.

The consequences of intestinal obstruction and distention are decreased luminal fluid resorption and increased intraluminal fluid secretion (e.g., intestinal distension, nausea, emesis), overall fluid and electrolyte abnormality from third-spacing of fluid into the interstitium and dehydration, and luminal fluid stasis and overgrowth of bacteria (i.e., foul-smelling vomitus). Intestinal obstruction and proximal distention alone cause significant crampy abdominal pain, but they do not necessarily cause abdominal tenderness to the same degree. Likewise, mesenteric vascular occlusion due to strangulation or closed-loop bowel ischemia causes significant pain but not the same degree of tenderness. Therefore, it is critically important that bowel strangulation or closed-loop obstruction be treated via surgical exploration for increasing abdominal pain alone, even if physical findings or laboratory tests are not diagnostic. One must never delay surgery waiting for the onset of significant abdominal tenderness, rebound tenderness, or systemic signs of inflammation (e.g., fever or increased leukocyte count), because these signs portend that the ischemic bowel may have already progressed to necrosis.

The emergency department physician reports that the patient's laboratory test and abdominal radiograph results are pending.

Which laboratory abnormalities are anticipated?
Signs of dehydration from emesis and third-spacing, such as mildly elevated hematocrit and normal or upper normal white blood cell count. Blood chemistries may show prerenal azotemia (blood urea nitrogen–creatinine ratio [BUN-Cr] above 20) and hypochloremic, hypokalemic metabolic alkalosis from ongoing emesis of acidic gastric juice.

What are the salient features of SBO on the KUB and upright abdominal radiographs?
Radiographic examination of a patient with SBO indicates (*a*) multiple loops of distended small bowel in a stepladder pattern, which (*b*) layer out on the upright film showing *air-fluid levels,* and (*c*) *absence of colonic air or stool.* Other findings, such as free air under the right diaphragm from bowel perforation, should be looked for as part of the routine radiographic evaluation.

Is it possible for the abdominal radiographs of SBO not to show any air-fluid levels?
Yes. Sometimes early in the course of SBO, effective emesis and relief of intraluminal fluid can give a normal-appearing bowel gas pattern. Also, completely fluid-filled loops of bowel can give a ground glass appearance on radiograph without the air-fluid levels.

What is the significance of loops of distended small bowel and air in the colon and rectum if they are visible on abdominal radiographs?
The possibility of *adynamic ileus* would increase in the differential diagnosis (discussed later).

If the abdominal radiographs show loops of distended small bowel, distended cecum and colon up to the descending colon, yet no rectal air or stool, what is the significance?
The possibility of *large-bowel obstruction* (LBO) increases in the differential diagnosis. However, colonic air does not rule out SBO, because it is sometimes seen in the early phase of SBO.

What causes LBO, how does one work it up, and what are the treatments?
Causes of LBO include sigmoid or cecal volvulus, obstructive colon cancer, obstruction from inflammatory reactions to diverticulitis or ulcerative colitis, fecal impaction or foreign body obstruction, sliding hernia, intraperitoneal adhesions (e.g., postsurgical adhesions, endometriosis), and in children, a host of congenital problems (e.g., Hirschsprung's disease, imperforate anus, meconium ileus). In addition to review of history, **workup** includes rectal examination and proctosigmoidoscopy to look for distal rectosigmoid disease. If the distal segment is normal in the presence of LBO, barium enema or colonoscopy is helpful to determine the more proximal colonic lesions. The **treatments** must achieve two therapeutic goals: relieving the obstruction and addressing the underlying problem. For example, in the case of a septic and metabolically deranged patient with obstructive colon cancer, the obstruction can be dealt with by placing a diverting colostomy proximal to the point of obstruction, and the definitive resection may be performed as a second procedure. Or, if the bowel preparation status and the patient's physiologic state are optimal, the cancerous segment may be resected and a primary anastomosis performed. A complete knowledge of the entire colon is necessary before beginning any definitive treatment for obstructive colon cancer. In cecal volvulus, on the other hand, the bowel may simply be untwisted and cecopexy performed. The management of LBO is very different from that of SBO, so it is important to distinguish the two in a patient with intestinal obstruction.

The abdominal radiographs show distended loops of small bowel with air-fluid levels. There is some air, though scant, in the colon. There is no free air under the diaphragm, and the chest radiograph is unremarkable. The laboratory test results are still pending. The working diagnosis is now small bowel obstruction.

What next step should be taken?
First, the patient's bowel must be decompressed with a nasogastric suction tube (e.g., Salem sump). Second, the patient should be dehydrated and needs aggressive intravenous (IV) fluid resuscitation. A urinary catheter should be inserted to monitor urine output. Boluses of IV fluid should be administered until the urine output becomes adequate (0.5 to 1 mL/kg/hour). If the patient is frail and elderly with a complicating cardiac disease, fluid resuscitation must be done with central venous pressure monitoring. Third and most important, a decision must be made as to whether this patient requires surgery.

How does a physician decide whether the patient is a candidate for surgery?
The decision to operate as compared with observation depends on one's index of suspicion for bowel strangulation, closed-loop obstruction, and ischemic bowel. It is difficult to make the diagnosis of strangulation and ischemic bowel with just history and physical examination. Clearly, abdominal pain associated with fever, leukocytosis, acidosis, peritoneal sign, and shock are all indications of bowel necrosis and necessitate surgical exploration. Generally speaking, even in the absence of these physical signs, unrelenting and increasing abdominal pain with obstipation and radiographic signs of SBO should indicate surgery. Unless there are extenuating circumstances to the contrary, complete bowel obstruction should *not* be dismissed without exploratory surgery.

What is the difference between complete and partial SBO?
Partial SBO is distinguished from complete SBO by passage of flatus through the rectum and radiographic presence of air or stool in the colon despite the loops of distended small bowel. These indicate partial blockage of the intestines, allowing distal passage of some air and fluid.

What is the significance of partial versus complete SBO?
Complete SBO is associated with a significant risk of strangulation and bowel ischemia. The incidence of necrotic bowel in patients with complete SBO has been reported to be as high as 30% (3). Patients with partial obstruction have a much lower incidence of ischemic complications. Accordingly, partial SBO may be treated conservatively, whereas a complete SBO requires timely operative intervention.

Does complete SBO always require operation?
No. For patients who have had multiple episodes of SBO and who have been successfully managed without operation, it may be worthwhile to try an initial period of conservative management with nasogastric decompression. In such patients, one should proceed to surgery if pain becomes worse or if obstipation continues for a period of 3 or 4 days without clinical progress. Generally speaking, however, the maxim "do not let the sun set or rise on bowel obstruction" holds true for complete SBO.

The patient undergoes insertion of the nasogastric tube and Foley catheter. He receives approximately 1 L of lactated Ringers solution intravenously, and he produces 80 mL of urine in the subsequent hour. When the patient is interviewed again, he reveals that he has just passed a large amount of flatus following the nasogastric tube insertion. In addition, the radiologist confirms that the patient has some air and stool in the colon. The radiologist asks whether he

should perform a contrast study of the upper gastrointestinal tract with small bowel follow-through to confirm passage of dye into the colon.

What is the role of contrast studies in the diagnosis of small bowel obstruction?
For a known complete SBO, there is no role for contrast studies. For a patient with unrelenting, increasing crampy abdominal pain, there is no role for contrast studies. Contrast studies should never substitute for clinical judgment to proceed to surgery. Contrast studies, which take up to 6 hours of bowel transit time, should never delay timely operation. However, contrast studies do have a role when there is not enough clinical indication for an immediate operation but symptoms of obstruction continue. Contrast studies can be helpful with such patients because the distinction between a complete and a partial SBO may not be so clear. Overall, however, the role of contrast studies in acute presentation of SBO is limited.

With the passage of flatus, Mr. Chapman reports that his abdominal pain has lessened. A working diagnosis of partial SBO is made, and the patient is admitted to the nursing floor for nasogastric decompression and observation. One hour later, the nurse from the floor states that there is no IV order.

How does one determine the IV fluid requirement for a 70-kg patient?
Fluid volume, sodium, and potassium requirements are determined separately. The following are rough estimations (4):

Daily fluid volume requirement
Adults: 35 mL/kg/day × 70 kg = 2450 mL/day
Children: 100 mL/kg/day for first 10 kg body weight (0–10 kg)
                   +50 mL/kg/day for second 10 kg body weight (10–20 kg)
                   +20 mL/kg/day for each kg >20 kg body weight (>20 kg)
Daily sodium requirement
Adults: 1.5–2 mEq/kg/day × 70 kg = 100–140 mEq/day
Children: 3.5 mEq/kg/day
Daily potassium requirement
Adults: 0.5 mEq/kg/day × 70 kg = 35 mEq/day
Children: 2–3 mEq/kg/day
Caloric replacement through peripheral IV
Adults: 100 g glucose per day produces protein-sparing effects; that
                   is, it minimizes endogenous muscle breakdown so that the
                   body can generate glucose (gluconeogenesis) for the brain
                   during the first few days of starvation (5).

The usual IV solution is 5% dextrose in water with 0.45% normal saline and 20 mEq potassium chloride at 100 mL/hour (D_5 1/2 NS + 20 KCl at 100 mL/hour). This order will provide the following:

- 120 g dextrose per day, which is presumably adequate for protein sparing and minimizing the nitrogen loss and muscle breakdown
- 2400 mL fluid per day, which is adequate volume replacement
- 184 mEq sodium per day, which is more than adequate for sodium replacement (some physicians prefer to give 25% NS instead, which would provide 92 mEq of sodium per day)
- Provide 48 mEq potassium per day, which is more than adequate for potassium replacement

Thus, **D_5 ½ NS + 20 KCl at 100 mL/hour** has become the usual IV order for a healthy 70-kg adult patient. However, each component of the IV therapy must change according to the following additional clinical factors:

- Third-space losses (increase fluid and electrolyte requirements)
- Operative blood and fluid losses (increase fluid and electrolyte requirements)
- Specific body secretory losses (increase fluid and electrolyte requirements)

Table 9.1 lists the specific secretory losses that must be replaced with supplemental IV therapy (6).

It is likely that this patient has had a period of gastric emesis resulting in severe salt and water deficits. Depending on the electrolyte pro-

Table 9.1. NORMAL CONTENT OF
GASTROINTESTINAL SECRETIONS

	Volume (mL/day)	Na (mEq)	K (mEq)	Cl (mEq)	HCO_3 (mEq)	pH
Gastric						
pH >4	2000	100	10	100	0	>4
pH 4	1500	60	10	130	0	<4
Duodenum	100–2000	140	5	80	0	<4–8
Bile	50–800	145	5	100	35	7.8
Pancreas	100–800	140	5	75	115	8–8.3
Small bowel	3000	140	5	104	30	7.8–8
Colon	200	80	30	40	40	
Feces	100	60	30	4	15	
Sweat		40	8	50		

file, the IV order must be modified accordingly from the standard solution. Table 9.2 lists commonly used IV fluid preparations. The nurse
also informs the physician that the laboratory has called her to report
the following serum test results:

Sodium, 130 mEq
Chloride, 96 mEq
Potassium, 3.1 mEq
Bicarbonate, 33 mEq
BUN, 38 mg/dL
Creatinine, 1 mg/dL
Hematocrit, 48%
White blood cell count, 9.2 K/mL
Platelet count, 354 K/mL

The patient receives D_5 NS + 40 KCl at 150 mL/hour.

How are this patient's blood chemistry abnormalities summarized?
Mr. Chapman's blood chemistry abnormalities are consistent with hypochloremic hypokalemic metabolic alkalosis due to hypovolemia from gastric
fluid emesis and third-spacing (Appendix 9.1).

What is the significance of the elevated BUN and creatinine level?
A BUN-creatinine ratio greater than 20:1 is typical of hypovolemia and prerenal azotemia.

Table 9.2.   COMPOSITION OF PARENTERAL FLUID
(ELECTOLYTE CONTENT, MEQ/L)

Solutions	CATIONS				ANIONS		Osmolality (mO)
	Na	K	Ca	Mg	Cl	HCO_3	
Extracellular fluid	142	4	5	3	103	27	280–310
Lactated Ringer's	130	4	3	–	109	28[a]	273
0.9% Sodium chloride	154	–	–	–	154	–	308
D_5 45% Sodium chloride	77	–	–	–	77	–	407
D_5W	–	–	–	–	–	–	253
M/6 Sodium lactate	167	–	–	–	–	167[a]	334
3% Sodium chloride	513	–	–	–	513	–	1026

[a]Present in solution as lactate that is converted to biocarbonate.
D_5W, 5% dextrose in water.
Reprinted with permission from Schwartz SI, Shires GT, Spencer FC, eds. Principles of Surgery. New
York: McGraw-Hill, 1994:75.

How does prerenal azotemia differ from renal failure on laboratory tests?
Table 9.3 compares renal failure and prerenal azotemia.

What is paradoxic aciduria?
In surgical patients, metabolic alkalosis commonly occurs because of naso-gastric suction of gastric acid and other compounding factors. It seems logi-cal that in the face of systemic alkalosis, the kidney would compensate by ac-tively secreting the bicarbonate ion and resorbing the hydrogen ion, producing relatively alkaline urine. However, the opposite is observed. In the face of hypochloremic, hypokalemic alkalosis compounded by physiologic stress, the kidney attempts to retain water and sodium. In exchange for avid sodium retention, the kidney excretes other cations, such as hydrogen ion, into the tubules. Thus, the urine becomes paradoxically acidotic.

What are the differential diagnoses for hyponatremia and hypokalemia? What are the re-spective treatments?
Appendix 9.1 covers electrolyte abnormalities; symptoms, signs, and complica-tions; differential diagnoses; causes; and treatments.

Over the next several hours, the crampy abdominal pain returns and acutely worsens. The patient is not passing flatus. Repeat abdominal radiographs show increased loops of small bowel with air-fluid levels and virtually no air in the colon. The patient is now writhing in pain and asks for pain medication.

What should be done for this patient now?
Although patients with partial SBO should have a period of observation on na-sogastric decompression, continued evidence of obstruction or worsening ab-dominal pain necessitates emergent surgery.

The patient is taken to the operating room for exploratory celiotomy. Preoperative antibiotic is administered.

Table 9.3.   PRERENAL AZOTEMIA VERSUS RENAL FAILURE

	Prerenal	Renal
Urine osmolality (mO/kgH_2O)	>500	<350
Urine sodium (mEq/L)	<20	>40
BUN/serum creatinine	>15	<10
Urine/plasma urea	>8	<3
Urine/plasma creatinine	>40	<20

Adapted with permission from Miller TR, et al. Urinary diagnosis indices in acute renal failure: a prospective study. Ann Intern Med 1978;89:47.

What is the optimal incision in this case?
When the cause of SBO is unclear and intraperitoneal adhesions are expected, a generous midline incision facilitates the best exposure and access to all quadrants of the abdomen.

What should the surgeon seek during exploration?
First, the cause of obstruction should be determined. Most commonly, it is due to surgical adhesions. If that is not the case, the physician should search for other causes, such as hernias or neoplasms. Second, the point of obstruction should be determined. This is the point at which the proximal dilated bowel collapses distally. Sometimes the transition zone is abrupt, as in the case of kinking or twisting, but it can spread over a segment, at which point the cause may be less certain. The possibility of multiple points and closed-loop obstruction must be entertained and ruled out. The entire bowel must be visualized. Third, evidence of bowel necrosis must be evaluated.

How can viable bowel be distinguished from the nonviable segment?
Although the pink peristaltic bowel is obviously viable and the bluish-black necrotic bowel is easily recognized to be nonviable, it can be difficult to distinguish ischemia from necrosis. The presence of peristalsis, the color of the bowel, and vigorous bleeding from cut edges are all clinical clues of viability. Intraoperative Doppler examination, fluorescein staining, and monitoring of the myoelectric activity of the bowel are all tests aimed at making the recognition of viable bowel easier. When bowel viability is questionable, the bowel may be left in place and the patient taken back to the operating room 12 to 24 hours later for a second look (6).

There are dense adhesions all over the peritoneum that require long tedious dissections to take down. Finally, in the left quadrant, clustered scar tissues tightly adhering around the midjejunum are discovered. The adhesions have kinked off the bowel lumen. The transition zone is acute at this point, with the proximal distended bowel and the distal collapsed segment apparent. After release of the scar, the bowel content passes freely into the distal segment. There is no evidence of bowel ischemia, and the rest of the bowel appears normal. The abdomen is closed, and the patient returns to the recovery room.

What are possible complications following surgery for SBO?
Recurrence, postischemic bowel stenosis, and other postsurgical complications such as wound infection, atelectasis, pneumonia, and urinary tract infection may follow surgery for SBO.

What is the incidence of recurrent SBO after the first episode from postsurgical adhesions is treated by celiotomy and lysis of adhesions?
The recurrence rate is probably 10 to 15%, which is higher than the incidence of the first episode.

What is the incidence of developing the first episode of SBO after an initial abdominal surgery?
Over a lifetime, the incidence of developing SBO following abdominal surgery is approximately 5%.

What is the risk of mortality from surgery for SBO?
The risk of mortality depends on the patient's comorbid factors (e.g., age, cardiopulmonary status), the preoperative hemodynamic and electrolyte derangement, and the extent of bowel ischemia, necrosis, and sepsis. Surgical mortality from uncomplicated SBO in a relatively healthy patient is less than 1%. However, the mortality from complicated septic SBO in compromised patients can be much, much higher, such that the overall mortality from surgical decompression of SBO averages 9 to 13% (2).

In the recovery room, the patient's vital signs are as follows: blood pressure, 90/50 mm Hg; heart rate, 140 beats per minute; temperature, 100.2°F. He is still on the ventilator and has not fully awakened from long operative anesthesia. The patient is receiving 50% F_iO_2 and 700 mL breaths (tidal volume) 10 times per minute as intermittent mandatory ventilation (IMV). His urine is dark brown and scant. The recovery room nurse informs the physician of the arterial blood gas (ABG) results: partial pressure of oxygen (PO_2), 160 torr; partial pressure of carbon dioxide (PCO_2, 28 torr; pH, 7.28; bicarbonate, 13 mEq.

What is the acid-base status of this patient, what are possible causes of his condition, and what is the treatment?
This patient has acute metabolic acidosis. (Appendix 9.2 provides a differential diagnosis.) Most likely, this is due to lactic acidosis from acute hypovolemic shock and hypoperfusion of distal organs. The treatment is volume resuscitation.

After 2 L of intravenous lactated Ringers solution, the patient's hemodynamic profile is improved, and the urine output increases to 100 mL/hour. The new ABG is normal: PO_2, 150 torr; PCO_2, 38 torr; pH, 7.38; bicarbonate, 23 mEq. However, as the patient awakens, he begins to breathe on his own in addition to the ventilator. The ABG results are then PO_2, 150 torr; PCO_2, 25 torr; pH, 7.50; bicarbonate, 22 mEq.

What is the patient's acid-base status, what are possible causes of his condition, and what is the treatment?
The patient has acute respiratory alkalosis. (Appendix 9.2 provides a differential diagnosis.) In this case, the patient hyperventilated as he awoke, and the ventilator maintained its support. The treatment is to decrease the minute ventilation or in this case to wean the patient from the mechanical ventilator.

The patient is weaned from the ventilator, and as he awakens and follows commands, he is extubated. He receives large volumes of intravenous fluid for the first 48 hours to maintain adequate urine output. On the fourth postoperative day, he complains of dyspnea. Chest radiograph shows a small left pleural effusion and mild pulmonary edema. The central venous pressure is 15 mm Hg. He appears to be in fluid overload. With IV furosemide around the clock, vigorous diuresis is achieved. While he is undergoing diuresis, the following lab-

Management Algorithm for Small Bowel Obstruction (SBO)

Algorithm 9.1.

oratory results are obtained: PO_2, 75 torr; PCO_2, 46 torr; pH, 7.48; bicarbonate, 33 mEq.

What is the patient's acid-base status, what are possible causes of his condition, and what is the treatment?
Mr. Chapman now has contraction metabolic alkalosis. (Appendix 9.2 provides a differential diagnosis.) This is a common sequela in a postsurgical patient who undergoes vigorous diuresis, losing both salt and water. Sodium is lost in the proximal tubule, much of which is resorbed in the distal tubule. Resorption of sodium in the distal tubule is counterbalanced by active excretion of hydrogen, which leads to acidic urine and metabolic alkalosis. The treatment is to decrease the diuretic dose, infuse saline as appropriate for the overall goal of volume status, and supplement potassium.

Mr. Chapman's IV furosemide dose is reduced, he receives IV potassium supplementation, and his fluid status returns to normal. He reports flatus on the fourth postoperative day; the nasogastric tube is discontinued. He is advanced on diet, and on sixth postoperative day, he is discharged home.

REFERENCES

1. Ellis H. Acute intestinal obstruction. In: Schwartz SI, Ellis H, eds. Maingot's Abdominal Operations. 9th ed. Norwalk, CT: Appleton & Lange, 1989:885–904.
2. Schwartz SI, Storer EH. Manifestations of gastrointestinal disease. In: Schwartz SI et al., eds. Principles of Surgery. 4th ed. New York: McGraw Hill, 1984:1021–1062.
3. Bulkley GB. Small bowel obstruction. Curr Surg 1986;43:57.
4. O'Brien WJ. Fluids and electrolytes. In: Berry SM et al., eds. Mont Reid Surgical Handbook. St. Louis: Mosby, 1997:17–19.
5. Shires GT, Shires GT III, Lowry SF. Fluids, electrolyte, and nurtritional management of the surgical patient. In: Schwartz SI, Shires GT, Spencer FC, eds. Principles of Surgery. New York: McGraw Hill, 1994:61–93.
6. Mast B, Dyke CM. Small bowel obstruction. In: Surgical Attending Rounds. Malvern, PA: Lea & Febiger, 1992:85–94.

Appendix 9.1. ELECTROLYTE ABNORMALITIES, SYMPTOMS AND SIGNS, CAUSES AND TREATMENT

Electrolyte Abnormality	Symptoms, Signs, and Complications	Differential Diagnosis	Treatment
Hyponatremia	Usually asymptomatic if mild (Na_s >125 mEq) or slow in onset. Neuromuscular effects: muscle spasms, hyperactive DTRs, seizures	Increased extracellular fluid: heart failure, renal failure, liver failure, malnutrition	(1) Treat underlying cause. (2) Asymptomatic: water restriction; symptomatic: hypertonic 3% saline (caution: overrapid correction of serum Na^+ level may cause central pontine myelinolysis).
		Normal extracellular fluid: SIADH, myxedema, adrenal insufficiency, hypothyroidism, stress, sickle cell disease	(1) Treat underlying cause. (2) Water restriction with or without diuretics.
		Decreased extracellular fluid: diuresis, adrenal insufficiency, renal tubular acidosis	(1) Treat underlying cause. (2) Saline infusion (total mEq Na^+ needed) = $(140 - Na_s)$ × (total body weight in kg) × (0.6)
		Pseudohyponatremia: hyperglycemia, hyperproteinemia, hyperlipidemia	Treat underlying cause
Hypernatremia	Thirst, fever, dry mucosal membranes, agitation, seizure, coma	DI (central neurogenic versus nephrogenic)	(1) Central DI responds to DDAVP; Nephrogenic DI does not respond to DDAVP. (2) Oral intake or IV infusion of free water.

continued

Condition	Cause	Signs/Symptoms	Treatment
	Hypovolemia from inadequate water intake, excessive excretory or secretory free water loss		If hypovolemic, free water repletion. (Correct less than 50% deficit in first 8 hours, then remaining 50% in 16–24 hours. If too rapid, cerebral edema occurs.) If hypervolemic, diuretics and hypotonic fluid.
	Excessive Na intake or infusion (e.g., iatrogenic sodium bicarbonate, IV drug vehicle) Hyperadrenalism, hyperaldosteronism		Same as above.
			Same as above. Note: Calculation of free water deficit $= \text{(Normal body water)} - \text{(Current body water)} = (TBW \times 0.6) - [(140 \times TBW \times 0.6)/Na_s]$.
Hypokalemia	Intracellular shift: alkalosis, rapid glucose metabolism associated with insulin administration in diabetic ketoacidosis, β-adrenergic agonists Potassium depletion through GI tract (diarrhea, emesis), diuretics, renal tubular disease, hyperaldosteronism	ECG changes (low-voltage QRS, T, ST waves; increased P or U waves); weakness; fatigue; decreased DTR; ileus; increased tendency for arrhythmias or digitalis toxicity; nephrogenic DI if severe	(1) Treat underlying cause (e.g., alkalosis). (2) Oral or IV potassium repletion (caution if renal failure present).
Hyperkalemia	Intracellular shift: acidosis β-adrenergic antogonists, reperfusion tissue necrosis, traumatic tissue necrosis	ECG changes (widened QRS, peaked T waves, first-degree heart block); bradycardia or asystole if severe; nausea; vomiting; diarrhea; weakness	(1) Treat underlying cause. (2) Exchange resin (e.g., Kayexalate). (3) IV insulin + dextrose 50% water. (4) Sodium bicarbonate. (5) IV calcium. (6) Diuretics if appropriate. (7) Dialysis if acute and severe.

Appendix 9.1.　ELECTROLYTE ABNORMALITIES; SYMPTOMS AND SIGNS; CAUSES AND TREATMENT

Electrolyte Abnormality	Symptoms, Signs and Complications	Differential Diagnosis	Treatment
		Pseudohyperkalemia: hemolysis, leukocytosis (>70 K), thrombocytosis (>1000 K)	Same as above
		Renal failure, adrenal insufficiency, spironolactone overuse, impaired renal tubular function, GI bleeding	Same as above
Hypocalcemia	Neuromuscular irritability [hyperreflexia, muscle cramps, periorbital twitching (Chvostek's sign), carpopedal spasm to relative ischemia (Trousseau's sign), tetany, seizure], decreased myocardial relaxation and contractility, ECG: prolonged QT interval	Hypoalbuminemia (normal ionized calcium), acute alkalosis, hypoparathyroidism, pancreatitis, hypomagnesemia, hyperphosphatemia, pancreatitis, sepsis, fat embolism, shock, renal failure, rhabdomyolysis, renal tubular acidosis Pseudohypoparathyroidism, anticonvulsants (phenytoin, phenobarbital), aminoglycosides	Acute: IV calcium chloride or IV calcium gluconate Chronic: calcium carbonate; lactate; glubinate; vitamin D; phosphate-binding antacids (improve calcium absorption)
Hypercalcemia	Stones, bones, moans, and groans: renal stones, osteolytic lesions, bone pains, psychiatric disorders, lethargy, confusion, abdominal pain with or without organ dysfunction (e.g., peptic ulcers or pancreatitis)	HAP SCHMIT, MD: Hyperparathyroidism, Addison's disease, Paget's disease, sarcoidosis, cancer (osteolytic bone metastasis, humoral hypercalcemia or malignancy, paraneoplastic syndrome), hyperthyroidism, milk-alkali syndrome, immobilization,	(1) Saline rehydration. (2) Furosemide. (3) Correct hypokalemia. (4) Mithramycin. (5) Calcitonin. (6) Glucocorticoids for malignancy. (7) Dialysis. (8) Also, treat underlying cause (e.g., parathyroidectomy for parathyroid hyperplasia).

	Symptoms	Causes	Treatment
Hypomagnesemia	Similar to hypocalcemia	thiazides, myeloma, vitamin D intoxication Malnutrition (alcoholism, starvation, malabsorption, GI fistulas), GI losses from chronic emesis or diarrhea, burns, pancreatitis, SIADH, diuresis, primary hyperaldosteronism, insulin treatment of DKA, hypoparathyroidism	Treat underlying cause. Replacement therapy: IV $MgSO_4$ or oral magnesium oxide. Monitor replacement progress with monitoring of DTRs and serum levels.
Hypermagnesemia	Nausea, vomiting, weakness, ECG changes (AV block and prolonged QT) Note on symptoms: (1) Serum levels >4 mEq, decrease of DTR. (2) Level >6 mEq hypotension and vasodilation. (3) Level >8 mEq, respiratory failure.	Renal failure, overdose of magnesium = containing antacids, severe acidosis, adrenal insufficiency, hypothyroidism, DKA, severe burns or crush injury, iatrogenic (treatment of eclampsia)	Treat underlying cause (generally, the same as the treatment of hypercalcemia).
Hypophosphatemia	Anorexia; weakness; tremors; decreased DTR; paresthesias; mental obtundation; rhabdomyolysis or hemolysis; impaired WBC, platelet, RBC functions, including decreased oxygen saturation due to decreased 2,3-DPG levels; decreased liver function	Reduced oral intake, nutritional recovery following starvation, alcoholism, acute renal tubular necrosis, anabolic state (treatment of DKA or nutritional recovery following starvation), alkalosis, decreased GI resorption due to vitamin D inadequacy	Treat underlying cause. Administer phosphate as needed [e.g., during nutritional phase following starvation (8 mM PO_4 for each 1000 calories)], IV phosphate if oral is unfeasible; fleets phosphate enema if oral or IV not available.

continued

Appendix 9.1. ELECTROLYTE ABNORMALITIES; SYMPTOMS AND SIGNS; CAUSES AND TREATMENT

Electrolyte Abnormality	Symptoms, Signs and Complications	Differential Diagnosis	Treatment
Hyperphosphatemia	Consequences of renal failure; acidosis, and consequent hypocalcemia; hypomagnesemia	Renal failure, hypoparathyroidism, acidosis, vitamin D intake, increased phosphate intake	Treat underlying cause. phosphate-binding antacid (e.g., Amphogel). Increase renal excretion with saline or acetazolamide. Renal dialysis as needed.

DKA, diabetic ketoacidosis; DDAVP, 1-deamino-8-D-arginine vasopressin; DI, diabetes insipidus; DTR, deep tendon reflex; GI, gastrointestinal; IV, intravenous; Na, serum sodium; ECG, electrocardiogram; SIADH, syndrome of inappropriate secretion of antidiuretic hormone; 2,3-DPG, 2,3-diphosphoglycerate; WBC, white blood cell; RBC, red blood cell; MgSO$_4$, magnesium sulfate; PO$_4$, phosphate.

Appendix 9.2. ACID-BASE ABNORMALITIES

Acid-Base	Primary Change**	Secondary Change**	Effect**	Cause	Treatment
Metabolic acidosis	↓ HCO_3	↓ PCO_2	Last two digits pH = PCO_2 $HCO_3 + 15$ = Last two digits pH	High anion gap: KUSSMAL: ketoacidosis (diabetic, alcoholic, nutritional), uremia, salicylates, spirits (ethanol, ethylene glycol), methanol, (par)aldehyde, lactate (ischemia from shock or hypoxia, hepatic insufficiency)	Treat underlying cause. If mild acidosis (pH >7.25), no treatment needed. If moderate-to-severe acidosis (pH <7.20), consider IV bicarbonate injections if absolutely needed.
				Normal anion gap with normal or high serum potassium: exogenous chloride infusion as in TPN, posthypocapnia, rapid hydration and dilutional acidosis, adrenal insufficiency, early uremia, carbonic anhydrase inhibitors (e.g. acetazolamide)	Give 1/2 of acute base deficit and recheck laboratory test. Acute base deficit = 50% × body weight (in kg) × (25 − serum HCO_3).
				Normal anion gap with low serum potassium: diarrhea, fistulas (small bowel, pancreas, biliary), ureteral diversions, renal tubular acidosis	

continued

143

Appendix 9.2. ACID-BASE ABNORMALITIES

Acid-Base	Primary Change**	Secondary Change**	Effect**	Cause	Treatment
Metabolic alkalosis	↑HCO_3	↑P_{CO_2}	$HCO_3 + 15 =$ Last two digits pH	Chloride responsive: excessive diuresis (acid loss through kidney tubules) or excessive vomiting (acid loss through emesis of gastric juice), contraction alkalosis, exogenous bicarbonate loading, villous adenoma Chloride unresponsive: severe potassium depletion, hyperaldosteronism, Cushing's disease, exogenous glucocorticoid injection.	(1) Treat underlying cause. (2) Correct hypovolemia with chloride solution (e.g., normal saline). Sufficient for most chloride-responsive causes. (3) Correct hypokalemia with IV or oral potassium as appropriate to renal function, especially if chloride unresponsive (4) Carbonic anhydrase inhibitor (Diamox) to increase renal excretion of bicarbonate. (5) Slow infusion of acid for chloride unresponsive refractory alkalosis. (6) H_2 antagonist to minimize acid loss through gastric tube.

continued

Respiratory acidosis				
Acute	$\uparrow PCO_2$	$\uparrow HCO_3$	Δ pH, 0.08 per 10 Δ in PCO_2	Hypoventilation and subsequent hypercapnia	(1) Treat underlying cause. (2) Increase ventilation; intubate if needed; increase ventilatory rate, tidal volume, pressure support.
Chronic	$\uparrow PCO_2$	$\uparrow\uparrow HCO_3$	$\leftarrow\Delta$ pH, 0.03 per 10 Δ in PCO_2		
Respiratory alkalosis				
Acute	$\downarrow PCO_2$	$\downarrow HCO_3$	$\Delta HCO_3 = 0.2 \times \Delta$ in PCO_2	Hyperventilation and subsequent hypocapnia	(1) Treat underlying cause. (2) Decrease ventilation; increase dead space (bag partially over mouth in anxious patient); decrease ventilatory rate, tidal volume, pressure support.
Chronic	$\downarrow PCO_2$	$\downarrow\downarrow HCO_3$	$\leftarrow\Delta HCO_3 = 0.3 \times \Delta$ in PCO_2		

PCO_2, partial pressure of carbon dioxide; PO_2, partial pressure of oxygen; HCO_3, bicarbonate; Δ, change; IV, intravenous; TPN, total parenteral nutrition.

**O'Brien WJ. Fluids and electrolytes. In: Berry SM et al., eds. Mont Reid Surgical Handbook. St. Louis:Mosby, 1997:20–31.

Appendicitis

K. Francis Lee

Tammy Jenkins is a 24-year-old woman who goes to the emergency department on Sunday evening with lower abdominal pain. The pain started on Saturday afternoon as a general discomfort in her abdomen. She attributed the discomfort to beer and chips she consumed at a football game, but she became concerned when she woke up Sunday morning with a sharp pain in her right lower abdomen. She had no appetite for breakfast and had increasing pain throughout the day.

In the emergency department, her temperature is 37.9°C. Abdominal examination shows a nondistended abdomen with hypoactive bowel sounds. There is involuntary guarding and rebound tenderness, and the right lower quadrant is exquisitely tender to palpation. The leukocyte count is 11.5 K with 78% segmentation. Serum electrolytes, blood urea nitrogen–creatinine ratio (BUN–Cr), bilirubin, and amylase are within normal limits. KUB radiograph shows normal gas pattern without any free intraperitoneal air. Urinalysis is unremarkable.

Is this presentation typical or atypical of appendicitis?
Appendicitis typically occurs in people in their second or third decade, is slightly more common in men than women (3:2), and usually affects previously healthy patients (1). The classic pain begins as a dull periumbilical discomfort, then settles in the right lower quadrant (RLQ) of the abdomen as a sharp pain occurring over a short time, as in the present case. Often, the typical case of appendicitis is diagnosed by the patient. However, roughly half of the time appendicitis presents atypically and eludes prompt diagnosis. Atypical cases can present in a variety of ways, and it is said that atypical acute appendicitis mimics many other causes of acute abdominal pain.

What are other possible diagnoses in this young woman?
In addition to appendicitis, there are a number of gynecologic causes that can cause RLQ pain. These include pelvic inflammatory disease, ectopic pregnancy,

ovarian cyst rupture, Mittelschmerz, endometriosis, ovarian torsion, and ovarian vein thrombosis. Other possible diagnoses include Crohn's disease, right colon diverticulitis, cholecystitis, perforated ulcer, and renal or ureteral calculi.

Ms. Jenkins reveals that she has had an active sexual life for the past several months and has had more than one partner. Her last period was 1 week ago. She has had midcycle pain before, but this pain seems to be different. Upon closer inquiry, she also reveals that she has had infections in her abdomen for which she has taken antibiotics. She denies any other gynecologic history, previous pregnancy, and personal or family history of inflammatory bowel disease. She asks if this can be another infection.

What are the salient clinical features useful for differentiation between pelvic inflammatory disease (PID) and appendicitis?
In a prospective study of 118 women at the University of California at San Francisco, several factors were found to be useful for differentiation of PID from acute appendicitis (2). These factors are usually associated with PID rather than appendicitis:

- Longer duration of symptoms
- Nausea, vomiting, or both
- History of venereal disease
- Cervical motion tenderness
- Adnexal tenderness
- Isolated peritoneal signs in RLQ abdomen

What is the chandelier sign?
The chandelier sign describes exquisite tenderness of the cervix during pelvic examination.

What data must one always obtain on history and laboratory examination when evaluating a young woman with abdominal pain?
It is necessary to obtain the following information from a woman in her child-bearing years who has abdominal pain:

Menstruation history. A suspiciously prolonged menstrual cycle may indicate an ectopic pregnancy. Midcycle pain and mucous discharge may signify *Mittelschmerz,* a syndrome of pain associated with ovulation.
Pregnancy history. A β-human chorionic gonadotropin (hCG) level should be ascertained to determine whether the woman is pregnant. Women who are in their third trimester of pregnancy may have atypical appendicitis, and therefore warrant a high index of suspicion.

Sudden RLQ or LLQ (left lower quadrant) pain without significant prodrome suggests *ovarian cyst rupture or torsion.*

What are the anatomic reasons that acute appendicitis may mimic a variety of abdominal diseases?
The appendix is a 10-cm hollow tube attached to the cecum. Its intraabdominal location depends on the way it is attached by the mesoappendix. Its tip can
point in any direction 360° from the cecal attachment (1). The symptoms vary
according to the location of the inflamed portion and the affected contiguous
structures. In 65% of appendicitis cases, the appendix is in the low cecal position, yielding the typical primary sign of sharp tenderness at McBurney's point.
In 30% of cases, it lies over the pelvic brim and as in the present case, may be
associated with midline lower abdominal tenderness or with various genitourinary symptoms. In 5% of cases, it lies outside the peritoneum behind the cecum
and the ascending colon, so that the tip may reach as high as the right upper
quadrant, in which case appendicitis may mimic cholecystitis (1).

What is the clinical significance of McBurney's point, and where is it?
Charles McBurney (1845–1914) was an American surgeon who in 1889 described the classic location of sharp pain on the spot "very exactly between an
inch and a half and two inches from the anterior spinous process of the ilium
on a straight line drawn from the process to the umbilicus" (1).

**Pelvic examination does not reveal cervical motion tenderness or purulent discharge. There is some discomfort in the right adnexal area.
The physician states that the main differential diagnosis is appendicitis versus PID.**

What are the therapeutic options for this patient at this point?
Ms. Jenkins may undergo surgery or expectant management.

**As the possibility of surgery is being explained to her, Ms. Jenkins
wants to know about the option of "video camera surgery through a
scope" that she has seen on television.**

What is the role of laparoscopic appendectomy in young women?
For the following reasons reported from randomized clinical trials, laparoscopic
appendectomy is preferable to the open approach in female patients in whom
the diagnosis is unclear. First, if the appendix is normal under laparoscopy, further intraperitoneal examination of the pelvic reproductive organs can be easily performed. Therefore, the chance of uncertain diagnosis after the procedure
is lower with laparoscopy (4 to 10%) than with the open technique (28% to
more than 50%) (3, 4). Second, the incidence of unnecessary appendectomy is

lower with laparoscopy than with the open approach (3, 5). Third, for women with chronic RLQ pain, laparoscopy can obviate unnecessary appendectomy in up to 90% of patients and lead to proper diagnosis and relief of chronic pain in up to 97% of patients (6).

Is postoperative pain less with the laparoscopic technique? Is the hospital stay shorter?
Studies have not always shown improvement in postoperative pain or length of hospital stay with laparoscopic appendectomy (4, 5). But there are far more clinical studies, some prospective and randomized, that report decreased postoperative pain and earlier return to normal activity (7–11).

Is the rate of perioperative complication higher with the laparoscopic approach?
Generally, no (8, 12).

Does laparoscopic appendectomy have the same role in acute inflamed appendicitis as in perforated appendicitis?
No. In perforated appendicitis, it seems that there is a trend toward a higher incidence of postoperative abscess formation following laparoscopic appendectomy than in open appendectomy (12). The rate of conversion from laparoscopic to open procedure is much higher in patients with perforated appendicitis.

In patients with perforated appendicitis, is there an alternative to immediate appendectomy?
Percutaneous drainage and interval appendectomy may be an alternative. If the appendiceal abscess is known to be well loculated and walled off on computed tomography (CT) and the patient is not septic, one may percutaneously drain the abscess cavity in lieu of immediate appendectomy, laparoscopic or open, and treat with antibiotics for a few weeks. The patient returns later to have the appendix resected when the inflammation has decreased. Reports indicate a success rate of 70 to 90%. The benefits of percutaneous drainage under radiologic guidance include precise anatomic identification of complex, multiloculated abscess; avoidance of operation for drainage without appendectomy; temporization of high-risk patients; and temporization of emergency appendectomy for an elective appendectomy (13). Interval appendectomy reportedly has been performed with the laparoscopic approach safely and effectively (14). However, not all surgeons support this approach, even for a confined appendiceal abscess; rather, open drainage with appendectomy is preferred.

Does laparoscopic appendectomy cost less than the open procedure?
This is controversial. Savings achieved by laparoscopic appendectomy (i.e., decreased length of hospital stay and reduced postoperative analgesic requirement) were offset by increased operating room supply cost and operative time

(15). In one study, these operating room costs resulted in greater hospital charges for the laparoscopic appendectomy (16). One may argue, however, that a patient's earlier return to work results in savings for society as a whole.

The patient agrees to a laparoscopic evaluation in the operating room and possible appendectomy. She was warned of a conversion from laparoscopic to open appendectomy. Before the operation, she asks what will happen if it is discovered that the appendix is not infected. Will her appendix be taken out anyway (incidental appendectomy)?

What are the arguments for and against performing an incidental appendectomy during this patient's laparoscopic examination?
It is controversial whether appendectomy in passing during a negative exploration is justified. The argument for incidental appendectomy is that the absence of the organ obviates any future question of appendicitis should the patient develop abdominal pain. The argument against incidental appendectomy is largely the risk of peritoneal or wound infection, especially during clean procedures in which resection through the appendiceal stump may spill the contents of the cecum. The controversy revolves around whether the postoperative infection rate is actually increased.

Many retrospective studies of open appendectomy report an increased rate of infection. However, a prospective study randomized 139 trauma patients with negative exploratory laparotomy; whether incidental appendectomy was performed depended on whether their hospital number was odd or even. There were no intraperitoneal infections in either group, and the wound infection rate was statistically insignificant (1.8% for incidental appendectomy group versus 3.6% for the control group) (17). These factors favor incidental appendectomy:

• Easy access to the appendix and technical feasibility
• Contaminated peritoneum (i.e., concomitant bowel content spillage)
• Young age
• Likelihood of future abdominal pains (e.g., history of PID, family history of Crohn's disease)

In this patient with a strong history of recurrent RLQ abdominal pain, an incidental appendectomy is justified.

The patient undergoes general anesthesia and endotracheal intubation for laparoscopy. With visualization through the infraumbilical laparoscope, dissection of the RLQ is performed through two 5-mm ports in the LLQ and left suprapubis. Densely inflamed tissue and desmo-plastic reaction in the right pericolic gutter comes into view. A perforated appendix

appears to be densely adherent to the cecum and lateral abdominal wall. After several futile attempts to dissect the base of the appendix, it is decided to convert to the open procedure. A 5-cm skin incision is made in the RLQ directly over the cecum and appendix.

What layers of the abdomen does a RLQ incision go through?
The incision will be made through the following layers in the following order: skin, subcutaneous fat, external oblique muscle and/or aponeurosis, internal oblique muscle, transversalis abdominis, and peritoneum.

When the peritoneum is opened, cloudy intraperitoneal fluid is noted. A culture and sensitivity sample of the fluid is sent to the microbiology laboratory. Further dissection reveals a gangrenous appendix with distal perforation in the pelvic brim.

How does one correlate Ms. Jenkins's signs and symptoms with the basic pathophysiology of acute appendicitis?
The pathophysiology of acute appendicitis is as follows:

1. Luminal obstruction due to lymphoid hyperplasia (60%), fecaliths (35%), foreign bodies (4%), or tumors (1%). Ms. Jenkins had a fecalith, shown on a radiograph of KUB.
2. Increase of intraluminal pressure due to mucous secretion
3. Obstruction of lymphatic drainage due to increased luminal pressure
4. Infection of static mucus by luminal bacteria (pus)
5. Mucosal ulceration (acute focal appendicitis)
6. Bacterial invasion of the appendiceal wall (suppurative appendicitis)
7. Ischemia of bowel wall because of compromised arterial blood supply secondary to venous thrombosis (gangrenous appendicitis)
8. Rupture of bowel wall secondary to ulceration, bacterial infection, and bowel ischemia (perforated appendicitis) (1)

Symptomatic transition from periumbilical dullness to RLQ sharp pain occurs when the inflamed appendix becomes contiguous with the parietal peritoneum, evoking sharp parietal pain rather than dull visceral pain.

What are the differences between uncomplicated appendicitis and perforated appendicitis in terms of morbidity and mortality? What are Ms. Jenkins's chances of developing complications?
The risk of mortality is 0.1% in patients with uncomplicated appendicitis, 0.6% in patients with gangrenous appendicitis, and 5% in patients with perforated appendicitis. With perforation, morbidity increases fourfold to fivefold, and wound infection increases 15 to 20%.

Does perforation of the appendix occur commonly among elderly patients with appendicitis?
Yes. The rate of perforation in the elderly is higher (30%) than in the general population for three main reasons. First, impaired structure and poor blood supply tend to cause early gangrene and early perforation. Second, there appears to be greater hesitancy to proceed with surgery in the elderly who have high perioperative risks (1). Third, appendicitis in the elderly presents atypically more often than in the general population.

Are there any other patient populations in whom diagnosis of appendicitis is particularly difficult and is associated with increased incidence of delayed diagnosis and perforation?
Yes, there are three other groups: infants and young children, young sexually active women of childbearing age, and pregnant women.

Why is it difficult to diagnose appendicitis in infants and young children? What is the incidence of perforation among children?
The rate of perforation in patients below 1 year of age is 100%; below 2 years, 70 to 80%; and up to 5 years of age, 50% (1). This correlation to age is because the younger the infant, the less well he or she can communicate abdominal discomfort. Another reason is that many nonsurgical pediatric diseases cause abdominal pain, leading to a greater tendency to delay surgical diagnosis and initially attempt medical therapy.

In children, what are the two most common medical conditions that mimic appendicitis?
The leading differential diagnoses are gastroenteritis and mesenteric lymphadenitis.

How is a pregnant woman suspected to have appendicitis managed?
Pregnant women suspected of having appendicitis are managed the same as nonpregnant women. Diagnosis and surgery must not be delayed because of the fear of the anesthetic's effects on the fetus. A retrospective study of 12 pregnant women with appendicitis showed that delay in treatment is common because of uncertainty in making the diagnosis and hesitancy to proceed with surgery. Patients without perforation had no complications. However, there was a 50% perforation rate, with death of one mother and three fetuses (18).

Does the presentation of appendicitis change during pregnancy?
Yes. The farther along in the pregnancy, the larger the uterus and the more atypical the pain. In the first two trimesters, the pain tends to be typically in the RLQ. During the third trimester, the appendix is displaced upward, and the pain tends to be in the right flank or even in the right upper quadrant (RUQ). Generally speaking, one may assume that in the first two trimesters, diagnosis of appendicitis should proceed in the same manner as in a nonpregnant woman. One must not regard appendicitis in early pregnancy any differently.

With some effort, the patient's appendix is bluntly dissected free from its dense adherence and brought out of the abdomen into the surgical field. The mesoappendix is ligated and divided. The appendix is then resected following double ligature around the stump. The pericolic gutter and the pelvis are copiously irrigated with warm normal saline.

Should a drain be placed in this patient's abdomen during the operation and left? What are the indications for drains after appendectomy?
Generally speaking, leaving a drainage tube is not indicated if there is no perforation, even if the appendix was found to be gangrenous. If an abscess is present, drainage is indicated. In the face of diffuse peritonitis, multiple prophylactic drainage tubes are *not* indicated; one should drain only the loculated areas. The most important measure is copious irrigation of the contaminated area with normal saline with or without antibiotics before closure.

What type of drainage tube should be used?
Most people use simple drainage such as a Jackson-Pratt (JP) drain.

What are the various types of surgical drains?
See Selected Topics at the end of the chapter for descriptions of various surgical drains.

There is no loculation or abscess cavity, so a drain is not considered necessary. The peritoneum and the muscular and fascial layers are closed. The subcutaneous tissue above the external oblique fascia is packed with Betadine-soaked gauze.

For Ms. Jenkins's case of perforated appendicitis, what is the best technique for wound closure?
Delayed primary closure is the best technique for closing this wound (see Chapter 2).

What is delayed primary closure? What are the types of wound closure?

Primary closure is healing by first intention, that is, to approximate the skin edges of the wound primarily in the operating room.

Secondary closure is healing by second intention, that is, to leave the wound open for chronic wound dressing changes. Secondary closure usually depends on granulation tissue for eventual skin closure.

Delayed primary closure is healing by third intention, that is, to delay approximating the edges of the wound by packing the wound with moist gauze until the third to fifth postoperative day, when there has been a decrease in the bacterial count within the wound. Delayed primary closure is used for moderately to severely contaminated wounds.

Dressing is applied to the wound, general anesthesia is reversed, and the patient is extubated. As the patient awakens from the operation, she receives intravenous analgesia and is sent to the recovery room in stable condition.

What step would have been taken if laparoscopic or open exploration had revealed the appendix and the cecum to be normal?
If the appendix appears normal, the abdomen must be explored systematically. The small intestine should be examined retrograde for regional enteritis or Meckel's diverticulum. The cecum and the ascending colon should be examined for any tumor, especially in older patients. Exploration is much easier with laparoscopy. However, it is possible to explore the majority of the abdomen through the RLQ skin incision. If difficulty arises because of inadequate exposure, the incision must be extended. The pelvic organs and genitourinary system are examined for the appropriate differential diagnoses. The peritoneal fluid should be cultured and sent to the microbiology laboratory. In the right upper quadrant, the duodenum and gallbladder should be examined. The stomach is examined for ulcer. Mesentery and omentum should be examined, as should any enlarged lymph nodes.

What is Meckel's diverticulum?
Meckel's diverticulum is an omphalomesenteric remnant that did not fully retract during embryonic development. It is present in approximately 2% of the population. Within 2 feet proximally of the ileocecal valve, Meckel's diverticulum causes clinical complications in approximately 2% of the patients who have it. It contains ectopic tissue in the mucosa, most commonly gastric cells. The most common complications are ulceration, perforation, bleeding, and obstruction. A narrow-necked diverticulum may be treated with wedge resection, but a broad-necked Meckel's diverticulum may require a full diverticulectomy and ileal anastomosis.

What would have been done if Crohn's disease of the terminal ileum had been discovered in this patient? What would have been done with the appendix?
There is controversy as to whether the appendix should be left alone in the face of Crohn's disease. Theoretically, appendectomy amidst severe granulomatous inflammation may increase the risk of complication (e.g., fistula formation). However, the literature has not yet clearly substantiated this. If the base of the appendix and the cecum are not involved in the inflammatory process, appendectomy is probably safe.

What would have been done if a tumor had been discovered in Ms. Jenkins's appendix? How often are tumors found in the appendix? What is the most common tumor of the appendix? What is the usual presentation of appendiceal tumor?
The most common type of appendiceal tumor is carcinoid, usually on the tip of the appendix. Carcinoid, comprising 77% of appendiceal tumors (19), was discovered in only 1.4% of 1000 consecutive appendectomies (20). If the carcinoid tumor is small, a simple appendectomy is adequate; if the tumor is large, a more extensive resection is indicated. A retrospective literature review noted that tumors larger than 2 cm had a much higher incidence of regional metastasis than smaller ones. For this reason, simple appendectomy for tumors smaller than 2 cm and right hemicolectomy for tumors larger than 2 cm is recommended (21). Primary adenocarcinoma of the appendix is exceedingly rare (0.1%) (20). The usual presentation of an appendiceal tumor is similar to that of appendicitis.

Postoperatively, Ms. Jenkins is ordered NPO (nothing by mouth) with intravenous hydration and antibiotics. The course is entirely unremarkable except that on the first postoperative day, she has a fever of 39.1°C.

What is the differential diagnosis of postoperative fever?
The five W's—*wind, water, wound, walk, wonder drugs*—is a popular mnemonic for common causes of postoperative fever. In the first 48 postoperative hours following abdominal procedures, atelectasis (wind) is the most common cause because pain prevents deep breathing. Urinary tract infection (water) occurs usually 3 to 5 days after surgery and is associated with indwelling Foley catheters and urinary symptoms. Wound infection occurs later, on postoperative days 5 to 7, and it is usually evident from local signs. Deep vein thrombosis (walk) can occur at any time; it is associated with calf tenderness and swelling. One must also consider superficial phlebitis from intravenous lines and line sepsis from central venous lines or hyperalimentation lines. Last, hypersensitivity to "wonder" drugs, such as antibiotics, can cause fever, rash, or pruritus at any time and is easily controlled by antihistamines and discontinuation of the culpable agents. In Ms. Jenkins's case, bacteremia from the RLQ abdomen is another possible source, although her clinical condition should improve after adequate irrigation and surgical drainage.

With vigorous respiratory therapy, including early walking and coughing, Ms. Jenkins's fever subsides. She receives a 3-day course of intravenous antibiotic therapy. The wound is closed after 4 days without any difficulty. Diet is advanced to clear liquids on postoperative day 2, then to regular diet on postoperative day 3. She is discharged on postoperative day 5 with a clinic appointment in 1 week.

SELECTED TOPICS

SURGICAL DRAINS

Each surgical drainage system is distinctive and may be described by a set of three features: location, type, and material.

Location

The location of the drain usually determines its name, as evidenced by the following examples:

Nasogastric (NG) tube
Esophagostomy tube
Gastrostomy tube
Duodenostomy tube
Jejunostomy tube
Long intestinal tube
Cecostomy tube
Biliary tube
Nephrostomy tube
Ureterostomy tube
Chest tube

Types

There are two general types of surgical drainage systems, **open** and **closed,** depending on whether the distal end of the drain communicates with the outside environment.

Open Drainage Systems

Most superficial abscess cavities are drained openly; the benefits include simplicity and age-old familiarity. In fact, open drainage of an abscess cavity with simple tubes is one of the oldest and most effective surgical techniques known. A major disadvantage is the possibility of retrograde infection into the body cavity because of free communication with the external environment. For areas where retrograde infection portends a serious complication (e.g., the splenic bed following splenectomy), it is best to use a closed drainage system with the hope of maintaining sterility.

Closed Drainage Systems

Closed systems may evacuate the fluid collection by either gravity or suction. Straight drainage by gravity suffices for some drains (e.g., urinary catheters). However, negative pressure applied on a drainage tube provides the additional benefit of facilitating closure of dead space. For example, the subcutaneous space in the axillae following axillary lymph node dissection may close and heal better with continuous suction applied to the drainage tubes. A special type of closed system may provide an additional port, enabling one to irrigate the body cavity while suctioning the irrigant. Another special type of closed drainage system may use a water seal at the distal end of the tube to protect against inadvertent influx of air or bacteria into the body cavity. A typical ubiquitous example is a chest tube.

Management Algorithm for Right Lower Quadrant Pain

RLQ PAIN

CLINICAL JUDGEMENT
History: Typical?
P.E.:   Tender abdomen?
Lab: Elevated WBC?
Other: Fever?
         Anorexia?

Diagnosis of appendicitis likely

Diagnosis of appendicitis uncertain

Diagnosis of appendicitis unlikely

CLINICAL JUDGEMENT

CLINICAL JUDGEMENT

Surgery

Observe

"Uncomplicating" factors (with good follow-up mechanism)

"Uncomplicating" factors (e.g. flat abdomen, young male)

"Complicating" factors (e.g. reproductive years, obesity, young female)

"Complicating" factors (e.g. elderly, pregnant, pediatric)

Appendectomy (Open laparoscopic)

Appendectomy (Open or laparoscopic)

Appendectomy (Laparoscopic)

Admission and serial evaluation

Admission and serial evaluation for further work-up

Discharge home

Algorithm 10.1.

Material

A drainage system is characterized by the material, often named after the company or the inventor. These include Foley catheter, Red Rubber Robinson catheter, Salem-Sump catheter, Penrose drain, Jackson-Pratt drain, and Hemo-Vac drain. If percutaneous drainage of a periappendiceal abscess is necessary, a closed drain system may be considered. In a patient with bladder atony, one may use a closed Foley urinary catheter, which is drained by gravity. A patient with gastric dilation usually receives a closed Salem-Sump nasogastric tube drained by wall suction. A patient with malignant gastric outlet obstruction may receive decompression through a closed Foley-gastrostomy drainage system.

REFERENCES

1. Condon RE. Acute appendicitis. In: Sabiston DC. Davis Christopher Textbook of Surgery. Vol. 13. Philadelphia: Saunders, 1986:967–982.
2. Bongard F, Landers DV, Lewis F. Differential diagnosis of appendicitis and pelvic inflammatory diseases. Am J Surg 1985;150:90–96.
3. Laine S, Rantala A, Gullichesen R, Ovaska J. Laparoscopic appendectomy: is it worthwhile? A prospective, randomized study in young women. Surg Endosc 1997;11:95–97.
4. Zaninotto G, Rossi M, Anselmino M, et al. Laparoscopic versus conventional surgery for suspected appendicitis in women. Surg Endosc 1995;9:337–340.
5. Reiertsen O, Larsen S, Trondsen E, et al. Randomized controlled trial with sequential design of laparoscopic versus conventional appendicectomy. Br J Surg 1997;84: 842–847.
6. AlSalilli M, Vilos GA. Prospective evaluation of laparoscopic appendectomy in women with chronic right lower quadrant pain. J Am Assoc Gynecol Laparosc 1995;2:139–142.
7. Hansen JB, Smithers BM, Schache D, et al. Laparoscopic versus open appendectomy: prospective randomized trail. World J Surg 1996;20:17–20.
8. Kluiber RM, Hartsman B. Laparoscopic appendectomy: a comparison with open appendectomy. Dis Colon Rectum 1996;39:1008–1011.
9. Richards KF, Fisher KS, Flores JH, Christensen BJ. Laparoscopic appendectomy: comparison with open appendectomy in 720 patients. Surg Laparosc Endosc 1996;6:205–209.
10. Ortega AE, Hunter JG, Peters JH, et al. A prospective, randomized comparison of laparoscopic appendectomy with open appendectomy. Laparoscopic Appendectomy Study Group. Am J Surg 1995;169:208–212.
11. Frazee RC, Bohannon WT. Laparoscopic appendectomy for complicated appendicitis. Arch Surg 1996;131:509–511.
12. Tang E, Ortega AE, Anthone GJ, Beart RW Jr. Intraabdominal abscesses following laparoscopic and open appendectomies. Surg Endosc 1996;10:327–328.
13. van Sonnenberg E, Wittich GR, Casola G, et al. Periappendiceal abscesses: percutaneous drainage. Radiology 1987;163:23–26.
14. Vargas HI, Averbook A, Stamos MJ. Appendiceal mass: conservative therapy followed by interval laparoscopic appendectomy. Am Surg 1994;60:753–758.
15. Fritts LL, Orlando R III. Laparoscopic appendectomy: a safety and cost analysis. Arch Surg 1993;128:521–524.

16. McCahill LE, Pelligrini CA, Wiggins T, Helton WS. A clinical outcome and cost analysis of laparoscopic versus open appendectomy. Am J Surg 1997;171:533–537.

17. Strom PR, Turkleson ML, Stone HH. Safety of incidental appendectomy. Am J Surg 1983;145:819–822.

18. Horowitz MD, Gomez GA, Santiesteban R, et al. Acute appendicitis during pregnancy: diagnosis and management. Arch Surg 1985;120:1362–1367.

19. Dunn JP. Carcinoid tumors of the appendix: 21 cases with a review of the literature. N Z Med J 1982;95:73–76.

20. Dymock RB. Pathological changes in the appendix: a review of 1000 cases. Pathology 1977;9:331–339.

21. Thirlby RC, Kasper CS, Jones RC. Metastatic carcinoid tumor of the appendix: report of a case and review of the literature. Dis Colon Rectum 1984;27:42–46.

Inflammatory Bowel Disease

Jan Wojcik

CROHN'S DISEASE

Danielle Katz is a 23-year-old nursing student who goes the emergency department complaining of several months of intermittent abdominal pain that has become more severe during the past several weeks. It occurs postprandially throughout the lower abdomen but appears to be mainly right sided. The pain is crampy and is usually associated with nausea. She notes some looseness of her bowel movements during the past 6 months. A review of systems reveals a moderate weight loss, increased malaise, and fatigue during the same period.

Physical examination reveals a thin, somewhat gaunt young woman who is normotensive and afebrile. The abdomen is mildly distended, and a sense of fullness is appreciated in the right lower quadrant. The bowel sounds appear to be hyperactive. Rectal digital examination reveals guaiac-positive stool and no masses. The laboratory values are remarkable for an elevated white blood cell (WBC) count of 14,700 mL^{-1}, hematocrit of 32.1 mg/dL, an albumin level of 2.7 g/dL, and an erythrocyte sedimentation rate of 63 mm/hour.

Plain radiographs of the abdomen reveal several moderately dilated loops of small intestine with rare air-fluid levels and air in the colon. A subsequent barium enema reveals a normal colon but a significant stricture in the distal ileum, which is proximally dilated.

What is the most likely diagnosis? How was this disease initially described?
At the 1932 meeting of the American Medical Association, Burrill B. Crohn described 14 cases of what he termed *terminal ileitis*. Later that year, 52 cases were reported in a classic paper by Crohn et al. (1). Its traditional name in American literature is regional enteritis; in Britain it is called Crohn's disease. Crohn's disease of the colon was first recognized as a separate entity by Lochart-Mummery and Morson in 1960 (2).

What causes Crohn's disease?
Although many investigators have sought an infectious agent in Crohn's disease, there has never been any conclusive evidence that such an agent will ever be isolated. For many years, there has been speculation that the immune system may be involved in the pathogenesis of the disease.

Ms. Katz is told that she may have inflammatory bowel disease. She reports that one of her nursing school friends has ulcerative colitis.

In terms of causation, how is ulcerative colitis different from Crohn's disease?
Ulcerative colitis may be caused by a transmissible agent that results in a theoretic immunologic response in the colon, although nobody has been able to elucidate a possible agent. Patients with ulcerative colitis also have a defect in the protective mucous glycoprotein secretion that is not present in patients with Crohn's disease (3).

Is there a genetic component in either Crohn's disease or ulcerative colitis?
In reported series of Crohn's disease patients, the percentage of people with a family history is 10 to 20% (4). The proband concordance rate among monozygous twins is 54% for Crohn's disease. Heredity may be quite strong in those who develop Crohn's disease at an early age. The hereditary link is much stronger in ulcerative colitis.

Does Crohn's disease occur more frequently in some parts of the world than in others?
Crohn's disease is common in northwestern Europe and North America. Low prevalence rates are reported in Hispanics and Asians. Areas of low incidence include Japan and southern Europe. Crohn's disease is infrequent in South America, Asia, and tropical Africa.

Is the geographic distribution of ulcerative colitis similar?
Yes, ulcerative colitis is most common in Scandinavia, the United States, Great Britain, Australia, New Zealand, and South Africa. In addition, ulcerative colitis appears five times as often in Jews as in non-Jews living in Western countries. As with Crohn's disease, there is a predilection for women, and there is a bimodal age distribution, with the greatest peak in the second and third decades and a minor peak in the elderly (5, 6). The term *ulcerative colitis* was in common use by the end of the Civil War. In 1885, Pitt and Durham described pseudopolyps as a complication of ulcerative colitis.

Ms. Katz becomes a bit anxious and asks for specific details about Crohn's disease.

What are the anatomic features of Crohn's disease?
The hallmark of Crohn's disease is its segmental distribution in the terminal ileum, often with rectal sparing but frequently with perianal disease. The transmural nature of the inflammatory process is characterized by deep fissures that penetrate adjacent structures, causing abscesses and fistulas. Fat wrapping of involved bowel segments and mesenteric lymphadenopathy are common stigmata. The principal microscopic features are noncaseating granulomas with multinucleate giant cells, microabscesses, fissures, a chronic inflammatory cell infiltrate, lymphoid hyperplasia, edema, and fibrosis. Identification of noncaseating granulomas is possible in 70% of cases; in the remaining 30%, the diagnosis is made by a combination of overall gross and microscopic features.

How is this different from ulcerative colitis?
Unlike Crohn's disease, ulcerative colitis is a continuous disease, maximally involving the rectum and spreading proximally. There are no true skip lesions; the involved segment in ulcerative colitis is contagious; and areas that may appear normal on endoscopic examination are always abnormal when examined microscopically. In 10 to 20% of patients with pancolitis, the ileum is also involved in a process that is indistinguishable from the colonic disease for 5 to 15 cm. Ulcerative colitis is predominantly a mucosal disease characterized by epithelial ulceration and regeneration. In active disease, polymorphonuclear infiltration with crypt abscesses is the hallmark of the disease. Depletion of the goblet cell mucin is characteristic, and its extent is related to the severity of the disease.

Clinically, how does one differentiate Crohn's disease from ulcerative colitis?
The features characteristic of Crohn's disease in the large intestine are rectal sparing; distal ileal involvement; focal aphthous ulcers; deep ulceration with a cobblestone pattern; and fistula, abscess, or stricture. In contrast, ulcerative colitis produces intermittent attacks of rectal bleeding in combination with granular mucosal disease.

What is the natural history of Crohn's disease?
Crohn's disease, unlike ulcerative colitis, rarely goes into complete remission. Once the disease becomes symptomatic, it tends to progress to its hallmark complications of obstruction, local sepsis, and fistulas. Patients with inactive disease may develop the mechanical complications but not usually sepsis, and the course of the disease is relatively benign. Active disease is associated with florid and diffuse small-bowel disease or active colitis that has associated metabolic sequelae and sepsis.

The survival rate in patients with Crohn's disease does not differ from that of the general population. Chronic active small-bowel disease tends to progress toward obstruction. The most common presentation of colonic disease is diarrhea and weight loss. Anorectal strictures tend to be progressive and may eventually require proctectomy. Anorectal fistulas have a variable course. Recurrence of Crohn's disease is almost inevitable, and recurrent disease tends to have the same presentation as the original episode. Recurrence is more common in perforating disease than in nonperforating (i.e., obstruction, bleeding) disease.

Ms. Katz wants to know whether there was evidence of obstruction on the barium enema study and what the radiograph showed. She is told that a mild to moderate degree of obstruction was seen in the terminal ileum, along with several other radiographic features.

What are the radiographic features of Crohn's disease?
Crohn's disease is usually demonstrated by the use of contrast radiographs. The diagnosis of small-bowel disease is best demonstrated either by upper gastrointestinal contrast study with modified follow-through examinations or by the use of enteroclysis studies. The classic string sign is usually from edema and spasm rather than fibrosis. Colonic disease can be demonstrated by double contrast studies. The general radiologic features can be best summarized as edema, ulceration, fibrosis, and fistulas. Fistulas are more common in small-bowel than in large-bowel disease. Traditionally, colonic Crohn's disease affects the proximal colon, usually with ileal involvement. Approximately 50% of patients with Crohn's disease have rectal disease. The coalescence of ulcerated areas leads to the formation of the cobblestone pattern. The terminal ileum is involved in 50 to 70% of patients with Crohn's colitis. Strictures in Crohn's disease tend to have tapered margins, in contrast with carcinomas, which have abrupt narrowing.

What are the radiographic features of ulcerative colitis?
Plain radiographs can be useful in patients with acute fulminant colitis, in whom the affected segments of the colon are widened and distended with air. Toxic megacolon usually affects the transverse colon but also may involve the sigmoid colon. Contrast radiology should never be used in patients with acute colitis because of concerns about septicemia, perforation, and megacolon. The earliest radiographic changes are an irregular mucosal line that is thick and indistinct. As the disease progresses, more severe superficial ulcerations or erosions appear. The presence and extent of ulceration correlates well with the disease activity. Eventually, the denuded mucosa is replaced by granulation tissue, leaving only islands of intact mucosa. These pseudopolyps are the result of severe colitis; they indicate an inflammatory process and virtually never become malignant. Although the rectum is usually the most involved structure, there is some relative rectal sparing in 20% of patients. Any stricture must be differentiated as benign or malignant.

What are the typical endoscopic features of Crohn's disease?
Endoscopy shows the mucosal surface in Crohn's disease as granular or nodular with friability, erosions, and aphthous ulcers. Discontinuous disease, especially with aphthous ulceration or serpiginous linear ulceration, is pathognomonic of Crohn's colitis. Aphthous ulceration is believed to be the first macroscopically recognizable sign of Crohn's disease. Deep linear ulcers give rise to a cobblestone pattern. True cobblestoning occurs only in patients with Crohn's disease. As a general rule, cobblestoning, discontinuous disease, and anal lesions suggest Crohn's disease.

How does this contrast with the findings in ulcerative colitis?
Endoscopy is essential for obtaining biopsies and making the diagnosis of ulcerative colitis. The findings at endoscopy are usually more pronounced than can be seen radiographically.

Is it always possible to classify a patient as having either Crohn's disease or ulcerative colitis?
No. Despite the differences outlined, in approximately 10 to 15% of cases there is doubt about diagnosis. Eventually, the patient's history dictates the final diagnosis. Recurrence in the small bowel, perianal disease, fistulas, and abscesses are hallmarks of Crohn's disease regardless of what the original biopsies may have indicated.

Ms. Katz is recommended to start medications right away.

What is the appropriate initial therapy for Crohn's disease?
Medical therapy should be the first-line treatment in patients with uncomplicated Crohn's disease. Corticosteroids have been beneficial for acute Crohn's disease. Azathioprine and 6-mercaptopurine have a steroid-sparing effect that may take months. Cyclosporine also has been shown to be somewhat useful in maintaining remission. Metronidazole has been used extensively in patients with perianal disease and to a certain extent in those with left-sided colonic disease (7). Sulfasalazine has a limited role in Crohn's colitis and no therapeutic benefit for ileal Crohn's disease. It does not appear to have a corticosteroid-sparing effect. Adverse reactions to the sulfapyridine moiety of sulfasalazine occurs in 15% of patients.

How does medical therapy differ for patients with ulcerative colitis?
As with Crohn's colonic disease, steroid therapy is initiated to control the disease, and as the steroids are reduced, sulfasalazine is added to prevent relapse. The active ingredient of sulfasalazine, 5-aminosalicylic acid, can be delivered orally or in enemas or suppositories. In contrast to Crohn's disease, the immunosuppressive agents have not been shown to have singular benefit.

How is sulfasalazine used?
Sulfasalazine consists of sulfapyridine bound to 5-aminosalicylic acid. It was first used in 1942, and clinical benefit was demonstrated by 1948. Unfortunately, sulfasalazine may be associated with dose-related side effects such as nausea, vomiting, headache, and malaise. Side effects rarely occur when the dose is less than 4 g/day. Sulfasalazine crosses the placental barrier and can impede the absorption of albumin-bound drugs. Most of the side effects of sulfasalazine are due to the sulfapyridine fraction of the molecule; therefore, pharmacologic research has concentrated on removing that moiety. Maintenance therapy with sulfasalazine usually consists of 2 g/day.

Are there any other therapies?
Metabolic surveillance should be carried out in anyone with inflammatory bowel disease. Electrolyte and nutritional abnormalities are common and should be aggressively sought. Complete bowel rest by total parenteral nutrition (TPN) has not been shown to reduce the colectomy rate or offer clinical benefit to patients with ulcerative colitis or Crohn's disease. Nutritional support should be carried out, however, to allow for repair of the diseased bowel.

Ms. Katz is prescribed a combination medical regimen with corticosteroids as the core agent. (For comparative dose-equivalency of corticosteroids, see Table 11.1.) In the ensuing several weeks in an outpatient setting, her symptoms improve steadily. One day, however, she complains of severe right lower quadrant pain, and she presents to the emergency department with a tight obstruction of the

Table 11.1.   BIOLOGIC ACTIVITY PROFILES OF
SYNTHETIC ANALOGS OF CORTISOL

Steroid	Potency	Equivalent Dose (mg)	Sodium Retention	Biologic Half-life (hours)
Cortisol	1	20.0	1.0	8–12
Fluorocortisol	10	–	125	–
Short-acting analogs				
Prednisolone	4	5.0	0.8	12–36
Methylprednisolone	5	4.0	0.5	12–36
Triamcinolone	5	4.0	0.0	12–36
Long-acting analogs				
Betamethasone	25	0.6	0.0	36–54
Dexamethasone	25	0.6	0.0	36–54

Adapted with permission from Tepperman J. Metabolic and Endocrine Physiology. Chicago: Year Book, 1980:193.

terminal ileum and evidence of complete small-bowel obstruction. Surgical consultation is obtained.

How should one proceed with the surgical management of a patient?
Certain principles should be adhered to in the management of patients with Crohn's disease. First, surgical treatment should be reserved for symptoms and not for radiologic findings. The presence of internal fistulas is not necessarily an indication for surgical intervention because not all internal fistulas cause symptoms. Fistulas most commonly develop in the distal ileum. Second, surgical treatment should avoid extensive small-bowel resection. Third, surgical management should avoid rendering patients incontinent. It often has been stated that incontinent Crohn's patients are the result of overaggressive surgeons, not of the disease itself. Last, surgical management is preferred for patients developing complications from medical therapy or sepsis from delayed surgery.

With nasogastric decompression and medical treatment, Ms. Katz's symptoms improve. Over the ensuing 2 weeks, she resumes a solid diet and has satisfactory bowel movements. However, 3 weeks after discharge she returns to the emergency department with obstructive symptoms. Radiologic workup indicates obstruction at the same area in the terminal ileum.

What are the indications for surgical intervention in Crohn's disease?
The principal indications for operating on a patient with Crohn's disease are complications, namely recurrent obstruction, abscess formation, severe colitis, anal destruction, or malignancy. Complications requiring urgent surgical intervention include profuse blood loss, free perforation, acute progressive ileitis, intestinal obstruction, and toxic dilation. An attempt should be made to avoid using suture material that might cause tissue reaction and promote the formation of strictures or recurrent disease at the site of anastomosis. Current techniques favor extramucosal polypropylene sutures or staples.

At this point, the surgeon recommends abdominal exploration to identify and treat the intestinal obstruction.

What type of incision should be used for a patient with Crohn's disease?
A midline incision is preferred for all operations in patients with Crohn's disease. It does not transgress possible stoma sites on the lateral abdomen, and it can be reopened relatively easily. Most patients with Crohn's disease have fewer adhesions than normal, but they can have significant intrabowel adhesions. It is usually advisable to have the patient in stirrups, because access to the vagina, anus, or rectum may be necessary.

In the operating room, exploration of the abdomen reveals a 6-inch area of terminal ileum that is densely inflamed, with fatty mesentery encroaching around the bowel. The area is tightly narrowed and is the obvious cause of bowel obstruction. An attempt is made to resect the least amount of small bowel, and a primary side-to-side anastomosis is made.

Why is small-bowel preservation so important?
More than 80% of patients with ileal Crohn's disease require surgical treatment. The likelihood of resection increases with the duration of follow-up. The risk of reoperation for recrudescence of Crohn's disease is approximately 50% at 10 years. Most patients need three or four operations in their lifetime, which makes small-bowel conservation essential.

Are there special techniques to promote small-bowel conservation?
Because small-bowel recurrence rates are independent of the extent of resection or lymphatic clearance, one need only resect to soft, pliable bowel. Although resection is the correct first surgical approach, stricturoplasty may be useful in the setting of recurrent disease accompanied by stricture formation (8). Strictures can be assumed to be symptomatic if the luminal diameter is less than 15 to 20 mm. One must make a longitudinal incision across the full thickness of the stricture and suture the opening at an orthogonal angle transversely. Extramucosal suturing in a single layer is preferred. Recurrence rates are approximately 2% in a 5-year period. Certain principles allow for the safe operation on a Crohn's disease patient:

• Surgical treatment should be used only for symptoms.
• Resection is not advisable for diffuse or acute disease.
• Surgical treatment should avoid rendering the patient incontinent.
• Surgical management must keep the safety of the patient foremost.

Are there any areas in the management of patients with Crohn's disease that require special consideration?
Yes, surgery has a limited role in the management of perianal Crohn's disease. Coexisting rectal disease is an unfavorable sign because most of those patients eventually require diversion. The use of metronidazole is advised, and any abscess must be drained. Establishing drainage is an essential means of preserving long-term function. Setons made from vessel loops and mushroom catheters are useful for establishing drainage. Anorectal fistulas should be opened only in the absence of rectal disease, only if the tract is superficial, and only if they are symptomatic. All other fistulas should be treated conservatively (9). Colonic disease portends a worse outcome than small-bowel disease. In addition, the more complex the fistula, the less likely it is to heal after a surgical fistulotomy.

Anorectal strictures rarely lend themselves to dilation, and most eventually require proctocolectomy because of the progressive disease.

What does one do in the setting of presumed appendicitis if acute ileitis is discovered instead at the time of laparotomy?
Acute appendicitis is exceedingly rare in patients with Crohn's disease; in fact, it is so rare that it is hard to justify a prophylactic appendectomy. If during laparotomy, the appearance is more consistent with acute ileitis, the procedure should be terminated, and medical therapy should be instituted postoperatively (10). If, however, the appearance is typical of chronic Crohn's disease, ileal resection with ileocolonic anastomosis is appropriate.

Ms. Katz recovers without any major complications except for postoperative atelectasis and fever. She receives pulmonary toilet and walks vigorously. On the third day after surgery, she passes flatus and begins to tolerate diet well. She is discharged on the sixth postoperative day, after which she is followed up by her internist. On medications, she enjoys a quiescent period without many abdominal symptoms.

About 3 months later, she is referred to the gastroenterologist for pain in the lower abdomen and bloody stool. Colonoscopic evaluation shows evidence of a severe inflammatory process in the right colon and in the midsigmoid colon. Ms. Katz requests to be seen by a surgeon, who discusses with her the merits of medical versus surgical treatment of Crohn's colitis.

Does the medical management of Crohn's disease differ with location?
Yes. There is no specific therapy for Crohn's disease in the true sense of the word. All therapy is directed at controlling symptoms rather than the disease. Although sulfasalazine has an effect on Crohn's colitis, it has no effect on small-bowel disease. Delayed-release medications have been used in ileocolonic disease and are effective at high doses. Corticosteroids are effective in the treatment of acute Crohn's disease, regardless of the location of the disease. In addition, 6-mercaptopurine and azathioprine have been used as corticosteroid-sparing agents and to treat recurrent Crohn's disease after multiple resections. There is a lengthy period before the agents exert their optimal effect. Cyclosporine may be useful in an acute setting. All these medications do have adverse side effects that should be discussed with the patient before treatment begins.

Are there any special considerations in the surgical treatment of colorectal Crohn's disease?

The proportion of patients requiring surgical intervention in Crohn's disease of the colon is slightly less than that in ileal disease, but nearly two-thirds of them require an operation. If the colon is involved, several overriding factors should be addressed:

• The likelihood of a permanent stoma if the disease is diffuse or involves the rectum
• The hazards of a total colectomy in a malnourished patient
• The high morbidity and mortality from intraabdominal sepsis

Those with right-sided disease have the highest operative rate; those with rectal disease have the lowest operative rate. Approximately 5 to 10% require an emergency operation for fulminant colitis. Between 40 and 50% of patients with colonic Crohn's disease eventually have an ileostomy. Of all patients with fulminant colitis, 20 to 30% will be found to have Crohn's colitis rather than ulcerative colitis. Surgical intervention is warranted whenever medical therapy fails to effect demonstrable improvement in signs and symptoms. Progressive dilation of the transverse colon to more than 5.5 cm is reason for concern. Any deterioration or lack of improvement within 72 hours while under maximal medical therapy mandates an urgent laparotomy.

The surgical options are limited in such situations, consisting mostly of subtotal colectomy and ileostomy. In the absence of rectal disease, an ileosigmoid anastomosis maximizes the rectal reservoir function and offers the best functional outcome. If there is rectal involvement, active perianal disease, or skip lesions in the small bowel, restoration of intestinal continuity is unlikely. Recurrence rates after ileorectal anastomosis are significantly higher than after proctocolectomy; hence proctocolectomy with ileostomy appears to be warranted. Steroids seem to have little influence on the eventual functional outcome. In the setting of a proctocolectomy, Crohn's disease may lead to delayed healing of the perineal wound, sometimes for up to a year.

Are there special complications associated with ileostomies?
Yes. The incidence of ileostomy dysfunction is high and may be associated with disease recurrence. Complications may include but are not limited to retraction, prolapse, and obstruction. Most ileostomy complications may be managed by local revision, but if recurrent Crohn's disease is the issue, a formal resection is mandated.

On the surgeon's recommendation, Ms. Katz undergoes aggressive medical treatment consisting of sulfasalazine enema and corticosteroids. Her symptoms wane, and once again she is relatively symptom free. She is quite satisfied with her medical and surgical care.

ULCERATIVE COLITIS

Barbara Leon is a 32-year-old woman who has had ulcerative colitis for 9 years. She is recovering from a 10-day hospital stay during which she was treated for a severe bout of acute ulcerative colitis. Ms. Leon would like to get a second opinion on the treatment she received for her acute colitis.

How is acute colitis treated in patients with ulcerative colitis?
Acute fulminating colitis often occurs without any history of disease. Optimal medical management is instituted with intravenous steroids, bowel rest, and repetitive examinations. Colonic dilation carries a poor prognosis, as it correlates with the depth of ulceration. Toxic dilation is often defined as the diameter of the transverse colon exceeding 5.5 cm. Some 30% of patients with toxic megacolon respond to medical management and avoid emergency colectomy. The counterpoint is that failure to heed the signs and symptoms of impending perforation is associated with a mortality of 35 to 75%.

There is compelling evidence that early colectomy is the single most important factor in maintaining low mortality in patients with acute fulminant colitis. The timing of the operation is crucial, and failure to respond clearly to maximal medical therapy over 72 hours is an indication for an emergency colectomy. Because the diagnosis of ulcerative colitis versus Crohn's colitis may not be firmly established, subtotal colectomy with ileostomy is the procedure of choice. The rectum should be divided above the pelvic brim so as not to open the pelvic planes of dissection with the associated risk of sepsis.

Ms. Leon is satisfied with the fact that she has recovered from her acute bout of colitis, but she wants to know what issues she should be concerned about now.

What are the concerns in chronic ulcerative colitis?
There is an increased risk of colorectal cancer in patients with ulcerative colitis. It is linked to the duration of the disease, the age of onset, and the severity of the first attack of the disease. The risk of cancer is significantly greater in those with pancolitis as opposed to those with predominantly left-sided disease. Whether there is a genetic predisposition to cancer in patients with extensive colitis is not known. The distribution of cancers probably does not differ from that of the sporadic carcinoma seen in the general population. The incidence of synchronous cancers in patients with ulcerative colitis is higher than that seen in sporadic disease. Detection of dysplastic areas is the key to early detection and treatment of chronic ulcerative colitis. An effective screening policy is essential, and the retained rectum after a colectomy without a proctectomy is often neglected.

How significant is the risk of malignancy in patients with chronic ulcerative colitis?
The increased risk of colorectal cancer in the setting of chronic ulcerative colitis is, as mentioned earlier, related to the extent of the disease, the age of onset, the severity of the first attack, and the duration of follow-up. The usual method of screening is surveillance colonoscopic examinations with appropriate biopsies, which are searched for dysplastic changes in the regenerative mucosa. Dysplasia is thought to be a marker for cancer. Because of the slow evolution of dysplasia and its patchy nature, biopsies should be multiple and repeated regularly. The optimal frequency of surveillance is not known. Most studies confirm that the risk of cancer is greater in those whose colitis extends at least into the right transverse colon as opposed to those with isolated rectosigmoid involvement.

The incidence of cancer arising in a patient who has had colitis for less than 10 years is negligible. The incidence after 15 years of extensive colitis rises to 3%, to 5% after 20 years of disease, and to nearly 10% after 25 years of disease. The risk of developing carcinoma is highest in patients who were diagnosed with ulcerative colitis before age 30 years. The best cohort study reveals that those diagnosed before age 30 had a risk of carcinoma 8 times that of the general population, and pancolitis raises that risk to a factor of 19. The incidence of synchronous lesions is greater among patients with chronic ulcerative colitis than in the general population. Contemporary reports indicate that the survival rate of colorectal cancers in patients with ulcerative colitis is comparable with that seen in persons with sporadic lesions.

What are the features of dysplasia?
Dysplasia is a histopathologic marker for patients who are likely to develop carcinoma. It is patchy and an imperfect marker, but it may help in the decision as to when to recommend a prophylactic colectomy. The following features are the cardinal signs of dysplasia:

• Variation in the size and shape of epithelial cell nuclei, which have prominent nucleoli and are hyperchromatic and distorted
• Possibly hyperchromatic cell cytoplasm
• Mucin at the base of the cell rather than at the apex, as is normal
• Abnormal mitosis in the upper third of the crypts
• Budding of the crypts (adenomatous changes)
• Elongation of the crypts (villous change)
• Loss of nuclear polarity (pseudostratification)

There are three gross features of dysplasia: polypoidal lesions, low elevated plaques, and stricture or ulcer (11). The low elevated plaques are the most difficult to detect during colonoscopy. Rectal biopsies for the detection of dysplasia or cancer are often negative, even in the presence of a malignancy, which limits its usefulness.

Ms. Leon is concerned that her disease was diagnosed when she was 23 years of age and that, in some episodes, her internist said that her entire colon was inflamed. In addition, she soon will be in her 10th year of ulcerative colitis. She asks whether she should undergo surgery to "get rid" of her disease.

What are the surgical options of patients with chronic ulcerative colitis?
One option is subtotal colectomy and ileorectal anastomosis. Although this procedure has fallen out of favor because of the use of restorative proctocolectomy, it still may have a role in the management of the elderly patient with long-standing ulcerative colitis. The subset of patients with relative rectal sparing are the best candidates for the procedure. It also can be used as a bridging procedure for adolescents who are not yet ready for a restorative proctocolectomy. The benefit of this procedure is preservation of anorectal control over bowel movement.

What are the disadvantages of subtotal colectomy and ileorectal anastomosis?
Caution must be exercised because the rectum may harbor disease, which may progress to become dysplastic or frankly malignant. Failure of the operation within 5 to 10 years is estimated at 20 to 50%. The anastomosis traditionally is done at the sacral promontory, with no pelvic dissection. If any part of the rectum has already been resected, a restorative proctocolectomy is favored.

What are other surgical options for patients with chronic ulcerative colitis?
As the cumulative clinical data have shown over the years, the restorative proctocolectomy with ileal pouch anal anastomosis has become the standard of care for patients seeking a cure without a permanent stoma. Parks and Nicholls first reported the procedure in 1978 (12). There is a reoperative rate of 15 to 25% and an overall failure rate of 5 to 15% after a median of 8 years. Also, there usually remains a small amount of mucosa at the top of the anal canal that is still at risk for carcinoma. Advanced techniques have led to the use of stapling to anastomose the pouch to the anal segment, obviating mucosectomy and its technical issues. Whether this will continue to be optimal in the long run remains to be assessed, but for now this has revolutionized the manner and time required to perform these procedures. The type of pouch created does not actually correlate with outcome. What is sought is a pliable, moderate-capacity pouch that is capable of distending and allowing the patient to defer the urge to defecate (Fig. 11.1). The common complications include pelvic abscess, intestinal obstruction, anal anastomotic stricture, and pouchitis.

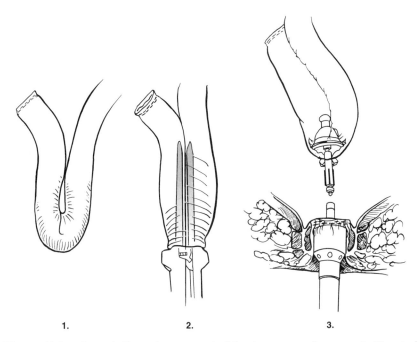

1.   **2.**   **3.**

Figure 11.1.   J-pouch ileoanal anastomosis following proctocolectomy. **1.** Terminal ileum configured in J shape. **2.** Stapled ileum into a J pouch. **3.** Ileoanal anastomosis using an end-to-end anastomosis (EEA) stapler. (Adapted with permission from Fazio VW, Tjandra JJ, Lavery IC. Techniques of pouch construction. In: Nicholls J, Bartolo D, Mortensen N, eds. Restorative Proctocolectomy. Oxford, UK: Blackwell, 1993.)

Is total proctocolectomy with an everted stoma (Brooke's ileostomy) also a surgical option for chronic ulcerative colitis?
This procedure has fallen out of favor for a variety of reasons. First and foremost is the issue of the permanent ileostomy. Second is the issue of a prolonged healing of the perineal wound, with wound failure rates ranging from 17 to 85%, even after a year. The third drawback relates to the sexual complications of proctocolectomy. Many women complain of dyspareunia at the perineal scar, and men note poor ejaculatory function. Finally, there is the permanency of the procedure, which is a difficult mental hurdle for young patients. Although this is almost never indicated as an emergency procedure, rectal bleeding may dictate an emergency proctocolectomy. The rate of revision of Brooke's ileostomy over 5 years ranges from 10 to 20%. It has a role in patients who have poor sphincter function or a low-lying rectal cancer, as well as those who are unwilling to commit themselves to the restorative proctocolectomy.

Is a total proctocolectomy with a continent ileostomy (e.g., Kock pouch) a surgical option for patients with chronic ulcerative colitis?
This procedure offers only historical interest because of its high reoperative rate (upward of 25 to 50% within 5 years) and poorer performance characteristics than the restorative proctocolectomy.

Ms. Leon decides to undergo restorative total proctocolectomy with a J-pouch ileoanal anastomosis. The operation is performed without difficulty. She has a relatively benign postoperative course and is discharged on the ninth postoperative day. Initially, she has more than 20 bowel movements per day, but over time this decreases to a manageable frequency of about four times per day. However, 6 weeks after the operation she presents with fever, blood-tinged diarrhea, and severe pain upon defecation. The surgeon diagnoses pouchitis.

What is pouchitis?
Inflammation of the ileal reservoir is a recognized complication of restorative proctocolectomy. Interestingly enough, this almost always occurs in the setting of ulcerative colitis, with familial adenomatous polyposis (FAP) being exceedingly rare. Within 5 years of creation of the pouch, approximately 35% of patients develop at least one episode of local inflammation leading to increased bowel movements, tenesmus, and bleeding. Two-thirds of these persons have only a single episode. Pouchitis can be classified as acute, acutely relapsing, subacute, or chronic. The cause is unknown. The endoscopic findings are hemorrhagic and edematous mucosa with very minute ulcerations. The inflammation may extend into the proximal ileum. A neutrophil infiltrate is revealed on biopsy. Treatment with metronidazole appears to be most effective, with a response rate of 80 to 90%. Pouchitis alone rarely necessitates pouch excision (13) (see algorithm at end of chapter).

With metronidazole and other symptomatic management, Ms. Leon's pouchitis resolves. Her bowel movements are once again manageable, and she is quite satisfied with her care. She is happy that she no longer has to deal with the inflammatory colon. However, she wonders whether there are other effects of ulcerative colitis that are cause for concern.

Are any other disorders associated with ulcerative colitis?
Hepatobiliary complications of ulcerative colitis or its treatment include fatty liver, gallstones, primary sclerosing cholangitis, primary biliary cirrhosis, biliary strictures, bile duct carcinoma, chronic active hepatitis, and intermittent cholestasis. These are its characteristics:

- There is a marked incidence of chronic active hepatitis in patients with ulcerative colitis.
- Gallstones occur more frequently if there has been an ileal resection.
- The incidence of cirrhosis varies from 1 to 5% and is usually associated with extensive colitis. Varices may develop, and, in the presence of an ileostomy, stomal varices can become a significant morbidity. If a colectomy is required, avoidance of a stoma should be a prime consideration, and a restorative proctocolectomy should be considered.
- Primary sclerosing cholangitis (PSC) is a rare disorder (affecting 1 to 4% of patients with inflammatory bowel disease) that affects all parts of the biliary tree in a chronic inflammatory process. It appears to be related to cross-reactivity of anticolon and antineutrophil antibodies; 70% of cases are associated with ulcerative colitis (14). Men are more commonly affected than women, and most patients are 25 to 45 years of age. Diagnosis is usually by endoscopic retrograde cholangiopancreatography (ERCP). There is no specific effective treatment, and patients may require liver transplant when liver failure supervenes. The diffuse and extensive nature of the disease usually prohibits the performance of any bypass procedures. Although PSC is a progressive disease, the rate of progression is quite variable. There is no evidence that colectomy affects the natural history of the disease.

Approximately 5 to 10% of patients with ulcerative colitis develop **cutaneous manifestations** at some point. The most common manifestations are erythema nodosum, pyoderma gangrenosum, exfoliative dermatitis, and vasculitis. These are its characteristics:

- Pyoderma gangrenosum is probably the most bothersome of the cutaneous manifestations, with an incidence of 1 to 5%. Approximately 50% of the patients who initially complain of pyoderma gangrenosum eventually are diagnosed with ulcerative colitis (15). Although it is not related to the severity of the colitis, pyoderma gangrenosum often rapidly improves upon colectomy. Rapidly enlarging deep areas of ulceration develop, usually over a lower limb, after initially appearing as a papule; it can also occur on the trunk. There is a predilection for areas previously traumatized, and the lesions tend to be extremely tender. Treatment of the underlying colitis is essential, and hyperbaric oxygen therapy offers some benefit. Retention of the rectal stump may prevent resolution of the lesions.
- Erythema nodosum occurs in 2 to 4% of patients with colitis and is more common in women than in men. Lesions, which generally present over the anterior surface of the tibia, consist of raised red tender nodules. Erythema nodosum usually improves after colectomy without any significant scarring. Its clinical course essentially parallels that of the colitis.

• Exfoliative dermatitis may occur as a complication of sulfasalazine therapy but also can result from severe colitis. It appears to resolve after proctocolectomy.

The incidence of **ocular lesions** in patients with ulcerative colitis varies from 1 to 12%, with episcleritis (predominantly in Crohn's disease) and uveitis being the most common.

Colitic arthritis is usually associated with asymmetric migratory arthropathy. The most commonly affected joints, in order, are the knees, wrists, and elbows. Treatment usually is conservative and related to symptoms.

Ankylosing spondylitis also is associated with ulcerative colitis and is 20 to 30 times as common as in the general population. There is a genetic patho-

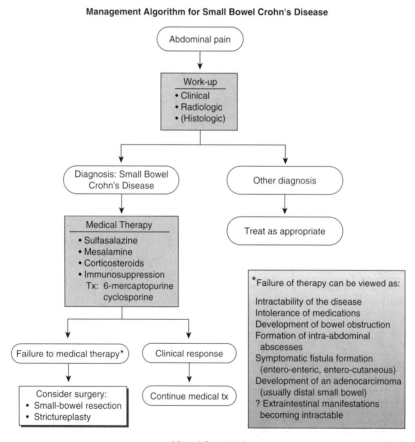

Management Algorithm for Small Bowel Crohn's Disease

Algorithm 11.1.

genesis and association with the HLA–B27 antigen. One or more vertebrae and a sacroiliac joint are inflamed. The development of a rigid spine often leads to pulmonary complications. Various nonsteroidal pain medications are used for the management of the associated pain, and physical therapy is indicated to minimize the disability. Surgical treatment of the inflammatory bowel disease has no influence on the course of the axial arthropathy.

Should ulcerative proctitis be considered as a part of the spectrum of ulcerative colitis, or should it be viewed in a different light?
Ulcerative proctitis, initially described by Thaysen in 1934, is quite different from ulcerative colitis. The risk of proximal extension into the sigmoid colon is less than 30% at 20 years of disease. The likelihood that surgery will be required is approximately 6% at 20 years of disease. Most patients respond to topical steroids or sulfasalazine. There appears to be a male preponderance, and it appears to occur in an older population. The inflamed mucosa begins at the dentate line and proceeds proximally for 5 to 15 cm. The histologic appearance is identical to that of ulcerative colitis. The presenting symptoms are bleeding, urgency, mucous discharge, and tenesmus. There are no general symptoms, as there are in colitis. Treatment is usually in the form of topical steroids, whether by enemas or foams. There is a spontaneous remission rate of 40%, making no treatment possibly a viable option. If no spontaneous remission has been noted within 6 weeks, a course of steroid enemas or suppositories is indicated.

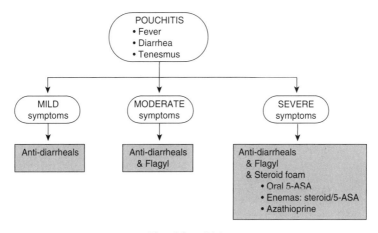

Management Algorithm for Pouchitis Following Ileoanal Anastomosis

Algorithm 11.2.

REFERENCES

1. Crohn BB, Ginzburg L, Oppenheimer GD. Regional ileitis: a pathologic and clinical entity. JAMA 1932;99:1323–1329.
2. Morson BC, Lockhart-Mummery HE. Crohn's disease of the colon. Gastroenterologia 1959;92:168–173.
3. Gold DV, Miller F. Comparison of human colonic mucoprotein antigen from normal and neoplastic mucosa. Cancer 1978;38:3204–3208.
4. Keighley MRB, Williams NS. Crohn's disease: aetiology, incidence and epidemiology. 1993;49:1592–1630.
5. Kirsner JB, Spencer JA. Family occurrences of ulcerative colitis, regional enteritis, and ileocolitis. Ann Intern Med 1963;59:133–144.
6. Corman ML. Nonspecific inflammatory bowel disease. In: Corman ML. Colon and Rectal Surgery. Philadelphia: Lippincott, 1989:741–887.
7. Farmer RG, Whelan G, Fazio VW. Long-term follow-up of patients with Crohn's disease: relationship between the clinical pattern and prognosis. Gastroenterology 1985;88: 1818–1825.
8. Alexander-Williams J. The technique of intestinal strictureplasty. Int J Colorect Dis 1986;1:54–57.
9. Allan A, Keighley MRB. Management of perianal Crohn's disease. World J Surg 1989; 12:198–202.
10. Strong SA, Fazio VW. Crohn's disease of the colon, rectum and anus. Surg Clin North Am 1993;73:933–963.
11. Nugent FW, Haggitt RC, Colcher H, Kutteruf GC. Malignant potential of chronic ulcerative colitis. Gastroenterology 1979;76:1–5.
12. Parks AG, Nichols RJ. Proctocolectomy without ileostomy for ulcerative colitis. Br Med J 1978;2:85–88.
13. Pemberton JH, Kelly KA, Beart RW Jr. Ileal-pouch anastomosis for chronic ulcerative colitis: long-term results. Ann Surg 1987;206:504–513.
14. LaRusso NF, Wiesner RH, Ludwig J, MacCarty RL. Primary sclerosing cholangitis. N Engl J Med 1984;310:899–903.
15. Mir-Madjlessi SH, Taylor JS, Farmer RG. Clinical course and evolution of erythema nodosum in chronic ulcerative colitis: a study of 42 patients. Am J Gastroenterol 1985; 80:615–620.
16. Thaysen TEH. Simple hemorrhagic proctitis and proctosigmoiditis. Acta Med Scand 1934;84:1–16.

Diverticular Disease of the Colon

Ciaran J. Walsh

DIVERTICULAR DISEASE

Helen Witt is a 65-year-old moderately obese woman who presents to the emergency department complaining of left lower quadrant abdominal pain associated with anorexia and nausea for the past 2 days. She says she had this type of pain once last year and was told she probably had diverticular disease. At that time, her symptoms settled down very quickly, no investigations were performed, and nothing more was done about her condition. On this occasion, her pain started gradually with intermittent gripping that became constant and more severe. She felt as though she had a fever and noted that going over the speed bumps on the way into the hospital caused her pain in the lower abdomen. Her history is significant for an appendectomy and open cholecystectomy many years ago, and recently her primary care physician prescribed ranitidine for a hiatal hernia diagnosed on upper gastrointestinal endoscopy. She is not diabetic. She denies any recent change in her bowel habit, blood from the rectum, or weight loss. She has no urinary frequency or dysuria and has no history of urinary tract infections.

On examination she looks a little flushed. Her temperature is 37.9°C, her pulse 92 beats per minute, and her blood pressure 156/88 mm Hg. Her abdomen is obese but not distended. Abdominal examination reveals local left lower quadrant tenderness and guarding but no palpable mass. The rest of her abdomen is soft and not tender. Her bowel sounds are normal. Digital rectal examination is normal. Her laboratory values are normal, as is her acute abdominal radiograph series. The emergency department staff members think she has acute diverticulitis, and they want to know what investigations should be performed and whether Mrs. Witt should be admitted.

What is diverticular disease?
It is a benign disease of the colon characterized by the development of pulsion-type outpouchings. These are really false diverticula because they consist of mucosa lined only by serosa. They most often occur between the mesenteric and antimesenteric taenia coli, where the colonic blood vessels pierce the muscle. They indicate herniation of the mucosa through weak points in the colon wall. They are most common in the sigmoid and left colon but may occur anywhere in the colon.

What is the difference between diverticulosis and diverticulitis?
Diverticulosis is diverticula in the colon. *Diverticulitis* is an infective complication of these diverticula.

What causes diverticulosis?
Diverticulosis most likely develops as a result of a low-fiber diet. As food becomes more refined and processed, the amount of dietary fiber decreases. This is particularly prevalent in Western societies, which consume only one-tenth the amount of fiber consumed 100 years ago, before refined diets were so prevalent. In rural Africa and other societies not exposed to a Western diet, diverticular disease is almost nonexistent (1). Rural Africans reportedly consume 60 to 100 g of fiber a day, whereas Americans consume only 10 to 15 g per day.

How does a high-fiber diet prevent diverticulosis?
Fiber increases stool weight, decreases whole gut transit time, and lowers colonic intraluminal pressure. A high-fiber diet requires less contraction by the bowel to propel the stool onward. There is less segmentation, and muscle hypertrophy does not occur.

What is the prevalence of diverticular disease?
Approximately 30 million Americans have diverticulosis. Only 1 to 2% of people younger than 30 years of age are affected; one-third of Americans older than 45 years are affected. The incidence rises with age; two-thirds of the population older than 85 years are affected (2). Most people are asymptomatic, but 15 to 30% eventually develop diverticulitis.

What is Saint's triad?
Saint's triad is the constellation of cholelithiasis, hiatal hernia, and diverticulosis.

What is the most likely diagnosis for Mrs. Witt? What is the differential diagnosis?
Acute diverticulitis with local peritonitis is the most likely diagnosis for this patient. She has had an appendectomy, so the most likely differential diagnoses are colon carcinoma, inflammatory bowel disease, and ischemic colitis.

What are the most common complications of diverticular disease?
Perforation (micro or macro) causing pericolic infection with formation of a phlegmon, pericolic abscess, fistula formation, and frank peritonitis are the most common complications of diverticular disease. Acute inflammation can also lead to ulceration or erosion into a colonic wall blood vessel (remember where on the bowel diverticula most commonly occur) and cause bleeding. Chronic inflammation may lead to stricture formation and colon obstruction. Small-bowel obstruction is a common but not frequently mentioned complication of acute diverticulitis. Up to 20% of patients with acute diverticulitis may have small-bowel obstruction as a result of a loop of small bowel getting snared in the inflammatory nest. This is to be distinguished from an ileus, which may develop as a result of acute diverticulitis.

What is the Hinchey classification of acute diverticulitis?
This is a classification of severity of acute diverticulitis (3). There are four stages. Stage 1 includes a pericolic abscess. Stage II includes a distant or remote abscess. Stage III includes purulent peritonitis. Stage IV includes fecal peritonitis. These classifications permit a realistic comparison of treatment outcomes and formulation of management guidelines for each stage of the disease. The basic pathophysiology of acute diverticulitis is perforation. Whereas microperforations seal and may lead to an abscess or phlegmon, a large perforation may cause fecal peritonitis.

What fistulas are associated with diverticulitis?
A fistula may develop between the inflamed colon and any surrounding structure. Colovesical fistulas are the most common, accounting for nearly 60% of fistulas associated with diverticular disease (4). Approximately 2% of patients with acute diverticulitis develop a colovesical fistula. They are more common in men than in women, probably because in women the uterus lies between the colon and the bladder. Colocutaneous fistulas are the next most common type associated with diverticulitis. Women who have had a hysterectomy may develop a colovaginal fistula.

What are the symptoms and signs of a colovesical fistula?
Dysuria (90%), pneumaturia (70%), and fecaluria (70%) are the most common symptoms. Chronic urinary tract infections may occur. There are no physical signs related to the fistula per se, although a third of patients have evidence of a systemic infection.

How is a diagnosis of colovesical fistula confirmed?
Barium enema, cystoscopy, or both may demonstrate the communication between the colon and bladder. Radiography of the urine after a barium enema is described. Often the fistula cannot be demonstrated and the diagnosis is made

on history. The patient may be asked to urinate while in the bathtub to see if bubbles appear in the water.

How should Mrs. Witt's diagnosis be confirmed? What investigation should be ordered?
The investigation of choice at this point is computed tomography (CT) of the abdomen and pelvis with intravenous and water-soluble oral contrast. This not only helps to confirm the diagnosis but also demonstrates the extent of the disease, including any abscess collections or free intraperitoneal air or fluid. In general, the diagnosis can be made clinically with sufficient confidence to permit treatment without more definitive investigation.

What are the criteria used to diagnose acute diverticulitis by CT?
Colonic wall thickening, stranding of pericolic fat, pericolic or distant abscesses, and extraluminal air are characteristics of diverticulitis seen on CT (5). Colonic diverticula seen on CT are not diagnostic of acute diverticulitis.

Should Mrs. Witt have a barium enema or colonoscopy?
Mrs. Witt definitely should not have a barium enema or colonoscopy. Both procedures could worsen the situation. Colonoscopy could blow open a sealed perforation. Barium enema could provoke free perforation and lead to extravasation of barium into the peritoneal cavity, causing barium peritonitis.

Mrs. Witt's CT shows significant thickening of the sigmoid colon, stranding of the pericolic fat with colonic diverticulosis, and a very small fluid collection in the pouch of Douglas.

Should the fluid be drained percutaneously? What should be done at this point?
The films should be reviewed with the radiologist. CT-guided percutaneous drainage is an excellent option for identifiable pericolic abscesses in patients with acute diverticulitis. The potential for CT-guided percutaneous drainage is one of the reasons CT is so attractive in patients with acute diverticulitis. Approximately 75% of peridiverticular abscesses can be drained in this way. The advantage is that it facilitates resolution of the sepsis without surgical drainage, and it permits a one-stage elective operation later. There is no evidence that Mrs. Witt has an abscess, so there is no merit in percutaneous drainage in her case.

While the physician is reviewing the CT, a staff member of the emergency department calls and says the cubicle is needed. They want to send Mrs. Witt home with antibiotics.

Is sending Mrs. Witt home with an antibiotic prescription appropriate?
No. Mrs. Witt should be admitted for bowel rest, intravenous fluids, intravenous antibiotics, pain relief, and observation. In general, outpatient manage-

ment is appropriate for patients who can tolerate diet, who do not have systemic symptoms, and who do not have peritoneal signs. Mrs. Witt fails to meet all of these criteria.

What percent of people with diverticular disease need surgery? Is Mrs. Witt likely to need surgery on this admission?
Approximately 1% of patients with diverticular disease eventually require surgery. Approximately 15 to 30% of patients admitted to the hospital with acute diverticulitis need surgery. Mrs. Witt is not likely to need surgery on this admission.

Mrs. Witt's condition settles quickly with conservative management, and she is sent home after 3 days with a prescription for a course of oral antibiotics.

How should Mrs. Witt be followed up?
Mrs. Witt should be seen in the clinic in a few weeks to make sure that the acute episode has settled. At that time, full assessment of her colon, either by flexible sigmoidoscopy and barium enema or by colonoscopy, should be arranged.

Mrs. Witt says she fears colonoscopy because her sister underwent colonoscopy and then needed an operation for a perforated colon. She agrees to a barium enema, which is performed 6 weeks after her acute attack. It confirms sigmoid and left-colon diverticulosis but is otherwise normal. There is no stricture or fistula noted, only minimal muscle hypertrophy and mild spasm.

What further treatment is advised for Mrs. Witt? Is she going to have another attack, and should she undergo surgery?
Mrs. Witt should be advised to continue with conservative treatment. After the acute inflammation has settled, she should start a high-fiber diet. Up to 45% of patients have recurrent symptoms after an attack of acute diverticulitis. Long-term dietary supplementation with fiber after a first attack of diverticulitis may prevent recurrent attacks in up to 70% of patients. With each recurrent attack, the patient is less likely to respond to medical treatment. In general, elective surgery is advised after two well-documented attacks of acute diverticulitis. However, if the first attack is complicated by abscess, stricture, obstruction, or fistula, surgery should be considered after the first attack. Mrs. Witt has not had two well-documented attacks, nor was this attack complicated by abscess, stricture, obstruction, or fistula.

What constitutes a high-fiber diet?
A high-fiber diet contains 20 to 35 g of fiber per day. This may be unpalatable to patients, and the fiber should be increased gradually (e.g., increase by 5 g per

week). These patients also should be advised to drink at least six glasses of non-caffeinated beverages a day.

Does age have any bearing on the treatment of patients with acute diverticulitis?
Yes. Diverticular disease tends to be most virulent in patients under 50 years of age. Acute attacks tend to be more severe than in older patients, and a higher percentage of these younger patients need surgery on the first admission. Moreover, many surgeons advocate elective surgery after one attack of acute diverticulitis in a young patient, even if the attack was uncomplicated.

Mrs. Witt says she does not like bran and cannot drink very much because she gets bloated. She really wants to consider an operation.

What elective operation is a surgeon likely to choose for her case? Would she need a stoma?
The elective operation of choice is a one-stage left colectomy with colorectal anastomosis. She had an uncomplicated attack and therefore is not likely to need a protecting stoma upstream of the anastomosis. *Refer to Algorithm 12.1 at the end of this chapter.*

PERITONITIS

Charles Moran is a 54-year-old man who goes to the emergency department complaining of severe lower abdominal pain. His history is unremarkable except for taking nonsteroidal antiinflammatory drugs for "rheumatism." He admits to having had three previous attacks of lower abdominal pain, similar to this although not as severe. On the first occasion, 7 years ago, he remembers having gripping left lower quadrant pain that settled spontaneously after 3 days. The next occasion was 5 years ago, at which time he went to his primary care physician. The physician wanted to send him to the emergency department, but Mr. Moran refused. He says the pain went away when he took the antibiotics his doctor gave him and stuck to fluids only by mouth.

His most recent attack was 2 years ago. He was on vacation overseas and developed severe left lower quadrant abdominal pain and fever. He said he had chills and felt so poorly that he had to go to the local hospital. He said they did CT and told him he had diverticulitis with an abscess on the bowel. He says they put "a tube in it under the scanner," administered intravenous fluids and antibiotics, and discharged him 5 days later. He has no records of his hospital admission. On direct questioning, he admitted to a change in his bowel habit during the past few months, saying his stools had become "like a pencil," more difficult to pass. He said that he had been feeling fine until this morning, when he was sitting on the toilet straining to pass a stool. He suddenly developed excruciating left lower quadrant abdominal

pain, which has now spread to the right side. He says that he has to lie very still or the pain gets worse. On examination, his face is pale, his pulse rate is 110 beats per minute, his blood pressure is 160/90 mm Hg, and his temperature is 38.7°C. A head and neck examination is normal. He is not jaundiced. Chest examination reveals reduced air entry in both bases. His abdomen is slightly distended, and he is very tender, with guarding in both the left and right lower quadrant. He has markedly reduced bowel sounds on auscultation. Digital rectal examination is normal. Laboratory values, including serum amylase level, are normal except for a WBC count of 17,000 with evidence of left shift. Urinalysis is normal. A chest radiograph is normal, without evidence of free air under the diaphragm. Abdominal films show a few dilated loops of small bowel in the lower abdomen.

What is this patient's diagnosis?
Mr. Moran has peritonitis. His history strongly suggests perforated diverticular disease.

If Mr. Moran has a perforated viscus, why is there no free air on the plain radiographs?
The emergency physician did not order an erect chest radiograph. Either an erect chest radiograph or a lateral decubitus abdominal film is required to demonstrate free air under the diaphragm. Furthermore, only 70 to 80% of patients with a perforated viscus have free air on preoperative radiographs.

What test should Mr. Moran undergo next?
Mr. Moran should have an exploratory laparotomy as soon as possible after adequate resuscitation and stoma marking.

Laparotomy confirms the preoperative diagnosis of perforated diverticular disease. There is diverticular disease throughout the left colon and a free perforation of the distal sigmoid with associated purulent peritonitis (Hinchey stage III).

What other disease must be considered at this time?
Perforated sigmoid colon cancer is a possibility in this patient. Both diverticular disease and colon cancer are common, and they may coexist. It can be very difficult to distinguish whether a phlegmon is caused by diverticulitis or sigmoid colon cancer, particularly in the presence of peritonitis.

What operation should Mr. Moran undergo?
The surgeon should perform Hartman's operation, a resection of the diseased sigmoid colon with an end left-sided colostomy and closure of the distal rectal stump (2).

Are there any other surgical options?
A one-stage resection and colorectal anastomosis, as would be performed during elective surgery for diverticular disease, is performed by some surgeons for patients with Hinchey stages I and II. It is not appropriate in Mr. Moran's case, because the risks of anastomotic breakdown are too high. The Hartman operation is the safer and more traditional approach. When the patient is fully recovered, intestinal continuity may be restored, usually 4 to 6 months after the initial procedure.

What are the complications of the Hartman operation?
Complications specific to this procedure include damage to the left ureter, stomal necrosis or retraction, disruption of the rectal stump suture line, and in the long term, failure to restore bowel continuity.

Sylvia Noro, a 69-year-old retired librarian, is brought to the emergency department by her daughter, who reports that Mrs. Noro passed a large amount of blood into the toilet bowl that morning and complained of being dizzy afterward. The patient denies any nausea, vomiting, or abdominal pain. She is uncertain whether she ever passed blood from the rectum in the past because she has very poor eyesight. She denies anal pain or prolapse of tissue in the rectum. She says that 10 years ago, she had surgery and radiation treatment for cancer of the cervix. Her only medicine is a "water tablet," which she takes each morning. She is not taking warfarin, aspirin, or other nonsteroidal antiinflammatory drugs. She does not smoke or drink alcohol. On examination, she looks pale, her pulse is regular at 98 beats per minute, and her blood pressure is 150/70 mm Hg when lying; when standing, her pulse is 110 beats per minute, and her blood pressure is 130/50 mm Hg. Her head, neck, and chest examinations are normal. There are no bruises, petechiae, or areas of abnormal skin pigmentation. She is not jaundiced. The abdomen is not distended and is completely nontender, with normal bowel sounds. There are no pulsatile masses, and peripheral pulses are all normal. Perianal examination is normal. She is able to tolerate digital rectal examination without any pain. There are no rectal masses, and anal sphincter tone is normal, but there is frank red blood on the glove. Urinalysis findings are negative; however, her urine is very concentrated.

Did Mrs. Noro have a significant bleed?
A little blood can look particularly impressive when mixed with the amount of water in a toilet bowl. However, Mrs. Noro most likely had a significant bleed. She gives a history of being dizzy, and she demonstrated orthostatic hypotension on examination in the emergency department. Orthostatic hypotension is common among the elderly, particularly those taking diuretic agents.

Why not measure her hemoglobin level and, if it is normal, send her home from the emergency department?
Mrs. Noro is tachycardic with a wide pulse pressure when lying down. In the context of her presentation, it would be dangerous to attribute her pulse and blood pressure to anything other than an acute bleed. Time and subsequent investigation may prove otherwise, but this is the safe approach. An acute bleed may not affect the hemoglobin level if there has not been time for equilibration of the intravascular volume. And, it would be dangerous to say that the bleed was not significant because the hemoglobin level was normal. Mrs. Noro should be admitted and worked up.

Is the color of the blood significant?
Although there are exceptions, knowing the color of the blood can help to narrow the possible sources of the blood loss. Blood from any site, no matter how old, can turn red when it is dropped into a bowl of water. Blood that is red on the glove is truly red. The descriptive terms of others may be misused. An example is the term melena, which should be reserved for the classic black, sticky, tarry, and foul-smelling stool caused by bleeding in the upper gastrointestinal tract. However, if the bleeding is particularly brisk or if the colon has been shortened by a colectomy, there may not be time for the bowel to produce typical melena. Maroon stools suggest distal ileal or right colonic blood, whereas true red blood usually comes from the left colon or anorectal area. The most common causes of massive bleeding from the upper gastrointestinal tract that present with red blood from the rectum are peptic ulcer disease, esophagogastric varices, gastrointestinal erosions, and an aortoduodenal fistula.

What is the initial working diagnosis?
Mrs. Noro most likely has bleeding in the lower gastrointestinal tract.

What is the differential diagnosis in this case?
The most likely alternatives are angiodysplasia (6) and diverticular disease. Considering her history, radiation proctitis is also a possibility. Other possibilities include hemorrhoids, inflammatory bowel disease, ischemic colitis, and a benign or malignant colonic neoplasm. Less likely causes are anal fissure, Meckel's diverticulum, and bleeding in the upper gastrointestinal tract. Mrs. Noro does not drink alcohol, has never smoked, does not take aspirin or other nonsteroidal antiinflammatory drugs, and has no history of aortic surgery.

Does the fact that the patient denies any pain associated with this episode help narrow the differential diagnosis?
The absence of abdominal pain is against ischemic colitis. Moreover, this patient has never smoked and has no stigmata of atherosclerotic vascular disease. The absence of anal pain makes bleeding from an anal fissure unlikely. Both

diverticular bleeding and bleeding due to angiodysplasia are usually painless, as is the bleeding caused by radiation proctitis.

Why isn't colorectal cancer high on the list of differential diagnoses?
This sort of brisk bleeding is uncommon in patients with colorectal malignancies. Patients with colorectal cancer usually present with more gradual or even occult blood loss. Colonic polyps can bleed briskly on occasion, particularly if the patient is taking warfarin.

Why is radiation proctitis part of the differential diagnosis?
Radiation therapy for carcinoma of the cervix in women and carcinoma of the prostate in men is the most common cause of radiation proctitis, which can cause very significant lower gastrointestinal tract bleeding. The fact that this is a first presentation and that Mrs. Noro's radiation treatment was 10 years ago does not preclude the diagnosis.

What is the first step in Mrs. Noro's management?
Mrs. Noro should have a large-bore peripheral intravenous line placed, have some crystalloid fluid to resuscitate her, and have blood drawn for the following tests: full blood cell count, platelet count, serum electrolyte levels, coagulation screen, blood type, and cross-match.

Is a nasogastric tube appropriate for this patient?
Yes. Although an upper gastrointestinal tract bleed is unlikely, a nasogastric tube helps to detect one. Blood in the nasogastric aspirate raises the possibility of upper gastrointestinal bleeding. Absence of blood in a bile-tinged nasogastric aspirate makes upper gastrointestinal bleeding very unlikely. Another indication of bleeding in the upper gastrointestinal tract is an elevation of the serum blood urea nitrogen (BUN) level out of proportion to the serum creatinine level.

Mrs. Noro's laboratory tests are all normal except the hemoglobin of 11.1 g/dL and a WBC count of 14.4.

How do Mrs. Noro's laboratory results help with the differential diagnosis?
The absence of coagulopathy suggests a primary lesion within the gastrointestinal tract rather than bleeding from the gastrointestinal tract as a manifestation of a systemic illness. The hemoglobin of 11.1 g/dL helps very little. The elevated white cell count is consistent with an acute bleed but does not narrow the differential diagnosis.

The patient remained stable in the emergency department with no further bleeding. Her pulse returns to 82 beats per minute with 500

mL of normal saline given over the hour that it took the laboratory
work to come back.

What is the next step in Mrs. Noro's care? What tests should be done first?
The next step is to start the search for the source of bleeding. Mrs. Noro should
undergo anoscopy and proctoscopy. Anoscopy reveals any hemorrhoids or anal
fissure. Digital examination does not diagnose hemorrhoids. Proctoscopy permits assessment of the mucosal lining of the rectum. Proctitis, whether caused
by radiation or by inflammatory bowel disease, can be identified, as can rectal
cancer. It is important to have suction and irrigation on hand so that blood or
clots can be removed to allow proper vision of the mucosa.

**Mrs. Noro's anoscopy and proctoscopy revealed red blood in the rec-
tum, which was easily evacuated. There was no evidence of proctitis,
and no bleeding source was identified.**

What is in the management plan now?
Lower gastrointestinal tract hemorrhage stops spontaneously with supportive
management alone in up to 90% of cases. Mrs. Noro should be admitted for
continued resuscitation and observation. When the bleeding stops, a
colonoscopy is performed after bowel preparation.

*Does the absence of signs and symptoms of diverticulitis mean that her bleeding is more
likely to be caused by angiodysplasia than by diverticular disease?*
No. Bleeding diverticulosis is rarely associated with inflammatory changes. It is
a different clinical scenario from that of acute diverticulitis.

*What investigations may be useful in a patient with a lower gastrointestinal tract hem-
orrhage?*
Aside from the investigations already mentioned, nuclear scintigraphy, angiography, and colonoscopy have all been beneficial. These patients should not have
a barium enema because barium precludes scintigraphy, confuses angiography,
and impedes colonoscopy.

**On the way to the nursing floor, Mrs. Noro passes a large amount of
red blood and clots from the rectum, and her blood pressure is now
90/40 mm Hg.**

How does this affect the treatment plan?
Mrs. Noro is now unstable, with evidence of a large lower gastrointestinal tract
bleed. She needs aggressive resuscitation and more urgent investigation. The
physician must make sure there is enough cross-matched blood for Mrs. Noro,
and at least 4 units should be kept in reserve.

What is the most likely diagnosis now?
Mrs. Noro most likely has diverticular disease or angiodysplasia.

How should Mrs. Noro be investigated now? Should she go straight to the operating room for a colectomy?
Every effort should be made to find the source of bleeding. Blind colectomies (i.e., without knowing the bleeding site) yield poor results. A segmental colonic excision may miss the source of bleeding, whereas subtotal colectomies and ileorectal anastomoses tend to have a poor functional outcome in this elderly population. Furthermore, these patients typically have comorbid medical conditions that put them at high risk for surgery.

What investigation should be performed at this time?
Nuclear scintigraphy, angiography, or both should be performed (7).

What are the two common forms of nuclear scintigraphy performed in the investigation of lower gastrointestinal tract hemorrhage?
Technetium-labeled sulfur colloid and technetium-labeled red blood cell are the two most common forms of nuclear scintigraphy used to detect bleeding in the lower gastrointestinal tract. Technetium-labeled sulfur colloid is cleared rapidly from the bloodstream and has limited value in the patient with intermittent bleeding. However, in the actively bleeding patient, such as Mrs. Noro, it is quicker to perform, is likely to be positive, and can direct selective angiography. Technetium-labeled red blood cell scans require a number of hours for completion and are less suitable in the unstable patient. However, these scans have the advantage of being able to detect intermittent bleeding because the labeled red blood cells remain in the vascular compartment for longer periods. Therefore, this scan is the technique of choice in the stable intermittently bleeding patient. It can detect bleeding rates as low as 0.1 to 0.5 mL/minute.

Mrs. Noro's sulfur colloid scan shows a lesion in the ascending colon.

What should be done next?
Mrs. Noro should now proceed to selective arteriography, which not only can accurately identify the source but also may be therapeutic.

Why not proceed directly to angiography and forgo the nuclear scan?
This is a reasonable strategy in the patient with a large bleed. Angiography requires a bleeding rate of 0.5 to 2 mL/minute to be positive. First doing a nuclear scan allows the physician to be more selective with the mesenteric vascular catheterization, and this has a number of advantages. First, if appropriate,

gel embolization can be performed. Also, a catheter can be introduced into the bleeding mesenteric vessel for selective vasopressin infusion.

Mrs. Noro is confirmed to have a bleeding diverticulum in the proximal ascending colon.

Should the radiologist remove the vascular catheter and send Mrs. Noro to surgery?
No. This type of lesion may respond to treatment with intraarterial vasopressin. This technique is successful in up to 70% of patients and avoids surgery in this high-risk group.

Despite vasopressin treatment, Mrs. Noro continues to bleed. She has now had 6 units of blood since admission.

What should be done next?
Mrs. Noro should proceed to surgery for a right hemicolectomy.

Does Mrs. Noro need an ileostomy or can she undergo a primary anastomosis?
Although she has not had a formal bowel preparation, resection and primary anastomosis of the right colon can be done safely. Many surgeons would also perform a primary anastomosis on left-sided bleeding lesions, although this is somewhat less conservative.

Is the course of bleeding diverticulosis in this patient typical of this condition?
No. As mentioned previously, most patients stop bleeding spontaneously (8). Most of those who do not stop spontaneously respond to angiographic intervention.

What is the role of colonoscopy in patients with major lower gastrointestinal tract hemorrhage?
Colonoscopy is technically difficult in these circumstances and is not the investigation of choice. Colonoscopy is better used for patients with intermittent bleeding who are stable enough to permit bowel preparation. Colonoscopy may be helpful intraoperatively in patients who proceed to surgery without localization of the bleeding site.

Mrs. Noro recovered uneventfully and was discharged home on the sixth postoperative day. She is tolerating a general diet.

What is the natural history of bleeding diverticulosis in patients not undergoing surgery?
Recurrent episodes of hemorrhage requiring a second admission to the hospital occur in 25% of patients. After a second episode, the chance of a third episode rises to 50%.

Management Algorithm for Diverticulitis

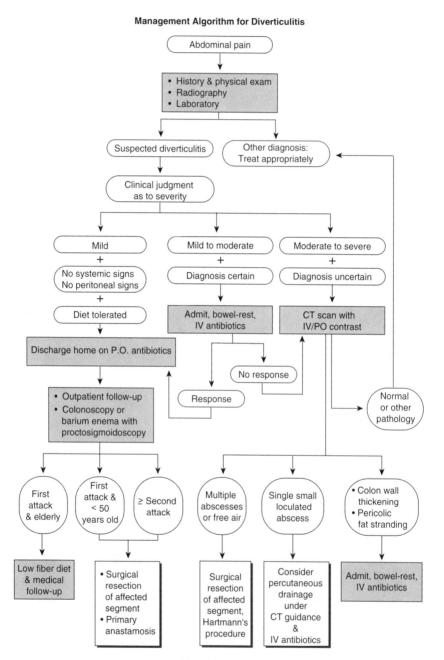

Algorithm 12.1.

Management Algorithm for Lower GI Bleed

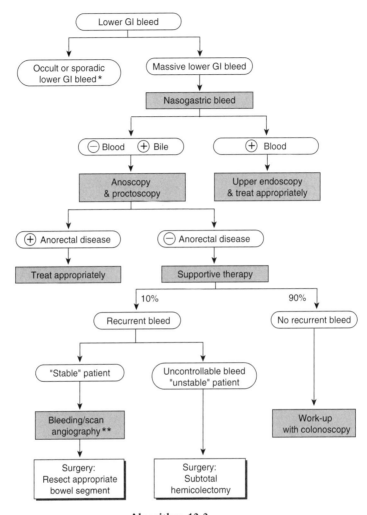

Algorithm 12.2.

REFERENCES

1. Painter NS, Burkitt DP. Diverticular disease of the colon: a deficiency disease of Western civilization. Br Med J 1971;2:450–454.
2. Roberts PL, Veidenheimer MC. Current management of diverticulitis. Adv Surg 1994;27:189–208.
3. Hinchey EF, Schaal PG, Richards GK. Treatment of perforated diverticular disease of the colon. Adv Surg 1978;12:85–109.

4. Colcock BP, Stahmann FD. Fistulas complicating diverticular disease of the sigmoid colon. Ann Surg 1972;175:838–846.
5. Hulnick DH, Megibow AJ, Balthazar EJ, et al. Computed tomography in the evaluation of diverticulitis. Radiology 1984;152:491–495.
6. Boley SJ, Brandt LJ. Vascular ectasias of the colon. Dig Dis Sci 1986;31(9 Suppl): 265–425.
7. Treat MR, Forde KA. Colonoscopy, technetium scanning and angiography in active rectal bleeding: an algorithm for their combined use. Surg Gastroenterol 1983;2:135–138.
8. Cheskin LJ, Bohlman M, Schuster MM. Diverticular disease in the elderly. Gastroenterol Clin North Am 1990;12:391–403.

13

Cancer of the Colon and Rectum

D. Lee Gorden and Todd M. Tuttle

Isaac Jones is a previously healthy 66-year-old man who arrives at the emergency department with a complaint of light-headedness when standing. When questioned, he describes passing black tarry stools at least three to four times in the past week. He has lost nearly 20 pounds in the past 6 months. He does not smoke, and he drinks alcohol only occasionally. His only medication is ibuprofen for mild arthritis.

What are the distinctions among melena, hematochezia, bright red blood per rectum, and heme positive when describing a patient's stools?
All these terms describe bleeding from the gastrointestinal tract (GI) tract.

Melena is the passage of tarry, reddish-black stools.
Hematochezia is a term for bloody stools.
Bright red blood per rectum implies bleeding from a distal source or a massive hemorrhage from a proximal source.
Heme-positive bleeding is bleeding that is not grossly visible; however, stools test positive on hemoccult cards.

The correct description of a patient's stools may give important clues as to the source and rate of bleeding.

At the initial physical examination, Mr. Jones's vital signs are as follows: blood pressure, 140/80 mm Hg; heart rate, 104 beats per minute; temperature, 37°C; respiratory rate, 12 breaths per minute. His chest is clear to auscultation bilaterally, and a mild, regular tachycardia is revealed. The abdomen is soft, not tender, and not distended, with normal bowel sounds. The rectal examination is significant, with hemoccult-positive melenotic stool in the vault. His neurologic examination produces normal findings.

Laboratory studies show a normal electrolyte profile. The white blood cell count is 7.4×10^3 cells/mm^3 (normal count, 4.5 to 11 cells/mm^3), hemoglobin level is 8.1 g/dL (normal level, 14 to 18 g/dL), with a mean corpuscular volume (MCV) of 72 fl (normal range 86–98 mm^3), and the platelet count is 240,000/mL (normal count 150,000 to 450,000/mL). Liver function test findings are within normal limits.

How is significant bleeding in the lower GI tract evaluated?
The most important steps in the initial evaluation of a patient with lower GI tract bleeding are a history and a thorough physical examination. Although this chapter focuses on the colon and rectum, an upper GI source of bleeding should also be considered. Numerous modalities are available to evaluate the colon and rectum, depending on the severity and suspected location of bleeding. Techniques include colonoscopy, flexible sigmoidoscopy or rigid proctoscopy, angiography, and radionucleotide-labeled red blood cell scanning (1).

Which conditions should be considered in the differential diagnosis of lower GI tract bleeding?
A British study ranks the following conditions, in order of decreasing frequency, as a cause of lower GI tract bleeding: diverticular disease, carcinoma of the colon, inflammatory bowel disease, colonic polyps, vascular ectasias, ischemic colitis, rectal ulcers, and hemorrhoids, together with several very rare disorders (2).

Mr. Jones is anemic, and the low MCV suggests that his blood loss results from a chronic, not an acute, process. He undergoes colonoscopy, which reveals a sessile fungating mass proximal to the hepatic flexure. The lesion is not amenable to endoscopic removal, and surgery is recommended.

What types of tumors occur in the colon and rectum?
Adenocarcinomas are the most common malignant colorectal tumors. Other malignant tumors are carcinoids, leiomyosarcomas, primary lymphomas, and metastatic tumors originating from other organs (3). The most frequently encountered neoplasms are adenomas and adenomatous polyps (discussed later in this chapter).

What are some important anatomic considerations of the blood supply to the colon and rectum?
Segmental resection for cancer requires knowledge of the arterial supply and venous drainage of the colon and rectum. The superior mesenteric artery gives rise to the ileocolic, right colic, and middle colic arteries. The ileocolic and right colic arteries are ligated and divided during a right hemicolectomy. To resect a lesion in the mid–transverse colon, the middle colic artery may have to be sacrificed. The inferior mesenteric artery gives rise to the left colic artery, one or

more sigmoid artery branches, and the superior hemorrhoidal artery, which supplies the upper half of the rectum. Blood supply to the lower rectum is via the middle and inferior rectal (hemorrhoidal) vessels that originate from the internal iliac (hypogastric) arteries. The anus is supplied by branches of the inferior rectal (hemorrhoidal) vessels that branch off from the pudendal arteries (from the internal iliac system). The rich network of anastomoses between the different blood supplies, which allows segmental resection, is extremely important. In particular, the marginal artery of Drummond provides collateral circulation between the left branch of the middle colic artery and the branches of the inferior mesenteric artery of the left side of the colon and rectum (Fig. 13.1). This

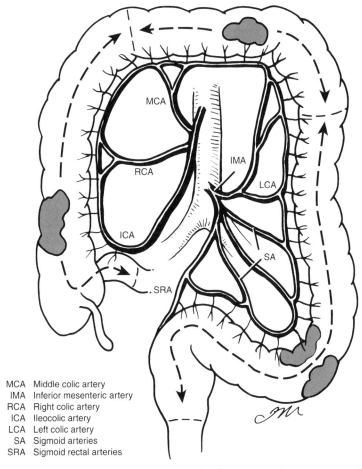

MCA	Middle colic artery
IMA	Inferior mesenteric artery
RCA	Right colic artery
ICA	Ileocolic artery
LCA	Left colic artery
SA	Sigmoid arteries
SRA	Sigmoid rectal arteries

Figure 13.1.   Anatomy of the colon. (Reprinted with permission from Nyhus LM, Baker RJ. Mastery of Surgery. Vol 2. JB Lippincott, 1992.)

is particularly important for an extended right hemicolectomy that includes part of the transverse colon and the middle colic artery (4).

The veins of the colon parallel the arteries, with veins of the same names that empty into the superior and inferior mesenteric veins. The superior and inferior mesenteric veins join the splenic vein, which drains into the portal vein to the liver.

How does lymphatic drainage from the colon and rectum occur?
The lymphatic drainage of the colon parallels the venous channels, which explains the metastatic lymphatic spread of colorectal cancer. Lymph nodes may be found in the colonic mesentery, the mesorectum, and the preaortic area. Low-lying cancers of the anal canal may spread to the deep inguinal nodes, and tumors of the anus may spread to the superficial inguinal nodes.

What are the surgical options for the treatment of colon and rectal cancers?
The surgical treatment of colon tumors depends on their location. For single lesions, a segmental resection is usually performed, whereas for synchronous lesions, a more extensive resection may be required. Standard surgical procedures according to the location of the tumor include right hemicolectomy, transverse colectomy, left hemicolectomy, and sigmoid colectomy, with the corresponding mesentery and mesenteric lymph nodes included in the resection. A surgical margin of at least 2 cm is desirable, both proximal and distal to the tumor (5).

Rectal cancers may be treated with transanal excision, low anterior resection, or abdominoperineal resection, depending on tumor size and location, depth of bowel wall penetration, and lymph node involvement. Excision of the mesorectum provides the best chance for cure. Patients with rectal tumors may be candidates for local resection if there is no evidence of fixation to adjacent structures, transmural invasion of the tumor, or nodal spread and if the histology of a biopsy specimen is favorable. Primary anastomosis of the bowel is routine unless there is obstruction with significant distention of the colon or perforation from a tumor. The exception is abdominoperineal resection, in which an end colostomy must be performed. For very low anastomoses, many surgeons recommend a temporary proximal diverting stoma to protect the distal anastomosis from the fecal stream. The technical considerations of the various procedures are not discussed in this chapter.

Mr. Jones is scheduled to undergo a right hemicolectomy.

Is any additional diagnostic or staging information required before surgery?
A preoperative chest radiograph must be obtained in all patients with a known colorectal malignancy to evaluate the lungs for nodules. The preoperative level of carcinoembryonic antigen (CEA), an important tumor marker, must also be

established so that subsequent levels can be monitored. Abnormal preoperative liver function tests in patients with colonic malignancy warrant further evaluation with computed tomography (CT).

In patients with rectal cancer, the most important step is preoperative determination of the stage of the patient's disease, including the depth of invasion of the tumor. Again, the history and physical examination, including a digital rectal examination and for women, a pelvic examination, are very important. Patients with rectal tumors should undergo CT of the abdomen and pelvis.

Endorectal ultrasound (EUR) is the most accurate method for staging local tumors. When performed by an experienced radiologist, this procedure can disclose the depth of invasion with an accuracy of 85 to 90% and predict any nodal metastases with an accuracy of 85%. EUR can help identify candidates for local therapy, patients who need radical surgery, and patients who would benefit from preoperative radiation therapy.

How should the bowel be prepared before colorectal surgery?
Three principles direct preparation of the colon for surgery: (*a*) mechanical preparation of the colon to cleanse it of stools, (*b*) intraluminal antibacterial treatment, and (*c*) systemic antibiotic therapy. The addition of oral antibiotics to the standard mechanical bowel preparation reduces complications after colonic surgery by as much as 40%. An accepted preoperative bowel preparation procedure is as follows:

1. The patient is maintained on a clear liquid diet for 24 hours before surgery.
2. A balanced electrolyte solution, such as Golytely, is used for mechanical cleansing and lavage of the bowel until the output is clear. A tap water or phosphate enema is a possible addition.
3. The patient is administered oral antibiotics 19, 18, and 9 hours before scheduled surgery. A widely used preparation is neomycin 1 g plus erythromycin 1 g with the possible addition of metronidazole. The use of parenteral antibiotics is somewhat controversial, but most surgeons recommend at least one dose of parenteral antibiotic, such as a second- or third-generation cephalosporin, within 30 minutes before incision to help reduce postoperative infection rates.

Mr. Jones undergoes a right hemicolectomy with no intraoperative complications. His postoperative course is uneventful.

What are the common staging systems for colon and rectal cancers?
Many staging systems have been devised and modified in an attempt to standardize and improve predictive outcomes. Two systems used frequently, the

Aster-Coller modification of Dukes' staging system and the tumor, node, metastasis system, are shown in Tables 13.1 and 13.2, respectively.

The pathology findings confirm that Mr. Jones has stage B1 adeno-carcinoma of the colon.

Which clinical or pathologic factors predict survival of patients with colorectal cancers? Factors that are important determinants of survival after treatment of colorectal cancer include the following:

• Vascular or lymphatic microinvasion
• Perineural invasion

Table 13.1.   ASTER-COLLER MODIFICATION OF DUKES'
STAGING SYSTEM FOR COLORECTAL CANCER

Stage	Description
A	Lesions limited to the mucosa
B1	Lesions limited by not penetrating the muscularis propria; no nodal disease
B2	Lesions penetrating the muscularis propria; no nodal disease
C1	Lesions limited to the bowel wall; nodal disease present
D	Distant metastases; part of the original Dukes classification, often mentioned but not included in the formal Aster-Coller system

Table 13.2.   TUMOR, NODE, METASTASIS STAGING
SYSTEM FOR COLORECTAL CANCER

Primary tumor (T)
T_0 No detectable tumor
T_1 Tumor invading submucosa
T_2 Tumor invading muscularis propria
T_3 Tumor penetrating muscularis propria into subserosa but not into serosa (when serosa is present)
T_4 Tumor penetrating serosa or invading a contiguous organ

Regional lymph nodes (N)
N_0 No regional node involvement with tumor
N_1 1–3 positive nodes
N_2 4 or more positive nodes
N_3 Central nodes positive

Distant metastasis (M)
M_0 No distant metastases
M_1 Distant metastases

- Lymph node metastases
- Deep bowel wall penetration
- Presence of signet ring cells
- Mucus content
- Neuroendocrine differentiation of the tumor
- Tumor ploidy

Would Mr. Jones benefit from either adjuvant chemotherapy or radiation treatment?
Adjuvant therapy is treatment of clinically inapparent microscopic disease. Chemotherapy improves the survival of colon cancer patients who have positive nodes (6). Chemotherapy would not be given postoperatively to Mr. Jones. Radiation therapy is used selectively for treatment of cancers of the colon only if the margins of the resection are positive or if the tumor has spread to adjacent organs.

How does the tumor stage influence survival of patients with colorectal cancer?
For patients treated with surgery alone, 5-year survival rates for the Aster-Coller stages are as follows:

Stage A, 90 to 100%
Stage B1, 75 to 100%
Stage B2, 70 to 90%
Stage C1, 49 to 76%
Stage C2, 45 to 56%

Do patients with rectal cancers benefit from adjuvant therapy?
As with patients with colon cancer, patients with node-positive rectal cancer benefit from chemotherapy. Patients with rectal cancer showing invasion (stage T3) benefit from adjuvant radiation therapy. However, whether preoperative or postoperative radiation is more beneficial is a subject of controversy. Recent evidence suggests that the outcome after radiation therapy may be improved by the addition of low-dose 5-fluorouracil (5-FU) to the treatment regimen; 5-FU acts as a radiosensitizer and potentiates the effects of the radiation therapy.

After discharge from the hospital, Mr. Jones requires follow-up and long-term surveillance for recurrence of colon cancer.

What factors influence tumor recurrence after surgery for colorectal cancer? What are the most common sites of recurrence?
Disease recurs in up to 50% of patients who have undergone a "curative" resection for colorectal cancer. These recurrences can be local, distant, or metachronous. Factors that influence recurrence are (*a*) stage of the initial tu-

mor, (*b*) histology, (*c*) gross tumor appearance, (*d*) vascular or perineural invasion, and (*e*) margin of resection of the primary tumor. The liver is the most common site of distant metastasis from colorectal cancer, with other likely sites of tumor recurrence being the lungs and the peritoneum. Transmural rectal cancers have a particularly high incidence of local recurrence.

Surveillance procedures that can aid in early detection of recurrences include the following:

1. History and physical examination. Weight loss and gastrointestinal bleeding are important indicators of possible recurrence.
2. Testing of the stool for occult bleeding. The value of this test is debatable, but it is probably most useful for detecting metachronous lesions.
3. Routine flexible sigmoidoscopy and colonoscopy.
4. Monitoring the levels of CEA. An elevated CEA level may be the first clue to tumor recurrence. Serum CEA levels, measured at scheduled intervals, should be compared with a baseline CEA level measured several weeks after the initial surgical resection. CEA is not a good screening marker for colorectal cancer in the general population, but it is useful in surveillance for recurrent disease.

A suggested follow-up schedule for patients with colorectal cancers is shown in Table 13.3.

At his 1-year follow-up visit, Mr. Jones is feeling well, but his alkaline phosphatase level is elevated, and his level of CEA is twice that of the measured baseline level. Colonoscopy shows no recurrence of tumor,

Table 13.3.   SUGGESTED FOLLOW-UP AFTER CURATIVE
RESECTION FOR COLORECTAL CANCER

	FREQUENCY (PER YEAR)		
Procedure	Years 1 and 2	Years 3 and 4	Years 5+
History and physical examination	3–4	2	1
Test for occult bleeding	3–4	2	1
Liver function testing	3–4	2	1
Determination of plasma CEA levels	3–4	2	1
Colonoscopy or barium enema	—	1	q 3 yr
Chest radiography	1	1	1

but CT of the abdomen reveals a single low-density lesion 3 cm in diameter in the left lobe of the liver.

What is the survival rate for patients with isolated liver metastases from a primary colorectal tumor?
Patients with untreated liver metastases have an expected median survival of less than 1 year. Systemic chemotherapy has not significantly improved the survival in this group of patients. Hepatic resection in patients with isolated lesions in the liver leads to a 25 to 35% 5-year survival, with a 30-month median survival.

What are the criteria for successful resection of liver metastases?
To be considered for resection of liver metastases from colorectal cancer, a patient must be medically fit to undergo a major operation. In addition, there must be no evidence of extrahepatic metastases, and the lesions must be completely resectable, with tumor-free margins. After liver resection, follow-up should include a physical examination, complete blood count, chemistry profile, chest radiography, and abdominal CT every 6 to 12 months, in addition to the routine follow-up for metachronous colon cancer.

Although there is some disagreement on this subject, the features of hepatic metastases that are associated with a poor prognosis include (*a*) more than four metastases, (*b*) positive margins at the time of resection of the tumor, (*c*) markedly elevated CEA levels, (*d*) lymph node–positive primary tumor, and (*e*) a short disease-free interval (less than 12 months) from the time of initial resection.

What are some causes of or predisposing factors for colorectal cancer?
Environmental risk factors include a high-fat, low-fiber diet and probably cigarette smoking. Diseases that predispose to cancer of the colon and rectum include ulcerative colitis and Crohn's disease. Patients who have had colorectal, breast, ovarian, or uterine cancer are at increased risk.

Molecular regulatory mechanisms play an important role in the pathogenesis of colorectal cancer. Oncogenes associated with colorectal cancer include K-*ras*, H-*ras* (most prevalent), N-*ras*, C-*myc*, and C-*src*. These mutated genes regulate the proliferation of tumor cells. In addition, the loss of tumor suppressor genes, including *APC, MCC,* and *DCC,* leads to decreased regulation of tumor cell growth. Identification of mutated genes may in the future be an important screening, staging, and surveillance tool in patients at risk for colorectal malignancies (7).

What is the importance of polyps in colorectal cancer?
Polyps of the colon and rectum may be divided into those that have potential for malignant degeneration and benign ones. The most common type, up to 90% of benign colonic polyps, are hyperplastic. Other benign polyps include

hamartomas, inflammatory polyps, and lipomas. Peutz–Jeghers polyps and juvenile polyps have very low malignant potential. Polyps with malignant potential may be associated with familial syndromes or sporadic. The most common are adenomatous polyps that are categorized according to type—tubular, villous, or tubulovillous—and the degree of dysplasia. The cancer risk for these polyps is related to size: less than 1 cm, 1 to 10%; 1 to 2 cm, 7 to 10%; and more than 2 cm, 35 to 53%.

Management Algorithm for Heme-Positive Stools

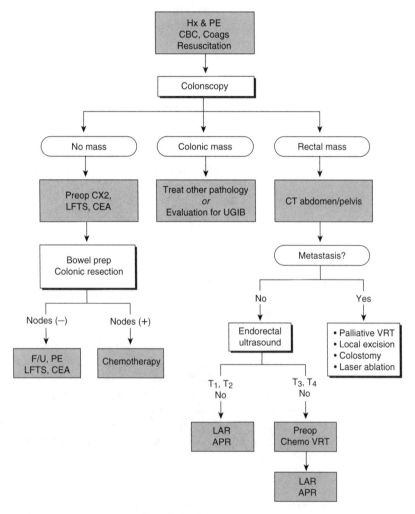

Algorithm 13.1.

What are the familial polyposis syndromes?

Familial adenomatous polyposis (FAP) is an autosomal dominant condition in which the patients are diagnosed by the presence of at least 100 adenomatous polyps in the colon and rectum. The incidence of malignant degeneration of polyps in these patients approaches 100% by the third or fourth decade of life. FAP is a general growth disorder associated with extracolonic manifestations, and this broad category is subdivided into groups with characteristic clinical manifestations. Thus, **Gardner's syndrome** is associated with osteomas of the skull and desmoid tumors, whereas **Turcot's syndrome** is characterized by brain tumors. Other extracolonic manifestations of FAP are gastric or duodenal polyps and periampullary cancers. Hereditary polyposis syndromes account for approximately 1% of colorectal cancers. Total proctocolectomy is recommended for FAP patients, who have a high lifetime risk of colorectal cancer.

Hereditary nonpolyposis colorectal cancer (HNPCC), also known as Lynch's syndrome, is inherited in an autosomal dominant manner, with high penetration and a young age of onset. In contrast to FAP, HNPCC is not characterized by numerous colonic polyps. It accounts for 1 to 6% of cases of colorectal cancer.

REFERENCES

1. Abrahms J, Cerra FB. Surgical Critical Care. St. Louis: Quality Medical Publishing, 1993.
2. Farrands PA, Taylor I. Management of Acute Lower Gastrointestinal Haemorrhage in a Surgical Unit Over a 4 Year Period. J Royal Soc Med 1987;80:79–82.
3. Sabiston DC. Textbook of Surgery. 14th ed. Philadelphia: Saunders, 1991.
4. Nyhus LM, Baker RJ. Mastery of Surgery. 2nd ed. Boston: Little Brown, 1992.
5. Cohen MC, Winawer SJ. Cancer of the Colon, Rectum, and Anus. New York: McGraw-Hill, 1995.
6. DeVita VT, Hellman S, Rosenberg SA. Cancer: Principles and Practice of Oncology. 4th ed. Philadelphia: Lippincott, 1993.
7. Maddoff RD. Colorectal Cancer Genetics. Bull Am Coll Surg 1996;81:26–32.

CHAPTER

14

Anorectal Disease

Daniel A. Saltzman and Todd M. Tuttle

Lucas Boyd is a 47-year-old man who seeks medical attention for a
10-day complaint of progressive rectal pain, perianal swelling, and
foul-smelling drainage. About 3 months earlier, a boil on his left buttock was drained in his physician's office. He now complains of a constant ache that is exacerbated by sitting and walking. He denies having fever, chills, constipation, diarrhea, or abdominal pain. Significant
aspects of his history include repair of a right inguinal hernia several
years earlier and hypercholesterolemia, for which he takes lovastatin.
He also has a 22-pack-year smoking history.

Mr. Boyd's vital signs are normal, and his temperature is 37°C. Findings of his head, neck, cardiovascular, and pulmonary examination
are also normal. His abdomen is flat, with normal bowel sounds, and
he has a well-healed, nontender right inguinal herniorrhaphy scar. Examination of the perianal region reveals a fluctuant tender mass measuring 3 × 2 cm in the left perianal region and a 4 × 2 cm mass in
the right perianal region, both masses draining a purulent discharge.
The overlying skin is indurated and erythematous. No rectal masses
are palpated, nor does the rectal vault feel tender when palpated. Stool
examination is negative for heme. Significant laboratory data include
a hemoglobin level of 13.2 g/dL, a white blood cell count of 7000,
and a normal platelet count. His serum electrolyte level is normal.

*What is the most likely diagnosis for Mr. Boyd's complaint on the basis of the history
and physical examination?*
Mr. Boyd has a perirectal abscess.

Where do perirectal abscesses originate?
A basic knowledge of anorectal anatomy is fundamental to understanding
perirectal disease (Figure 14.1). The rectum is the distal 12 to 15 cm of the large
intestine. The anal canal, the terminal end of the alimentary tract, measures ap-

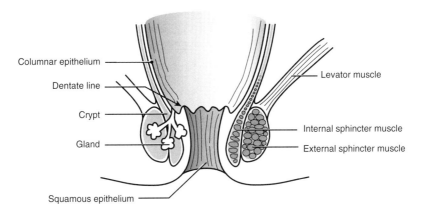

Figure 14.1.   Anatomy of the anal canal.

proximately 4 cm. The rectal wall consists of mucosa, submucosa, and two complete muscular layers: the inner circular and the outer longitudinal. In the anal canal, the internal sphincter is the continuation of the inner circular smooth muscular layer. The external sphincter, the continuation of the outer longitudinal skeletal muscular layer, consists of three parts: subcutaneous, superficial, and deep muscle. The superior border of the external sphincter fuses with the puborectalis muscle and forms a sling originating at the pubis and joining behind the rectum. The intersphincteric plane, the space between the internal and external sphincters, is a fibrous continuation of the longitudinal smooth muscle of the rectum. Normally, 6 to 10 anal glands lie in this intersphincteric space. Each gland has a duct and discharges into an anal crypt at the dentate line. Infection originating in these glands is the primary cause of perirectal abscess and fistula in ano.

What is the dentate line, and what is its anatomic significance?
The dentate line is an important surgical landmark at the union of the embryonic ectoderm with the gut endoderm. The line is recognizable as the line demarcating the transitional epithelium below and the rectal mucosa above. The columns of Morgagni begin at this line and extend cephalad. The dentate line divides the nervous system, vascular supply, and lymphatic drainage of the anal canal into two routes (Table 14.1).

What is the typical presentation of a perirectal abscess?
Pain is the most common symptom, and swelling is present in 95% of patients. However, only 12% of patients have a purulent discharge, and only 18% have fever (temperature higher than 38°C). The male-to-female ratio is approximately 2:1; the peak incidence is in the third and fourth decades (1).

Table 14.1. ANATOMIC SIGNIFICANCE OF
THE DENTATE LINE

	Above Dentate Line	Below Dentate Line
Innervation	Autonomic	Somatic
Venous blood supply	Superior rectal vein into inferior mesenteric, portal system	Middle rectal vein into internal iliac vein; inferior rectal vein into internal pudendal vein
Lymphatic flow	Inferior mesenteric, internal iliac lymph nodes	Inguinal lymph nodes

How does the original infection of the anal glands spread?

An **intersphincteric abscess** results from infection in the anal glands between the internal and external sphincters. Fecal coliforms are typically the offending organisms. As the abscess enlarges within the intersphincteric plane, it can spread in any of several directions.
A **perianal abscess** results when pus spreads downward between the two sphincters, and it manifests as a tender swelling at the anal verge. This is the process responsible for Mr. Boyd's clinical condition.
An **ischiorectal abscess** is formed if the growing intersphincteric abscess penetrates the external sphincter below the puborectalis. Infection can spread into the fat of the ischiorectal fossa, and the abscess can become quite large.
A **supralevator abscess** develops when an intersphincteric abscess expands upward between the internal and external sphincters.

Which types of perirectal abscesses are most common?
The frequencies of perirectal abscesses, in decreasing order, are as follows: perianal, ischiorectal, intersphincteric, and supralevator.

What is the differential diagnosis of a perirectal inflammatory process?
The differential diagnosis includes pilonidal abscess, hidradenitis suppurativa, infected sebaceous cyst, folliculitis, periprostatic abscess, Bartholin gland abscess, inflammatory bowel disease, actinomycosis, and tuberculosis.

Mr. Boyd is admitted to the hospital and receives cefoxitin 1 g intravenously before surgery. Anoscopy is performed with the patient under spinal anesthesia, and no internal opening is found. The bilateral perianal abscesses are incised and drained, and the wound is packed with Betadine dressing. Mr. Boyd's postoperative care includes sitz

baths, dressing changes, and analgesia. He is discharged the day after surgery.

Are incision and drainage alone appropriate treatment for a perirectal abscess?
For most patients, particularly those with perianal abscesses, incision and drainage alone are adequate. The primary opening of the anal crypt is rarely identified; the rate of identification was only 34% in one series. The intersphincteric abscess is treated by looking at the bulging area with the anoscope and then performing an internal sphincterotomy over the abscess. Supralevator abscesses are drained through the appropriate ischiorectal space or through the rectum. Horseshoe abscesses (those surrounding the rectum) are drained through the rectum, with counter drains placed in each ischiorectal space.

Mr. Boyd's recovery is uneventful, but 6 months later he returns with a complaint of persistent painless perirectal drainage. A physical examination reveals bilateral perianal incisions, left perianal induration, and an external opening that is draining purulent discharge from the left perianal incision.

What is a fistula in ano?
A fistula is an abnormal communication between two epithelium–lined surfaces. A fistula in ano has its external opening in the perirectal skin and its internal opening in the anal canal at the dentate line.

Mr. Boyd presented with painless discharge. Is pain a common manifestation of fistula in ano?
Pain is rare with fistula in ano. Patients more commonly complain of perirectal itching, irritation, and discharge (2).

What is the pathogenesis of fistula in ano?
A fistula in ano forms during the chronic phase of an acute inflammatory process that begins in the intersphincteric anal glands. As previously discussed, extension of the acute inflammation can result in a supralevator, ischiorectal, or perianal abscess. With chronic inflammation, the abscess communicates with the external surface, forming supralevator, transsphincteric, or intersphincteric fistulas (3).

What is the incidence of fistula in ano after incision and drainage of a perirectal abscess?
Approximately 40% of patients develop fistula in ano after treatment of a perirectal abscess (4).

How is the internal opening of a fistula in ano located? What is Goodsall's rule?
Goodsall's rule relates the location of the internal opening to the external opening of a fistula in ano. If the anus is bisected by a line in the frontal plane, an

external opening anterior to the line connects to an internal opening via a short direct tract. However, if the external opening is posterior to this imaginary line, the fistula tract follows a curved route to an internal opening in the posterior midline. An exception is an external opening that is anterior to this imaginary line and more than 3 cm from the anus, in which case the tract may curve posteriorly and end in the posterior midline (5).

What other diseases are included in the differential diagnosis of fistula in ano?
Other disease processes that can cause fistula in ano include Crohn's disease; diverticulitis with perforation and fistula to the perineum; hidradenitis suppurativa; pilonidal cyst; malignancy of the distal rectum, anal canal, or perianal skin; tuberculosis; and actinomycosis.

What is the appropriate treatment for a patient, such as Mr. Boyd, who has an intersphincteric fistula?
The principle of treatment is to lay the fistula tract open, and therefore internal sphincterotomy is the treatment for an intersphincteric fistula. Deep or high fistulas may require a two-stage operation to prevent incontinence. In the first stage, a seton or silk suture is placed around the sphincter to stimulate fibrosis adjacent to the sphincter muscle. In the second stage, which is performed 6 to 8 weeks later, the intersphincteric portion of the fistula tract is laid open.

Mr. Boyd undergoes an internal sphincterotomy without complications, and the follow-up examination indicates he is progressing well.

What is an anal fissure?
An anal fissure is a tear in the anal canal, frequently associated with sudden pain or bleeding during defecation. The fissure occurs in the posterior midline and may be associated with skin tags or a sentinel pile. Stool softeners prevent recurrence. Chronic anal fissures may require a lateral internal sphincterotomy (6).

What are hemorrhoids?
The upper anal canal is lined by anal cushions consisting of three thick vascular submucosal bundles that always lie in the left lateral, right posterior lateral, and right anterior lateral positions. The function of these cushions is not entirely clear, but they aid in continence and engorge during defecation to protect the anal canal from abrasions. Hemorrhoid is the pathologic term for a downward displacement of the anal cushions, which causes dilation of the venules.

What are the most common presenting symptoms of a patient with internal hemorrhoids?
The most common manifestation of internal hemorrhoids is painless rectal

bleeding, often during a bowel movement. Patients often notice bright red blood in the stool, on the toilet tissue, or in the toilet. Prolapse of an internal hemorrhoid may produce moisture in the anal region or a mucous discharge that causes itching. Pain is not a common symptom of internal hemorrhoids unless thrombosis or infection is also present (7). The standard classification of hemorrhoidal disease, as outlined by Buls and Goldberg, is presented in Table 14.2 (8).

If a patient presents with rectal bleeding and internal hemorrhoids are found, can the workup be considered complete?
Although internal hemorrhoids are the most common cause of rectal bleeding, it is prudent to exclude other causes of rectal bleeding. Anoscopy is the procedure of choice for diagnosing internal hemorrhoids, but proctoscopy or flexible sigmoidoscopy is required to rule out other sources of rectal bleeding, such as cancer and inflammatory disease. For older patients and those with atypical symptoms, a complete colonic evaluation is necessary to exclude colonic disease.

Does portal hypertension cause hemorrhoids?
No. The incidence of hemorrhoids in the adult population with portal hypertension is no higher than in the normal population (9).

What are the major complications of endoscopy? To what extent can the colon and rectum be accessed by the various colonoscopic instruments?
The major complications associated with endoscopy are perforation and hemorrhage, which occur in fewer than 1% of procedures (10). Table 14.3 lists the length of colon that can be examined by the various colonoscopic instruments.

What is the preferred treatment for external and internal hemorrhoids?
External hemorrhoids are best treated with analgesia and warm soaks. However, if the pain is severe, the thrombosed hemorrhoid must be excised. Mild bleeding and protrusion of internal hemorrhoids can be controlled with conservative

Table 14.2. CLASSIFICATION OF HEMMORRHOIDAL DISEASE

Class of Hemmorrhoid	Attributes
First degree	Does not protrude through anal orifice
Second degree	Protrudes on straining; spontaneously reduces
Third degree	Protrudes; requires manual reduction
Fourth degree	Protrudes; cannot be reduced manually; often requires urgent operation

Table 14.3. ENDOSCOPY OF THE
COLON, RECTUM, AND ANUS

Instrument	Length of Colon, Rectum Examined
Anoscope	Anal canal and distal rectum
Rigid proctoscope	Rectum (20–25 cm)
Flexible sigmoidoscope	Rectum and sigmoid colon (55–60 cm)
Colonscope	Entire colon and terminal ileum

treatment that includes avoiding constipating foods, increasing the fiber content
of the diet, and using hydrophilic bulk stool-forming agents. These measures
alone can often resolve all symptoms. Rubber band ligation, a simple outpatient
procedure, can be used to treat patients with first- and second-degree hemorrhoids. Third- and fourth-degree hemorrhoids and mixed internal-external hemorrhoids require hemorrhoidectomy.

**Keri Jones is a 22 year-old woman who has had pain in the region of
the buttock for 4 months. The pain often resolves after she feels
drainage between her buttocks. On physical examination, a fluctuant
and indurated mass is observed in her postsacral intergluteal region,
approximately 5 cm from the anus. The anus is not involved.**

What is causing Ms. Jones's symptoms?
Ms. Jones has pilonidal disease, a hair-containing sinus or abscess that usually
involves the skin and adjacent tissues in the intergluteal region. Most patients
have pain, swelling, and drainage when these sinuses become infected. Most investigators believe this condition is caused by the ingrowth of hair, although
whether it is acquired or congenital is not known. Pilonidal disease can occur
at any age but is most prevalent between adolescence and the third decade of
life. Recurrent infections are common.

How is pilonidal disease treated?
Treatment depends on the phase of disease at presentation. A **pilonidal abscess** is best treated by incision and drainage. However, for a **pilonidal cyst,**
results of treatment remain imperfect, although numerous methods have been
reported. The simplest methods of treatment are incision, drainage, and curet-
tage, with secondary healing (11) or cyst excision and closure.

**Maurice Sellers is a 32-year-old homosexual man who has been com-
plaining of perirectal pain, bleeding, and occasional discharge. He has**

also noticed numerous perianal growths. A proctoscopic examination reveals numerous anal warts in the perianal region and in the anal canal.

How can Mr. Sellers's problem be treated?
Mr. Sellers has condylomata acuminata of the anorectum. This disease is caused by the human papillomavirus, and anal intercourse is the most common means of transmission. Condylomata acuminata is often associated with other sexually transmitted diseases, and therefore, examination and testing for herpes or chlamydial infection, gonococcal proctitis, anorectal syphilis, and AIDS is prudent. If the warts are small and few, anal condylomata are usually treated in the office with bichloracetic acid or podophyllin. For numerous and large anal warts, excision with electrocoagulation is effective. The successful use of adjuvant interferon has been reported for severe cases of anal condylomata. Infection with human papillomavirus types 16 and 18 is associated with malignant degeneration (12–14).

Which neoplasms occur in the anorectal region?
Squamous cell carcinoma of the anus, basal cell carcinoma of the anal margin, Bowen's disease, extramammary Paget's disease, anal melanoma, adenocarcinoma of the anal canal, and metastatic tumors can occur in this region.

What are the complications of anorectal surgery?

Postoperative bleeding is one of the most common complications after anorectal surgery, particularly after hemorrhoidectomy. In a recent series of 2038 consecutive hemorrhoidectomies, the incidence of early postoperative bleeding was 1.9%. In most instances, early postoperative hemorrhage is caused by inadequate hemostasis at the time of operation. Late bleeding characteristically occurs between 7 and 10 days after surgery, when the suture is almost completely dissolved.

Incontinence may result after the division of the sphincteric muscles during extensive fistula surgery. Sphincteroplasty may be indicated if improvement is not seen with sphincteric exercises.

Anal stricture, an infrequent and late complication of anorectal surgery, manifests as progressive constipation and decreased caliber of stools. Initial treatment should consist of bulk laxatives and stool softeners, but anoplasty may be required if painful stenosis persists.

Other complications of anorectal surgery include urinary retention, infection, anorectal suppuration, anal pruritus, constipation, and fecal impaction (15).

Management Algorithm for Anorectal Pain, Drainage, or Bleeding

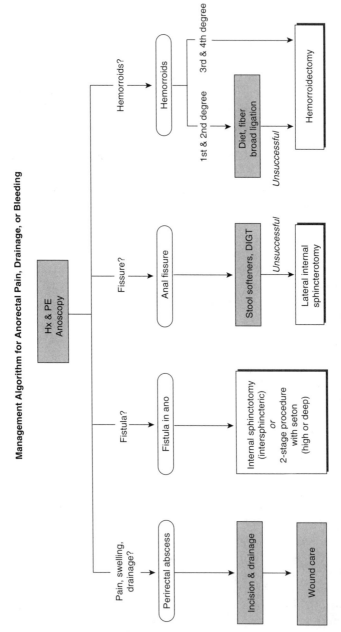

Algorithm 14.1.

REFERENCES

1. Ramanujam PS, Prasad ML, Abcarian H, Tan AB. Perianal abscess and fistulas: a study of 1023 patients. Dis Colon Rectum 1984;27:593.
2. Garcia-Aguilar J, Belmonte C, Wong WD, et al. Anal fistula surgery: factors associated with recurrence and incontinence. Dis Colon Rectum 1996;39:723.
3. Parks AG, Gordon PH, Hardcastle JD. A classification of fistula-in-ano. Br J Surg 1976; 63:7.
4. Scoma JA, Salvati EP, Rubin RJ. Incidence of fistulas subsequent to anal abscess. Dis Colon Rectum 1974;17:357.
5. Goodsall DH. Diseases of the Anus and Rectum. London: Lonmans, 1900.
6. Fry RD. Kodner IJ. Anorectal disorders. Clin Symp 1985;37:1.
7. Ganchrow MI, Mazier WP, Friend WG, Ferguson JA. Hemorrhoidectomy revisited: a computer analysis of 2038 cases. Dis Colon Rectum 1971;14:128.
8. Buls JC, Goldberg SM. Modern management of hemorrhoids. Surg Clin North Am 1978;58:469.
9. Jacobs DM, Bubrick MP, Onstad GR, Hitchock CR. The relationship of hemorrhoids to portal hypertension. Dis Colon Rectum 1980;23:567.
10. Damore LJ, Rantis RC, Vernam AM, Longo WI. Colonoscopic perforation. Dis Colon Rectum 1996;39:1308.
11. Hodgson WJ, Greenstein RJ, A comparative study between z-plasty and incision and drainage or excision with marsupialization for pilonidal sinuses. Surg Gynecol Obstet 1981;153:842.
12. Gal AA, Meyer PR, et al. Papillomavirus antigens in anorectal condyloma and carcinoma in homosexual men. JAMA 1987;257:337.
13. Fleshner PR, Freilich MI. Adjuvant interferon for anal condyloma. Dis Colon Rectum 1994;37:1255.
14. Wexner SD. Sexually transmitted diseases of the colon, rectum, and anus: the challenge of the nineties. Dis Colon Rectum 1990;33:1048.
15. Schoetz DJ. Complications of anorectal operations. Surg Clin North Am 1983;63:1249.

15

Cholelithiasis and Acute Cholecystitis

Viriato M. Fiallo

Consuelo Rodriguez is a 40-year-old woman with right upper quadrant pain that started 2 months ago. The pain is precipitated by fatty meals; it begins approximately 60 minutes after eating and lasts for several hours. On occasion, she feels the pain in the inferior aspect of the scapula, the shoulder, and the epigastrium. She frequently feels nauseous with the pain, and she has occasional emesis. Her primary care physician orders an ultrasound of the right upper quadrant that shows multiple stones in the gallbladder. The patient is referred to be evaluated for surgery.

Can cholelithiasis cause any other symptoms?
A significant number of patients with cholelithiasis do not have postprandial pain but instead have dyspepsia, vague upper gastric discomfort, or even mildly increased flatulence as primary symptoms (1).

How many types of gallstones are known?
There are three types of gallstones: cholesterol, pigmented, and mixed. Approximately 10% of stones are pure cholesterol, 15% are pigmented, and the remaining 75% are mixed (1).

What are the factors in the formation of gallbladder stones?
Factors in the formation of cholesterol stones include supersaturation of bile acid micelles, formation of abnormally high-cholesterol–containing biliary vesicles, and ileal disorders or ileal resections. The gallbladder also plays a role in the pathogenesis of cholesterol stones by favoring nucleation (the process by which cholesterol monohydrate crystals form and agglomerate) and crystal growth by abnormal absorption or secretion, by a defective surface pH, or by providing essential nucleating factors including mucin, desquamated cells, bacteria, and reflux intestinal contents (1–3).

Are stones the only cause of symptoms related to gallbladder disease?
No. Functional disorders of the gallbladder and the sphincter of Oddi can give rise to clinical manifestations similar to those of cholelithiasis. These motility disorders have been called chronic acalculous cholecystitis, or gallbladder dyskinesia. The most specific test for these disorders is cholecystokinin-enhanced cholescintigraphy with assessment of gallbladder ejection fraction. An ejection fraction less than 35% is considered abnormal (4). Other than biliary dyskinesia, undetectable small stones or cholesterolosis also can be symptomatic. For these patients, duodenal drainage studies demonstrating abnormal bile-containing cholesterol or calcium bilirubinate crystals have been useful. Approximately 80% of patients with abnormal cholecystokinin-cholescintigraphy or abnormal duodenal drainage studies have significant improvement of their symptoms after cholecystectomy (1).

What is the significance of biliary sludge?
A recent study looked at the clinical significance of gallbladder sludge. Diagnosis of gallbladder sludge was made by ultrasound in 286 patients followed up for a mean of 20 months. Although sludge disappeared spontaneously within a relatively short time in 71% of the patients, gallbladder sludge was significant because cholelithiasis or other complications occurred in 19% of the patients. Acute calculus cholecystitis developed in 7.1% of the patients (5).

Are there any conditions associated with the formation of gallstones?
An increased incidence of gallstone disease has been observed in elderly patients, certain ethnic groups, women, immediate family members of a patient with cholelithiasis, obese patients, diabetic patients, cirrhotic patients, patients with truncal vagotomy, and patients receiving long-term total parenteral nutrition (1).

What is the natural history of gallstones?
Asymptomatic patients with gallstones generally have a benign course. Approximately 2% of asymptomatic patients with gallstones develop symptoms every year. One study of 123 patients with asymptomatic cholelithiasis and an actuarial follow-up period of up to 20 years shows that only 5.7% of these patients developed severe complications, including obstructive jaundice, acute cholecystitis, gallstone ileus, and pancreatitis. Of these patients, 13% eventually developed mild symptoms that required elective cholecystectomy (2, 6, 7).

Should asymptomatic gallstones be treated?
It is a general practice not to treat cholelithiasis until symptoms develop. The morbidity and mortality rates of asymptomatic patients treated with observation versus cholecystectomy are similar (8). However, certain conditions warrant a prophylactic cholecystectomy. This includes children with gallstones, because they almost always develop symptoms. Patients with sickle cell disease

pose diagnostic difficulties, and approximately 25% of these patients develop symptoms. Calcified gallbladder is also an indication for cholecystectomy because approximately 50% of these patients have an associated gallbladder cancer. Stones larger than 2.5 cm are frequently associated with acute cholecystitis, and a prophylactic cholecystectomy may be warranted. A nonfunctioning gallbladder also is an indication for a cholecystectomy because it indicates advanced disease, with development of symptoms in 25% of patients (8, 9).

Is diabetes mellitus an indication for prophylactic cholecystectomy?
A recent prospective study of non–insulin-dependent diabetic patients who were followed for 5 years showed a cumulative percentage of 10.8% for development of symptoms and 4.2% for development of complications (9). Another prospective review comparing diabetic and nondiabetic patients who underwent cholecystectomy did not show a difference in the incidence of perforation, wound infection, overall morbidity, or mortality (1). Therefore, in general, prophylactic cholecystectomy in an asymptomatic diabetic patient may not be recommended (2, 10). However, consideration of individual factors such as age and comorbidities is important, and surgery may be appropriate in selected asymptomatic diabetic patients.

What are the possible complications of untreated symptomatic cholelithiasis?
These complications include acute cholecystitis, obstructive jaundice, acute cholangitis, gallstone ileus, and gallstone pancreatitis. Fewer than 1% of patients with initial complication of cholelithiasis have a fatal outcome during that hospitalization (1).

Now that Mrs. Rodriguez has a good understanding of the pathogenesis of gallstones and the possible complications of cholelithiasis, she wants to know her treatment options.

What are the treatment options for symptomatic cholelithiasis?
The treatment options include operative management consisting of open or laparoscopic cholecystectomy, percutaneous cholecystostomy, extracorporeal shock wave lithotripsy (ESWL), oral gallstone dissolution agents, and contact dissolution agents through a percutaneous approach with methyl *tert*-butyl ester (MTBE).

How effective are the nonoperative options in the management of symptomatic cholelithiasis?
ESWL is usually combined with oral bile acid dissolution. Complete stone clearance rates vary from 60 to 90%. The factors that determine the complete clearance of the stones are the isodensity with bile and the computed tomography (CT) score (Hounsfield units below 75). The main causes of failure are acquired stone calcification and impaired gallbladder motility (11). When cal-

culated by actuarial analysis, the probability of stone recurrence has been 5.5 to 7% after 1 year, 11 to 12% after 2 years, 13% after 3 years, 20% after 4 years, and 31% after 5 years (11, 12). Gallbladder emptying is an important factor in the recurrence of gallstones. One study showed that the recurrence rate was 53% at 3 years when the gallbladder ejection fraction was less than 60% but only 13% in patients with an ejection fraction above 60% (13). The cumulative risk of gallstone recurrence by actuarial analysis has been shown to be 23, 34, 55, and 70% at 1, 2, 3, and 4 years, respectively, after complete direct contact dissolution with MTBE (14).

When are nonsurgical options indicated?
These modalities are indicated for symptomatic patients who are poor risks for laparoscopic cholecystectomy. Most protocols for ESWL are limited to symptomatic patients with one to three radiolucent stones with a diameter of 30 mm or less and a functioning gallbladder according to oral cholecystography (OC). ESWL is safe and effective for patients with a single stone not more than 20 mm in diameter, but the efficacy for larger single stones and multiple stones is poor (12, 14, 15).

For cholelithiasis, how should symptomatic gallstones be treated?
The preferred method of treating symptomatic gallstones is laparoscopic cholecystectomy. It has the advantages of little postoperative discomfort, short hospital stay, and short postoperative disability. This procedure can be performed safely with an overall morbidity that ranges from 3 to 10%, and mortality rates are 0 to 0.1%. Injury to the bile ducts occurs in 0.2 to 0.6% of patients undergoing this procedure. The incidence of complication decreases with increase in the experience of the surgeon and with careful attention to laparoscopic surgical technique. The incidence of major bile duct injury can decrease to rates comparable with those of open cholecystectomy.

What are the chances of having calculi in the common bile duct (CBD) in routine cholecystectomy?
CBD stones are found in 8 to 15% of patients undergoing cholecystectomy for symptomatic cholelithiasis (1). The incidence seems to be greater in patients older than 60 years of age (25%).

Should intraoperative cholangiography be performed routinely during laparoscopic cholecystectomy?
This topic is controversial. Advocates of routine intraoperative cholangiography during laparoscopic cholecystectomy argue that this practice gives a better definition of the anatomy by providing a road map for the surgeon and by identifying anomalous insertion of the cystic duct or other anatomic aberrations of the bile ducts. Only those performing it routinely get the proficiency in cannulating

the cystic duct and in interpreting the fluoroscopic images. Also, a routine intra-operative cholangiogram allows the surgeon to detect an injury to the bile tract early during operation, allowing a prompt repair and reducing the morbidity associated with delayed diagnosis and repair of injuries made to major bile ducts (2, 16). Other surgeons argue against the routine use of cholangiography because of the technical aspects of the procedure, wasted time and expense, false-positive studies (4%), and the fact that it has not been proven that routine intraoperative cholangiography prevents bile duct injury (1, 16, 17).

In what circumstances should an intraoperative cholangiogram be performed?
An intraoperative cholangiogram should be performed if there is cholangitis, pancreatitis, or a history thereof; if preoperative evaluation shows a dilated or thick CBD; if there are multiple small stones in the gallbladder and the cystic duct; or if the liver function tests are abnormal. An intraoperative cholan-giogram also should be performed if the surgeon is unable to identify all the structures of the triangle of Calot.

Mrs. Rodriguez agrees to have her gallbladder taken out via lap-aroscopy. While waiting for surgery, she develops severe, constant right upper quadrant pain accompanied by nausea and vomiting. The pain increases rapidly in intensity and is referred to the epigastrium, the right shoulder, and the tip of the scapula.

What is wrong with Mrs. Rodriguez?
The patient may have acute cholecystitis or biliary colic. Biliary colic causes pain that reaches a plateau lasting minutes to hours. In patients with acute cholecystitis, the pain persists after several hours and may last days. With time, the pain tends to localize more in the right upper quadrant because of the in-flammation irritating the peritoneum (1).

What causes the inflammation of the gallbladder in acute cholecystitis?
It is believed that the initial inflammatory process is a biochemical phenome-non as opposed to an infectious event. The mediators that have been shown to cause cellular injury and inflammation are the bile acids, lithogenic bile, pan-creatic juice, lysolecithin, phospholipase A, and prostaglandins. The bacterial invasion is a secondary process (1).

During physical examination, Mrs. Rodriguez is found to have a ten-der right upper quadrant with mild guarding and a positive Murphy's sign. Her temperature is 37.8°C orally. Laboratory examination re-veals a leukocyte count of 10,000/mL, normal electrolyte levels, and a total bilirubin of 1.8 mg/dL. Plain radiograph of the abdomen shows a normal bowel pattern but no stones.

What is Murphy's sign?
A classic physical sign of cholecystitis, Murphy's sign is elicited by pressing the right upper quadrant with one's hand and asking the patient to inspire. The sign is present when the patient suddenly stops the inspiratory effort because of the exquisitely painful contact of the inflamed gallbladder with the examiner's hand.

What is the significance of a palpable mass in the right upper quadrant when acute cholecystitis is suspected?
The palpable mass may represent hydrops (mucocele) or a pericholecystic abscess. Hydrops occurs when a gallbladder obstructed by an impacted stone fills with a clear or white mucoid material. The wall usually is not inflamed. The mucoid fluid results from altered secretion of the gallbladder epithelium. Symptoms suggesting cholecystitis may or may not be present (1, 2). In the case of pericholecystic abscess, the patient usually is toxic. Empyema, pus in the lumen of the gallbladder, frequently accompanies this condition. The abscess is secondary to a subacute perforation of the inflamed gallbladder. Intervention in the form of cholecystectomy or cholecystostomy is mandated.

Does the lack of an elevated white blood cell count and high fever rule out acute cholecystitis?
No. A recent retrospective study of 100 consecutive patients seen in the emergency department suspected of having acute cholecystitis revealed that only Murphy's sign had a high sensitivity (97.2%) and a high positive predictive value (93.3%) in diagnosing acute cholecystitis compared with biliary scintigraphy (18). These results are similar to those of another retrospective study of 198 patients showing that patients with acute cholecystitis (confirmed at surgery) frequently lacked fever and leukocytosis (19).

Does a negative abdominal radiograph rule out gallstones?
No. Because gallstones consist largely of the radiolucent cholesterol pigments, only 15% of them are radiopaque. In contrast, kidney stones are 85% radiopaque, a consequence of the higher composition of calcium in kidney stones.

What is the significance of air in the gallbladder revealed by plain radiograph?
Emphysema of the gallbladder is a result of infection by gas-producing organisms (e.g., clostridia) and is a surgical emergency. It also may arise from a fistula between the intestine and the gallbladder, allowing air into the latter.

How does ultrasound compare with radionuclide imaging, such as hepatoiminodiacetic acid (HIDA) scan? In which situations is one preferred over the other?
Ultrasound is simple, fast, and 95% accurate for demonstrating gallstones (i.e., cholelithiasis) (20). However, it cannot demonstrate as well the acute infection of the gallbladder (accuracy, 79 to 86%) (21). Ultrasound diagnosis of acute

cholecystitis is inferred from the ultrasonic images of thickened wall, pericystic fluid, and the presence of intracavitary sludge or stones, intramural gas, and sloughed mucosal membrane. However, a radionuclide scan has almost 100% sensitivity for diagnosing acute cholecystitis (21). Intravenously injected isotopes (e.g., HIDA) are secreted into the bile, revealing the biliary tract. The test is reliable with the serum bilirubin level of up to 8 to 10 mg/dL; above those levels, the reliability decreases. The gallbladder is usually visible within 20 to 30 minutes. Failure to reveal the gallbladder implies obstruction of the cystic duct and infection of the organ. Acute cholecystitis is highly likely if the gallbladder is not visible at 1 hour and is certain if the gallbladder is not visible at 4 hours. Acute cholecystitis is mostly a clinical diagnosis, so ultrasound is an adequate test to demonstrate it in a patient with a high clinical suspicion. In patients whose clinical presentation for acute cholecystitis is equivocal or in whom preoperative diagnosis is mandatory because of a significant surgical risk, HIDA scan is more appropriate because of its higher accuracy.

What is the role of oral cholecystogram (OCG) in the evaluation of acute cholecystitis? What is its accuracy?
OCG is just as accurate (95%) as ultrasound for diagnosing gallstones and is more accurate for acute cholecystitis (22). However, with serum bilirubin levels greater than 1.5 to 2 mg/dL, the test is unreliable. Because the test must be given over 24 to 48 hours, it is logistically inconvenient in acute settings and has been largely replaced by ultrasound or HIDA scan. OCG has a very limited role. In the chronic setting, it may have a role in conjunction with other gastrointestinal tests, such as barium enema, in which the patient is prepared 2 to 3 days in advance.

What is the problem with the HIDA scan?
It can have false-positive results, especially in critically ill patients on total parenteral nutrition with prolonged fasting and in patients with acute pancreatitis.

Can the specificity of HIDA scan be improved in these circumstances?
Yes. Pretreatment with cholecystokinin is helpful in the presence of functional resistance to tracer flow into the gallbladder (23). Administration of intravenous morphine causes spasm of the sphincter of Oddi, therefore causing reflux of bile with radionuclide in the gallbladder. This technique is recommended when the gallbladder is not visible after 1 hour (23). Morphine also increases the visibility of gallbladder in patients pretreated with cholecystokinin (24).

Mrs. Rodriguez has a mildly elevated total bilirubin.

What does this test result mean in her case?
Because the patient does not have a history of liver disease, the two possible explanations are the presence of a stone or stones in the CBD and Mirizzi's syndrome.

What is Mirizzi's syndrome?
Mirizzi's syndrome is characterized by obstruction of the common hepatic duct (CHD) or CBD due to contiguous inflammation in the gallbladder or cystic duct or compression of the CHD by an impacted large stone in the adjacent cystic duct. The chronic inflammation can result in a stricture. Mild jaundice is present in up to 20% of patients with acute cholecystitis (1). It is usually the result of contiguous inflammation.

Can acute cholecystitis occur in the absence of cholelithiasis?
Yes. The condition known as acalculous cholecystitis comprises 4 to 8% of cases of acute cholecystitis (25). Classically, this condition is found in critically ill patients. Recent evidence suggests that the incidence is increasing and that it can be found outside the critical care setting. Most of these patients suffer from atheromatous vascular disease or diabetes mellitus (2). Risk factors include blood volume depletion, prolonged ileus, opioid administration, total parenteral nutrition, severe trauma, sepsis, severe burns, and starvation. The inflammation may arise from prolonged distention of the gallbladder or stasis and inspissation of bile, with subsequent mucosal injury and thrombosis of the vessels of the seromuscular layer of the gallbladder (2). A recent microangiographic study of 15 patients with acutely inflamed gallbladders showed poor and irregular capillary filling in acalculous cholecystitis versus dilation of arterioles and regular filling of capillaries in calculous cholecystitis (26).

Where do biliary fistulas most commonly form? What are some of the complications?
Fistulas are formed frequently between the gallbladder or the CBD to the skin (e.g., biliary cutaneous), duodenum (e.g., cholecystoduodenal), and pleura. Problems with fistulas are infection (e.g., cholangitis from the retrograde infection from the bowel, peritonitis from bile leakage, or infection of the affected organ), electrolyte abnormalities (e.g., from the continual loss of electrolytes in the bile, most commonly resulting in hyponatremia), malabsorption syndrome (from the lack of bile, which is critical in the intestinal absorption of fat and fat-soluble vitamins), and gallstone ileus.

What is the radiographic interpretation of air in the gallbladder, dilated proximal loops of bowel, and a calcified mass in the right lower quadrant of the abdomen?
The interpretation includes the diagnosis of gallstone ileus, which occurs when a large stone formed in either the gallbladder or in the CBD passes through a biliary-enteric fistula. In the intestine, it may cause obstruction at a narrow lumen, most commonly at the ileocecal valve, which causes dilation of the proximal bowel.

What is the proper treatment of gallstone ileus?
Gallstone ileus is treated surgically. The gallstone is removed through a small enterotomy. Concomitant cholecystectomy and repair of the fistula are indi-

cated because the patent biliary-enteric fistula may cause recurrent episodes. However, if the patient is too ill, the definitive therapy may be performed later. Enterolithotomy alone has a mortality rate of 5%, in contrast to a mortality rate of 15% for enterolithotomy and cholecystectomy (1).

If inflammation of the gallbladder and the surrounding tissue is anticipated in the setting of acute cholecystitis, is laparoscopic cholecystectomy technically feasible? Is it a good choice?
Yes. With increasing experience, laparoscopic cholecystectomy can be performed safely with complication rates and mortality rates comparable with those of open surgery for acute cholecystitis (27–31). Acute cholecystitis has a higher conversion rate and incidence of accidental opening of the gallbladder than does laparoscopic cholecystectomy for chronic disease (31, 32).

What are the factors that determine the conversion to an open cholecystectomy?
The two main factors determining conversion from laparoscopic to open operation for acute cholecystitis are any gangrenous cholecystitis and the timing of the operation (27–29, 31). Conversion rates are lower if the operation is performed within 96 hours of the start of the attack (27, 28). The operation should be performed as soon as possible after admission to prevent the development of significant inflammation, which increases the technical difficulty of the procedure (29, 31).

Mrs. Rodriguez, a well-informed patient, raises the point that perhaps she should see a gastroenterologist first, especially if there is any doubt that there is a stone in her CBD.

Should Mrs. Rodriguez undergo a preoperative endoscopic evaluation of her biliary anatomy? What is the role of endoscopic retrograde cholangiopancreatography (ERCP) in the era of laparoscopic cholecystectomy?
A study of one series of selected patients shows that the positive yield for CBD stones during ERCP ranged from 14 to 55%, with an average of 35%. The clearance of CBD stones varies between 74 and 100%. This indicates that 65% of patients have a negative study with its attendant costs, additional hospitalization, and inherent risk of unnecessary complications. Evidence in the literature suggests that the highest yield for preoperative ERCP detection and treatment of CBD stones is in patients who are jaundiced, whose ultrasound shows CBD stones, who have acute cholangitis, and who have worsening gallstone pancreatitis. Patients with a moderate risk of having CBD stones are those with a CBD diameter of 8 mm; those with worsening liver function tests, particularly bilirubin, alkaline phosphatase, serum glutamic-oxaloacetic transaminase (SGOT), and serum glutamate pyruvate transaminase (SGPT); and high-risk elderly patients, because of the possibility of prolonged operation. Patients with less than a 2% risk of having CBD stones are those with no history of jaun-

dice, normal bile duct diameter in ultrasound, and normal liver function studies (33).

Mrs. Rodriguez agrees to have her gallbladder taken out with laparoscopy without ERCP. A 10-mm trocar is placed inferior to the umbilicus with the open technique. The abdomen is insufflated with carbon dioxide, and the laparoscope is introduced into the abdominal cavity. Another 10-mm trocar is placed below the xiphoid process under direct visualization with the laparoscope. Then 5-mm trocars are placed below the costal margin at the midclavicular line and the anterior axillary line. An edematous and friable gallbladder wall is found, as are adhesions to the omentum.

What are the important technical steps of performing the laparoscopic cholecystectomy in this situation?
If the gallbladder is so distended that it is difficult to grab the fundus, it should be drained of bile (or mucoid material in the case of hydrops) to allow good placement of the grasping forceps. The fundus should be retracted over the liver and another grasping forceps used to grab the ampulla. The ampulla should be retracted away from the liver, exposing the triangle of Calot. The most important step is to identify all of the structures in the triangle, including the cystic duct, the cystic artery, the junction of the cystic duct and the gallbladder, and the junction of the cystic duct with the CBD. The major contraindication to the laparoscopic approach is the failure to expose all of the structures in the triangle (2).

Where is the cystic artery? What is the triangle of Calot?
It is important to attempt to ligate the cystic artery first so that the subsequent dissection upon the gallbladder is relatively bloodless. The cystic artery is usually found in the triangle of Calot. The boundaries of the triangle of Calot are the cystic duct, the right border of the common hepatic and right hepatic ducts, and the inferior border of the liver.

What are the common variations of the arterial supply of the gallbladder?
The cystic artery arises from the common hepatic artery in 95% of cases. In the remaining cases, the variations include origination from the gastroduodenal artery, two cystic arteries, and coursing of the cystic artery anterior to the common hepatic duct instead of posterior (34).

What are the common anomalies of the biliary tree?
Usually, the cystic duct originates from the middle to the upper part of the common hepatic duct. However, common variations include origination from as high as the right hepatic duct to as low as just proximal to the ampulla of Vater;

spiral anterior or posterior insertion to the common hepatic duct; and absent, short, or long cystic ducts (34).

What are accessory bile ducts? What are the sinuses of Luschka?
Accessory bile ducts are common; reported incidence ranges from 1 to 33%. They are bile ducts from the liver that course adjacent to the gallbladder and empty into a larger distal duct. Some of the smaller ducts (e.g., sinuses of Luschka) may empty directly into the gallbladder. Performing cholecystectomy without recognizing them may result in cutting across these ducts, which leads to persistent drainage of bile into the subhepatic bed and causes biloma or abscess.

What are the valves of Heister, and what is their significance?
The valves of Heister are mucosal folds (not true valves) in the cystic duct that may complicate attempts to pass a probe or a cholangiogram catheter into the gallbladder. During the laparoscopic exploration, all of the structures in the triangle of Calot are identified. An intraoperative cholangiogram is obtained because of the mild elevation of the total bilirubin. The cholangiogram reveals two small filling defects in the distal CBD.

At this point, what are the options for dealing with CBD stones?
Laparoscopic CBD exploration, laparoscopic antegrade sphincterotomy, open CBD exploration, and postoperative ERCP may be performed to remove the CBD stones (35). The precise indications for laparoscopic exploration, open CBD exploration, and postoperative ERCP have not been clearly established. The laparoscopic transcystic exploration is performed after cannulation and dilation of the cystic duct with a balloon catheter or a ureteral dilator. The stones are dealt with under fluoroscopic or ureteroscopic guidance by flushing, pushing through the ampulla, basket retrieval, or electrohydraulic lithotripsy. The transcystic approach is preferred when stones are less than 6 mm in diameter, when the diameter of the cystic duct is greater than 4 mm, when the diameter of the CBD is less than 6 mm, and when the cystic duct entrance is lateral (36).

Laparoscopic choledochotomy with CBD exploration is preferred in the case of multiple stones, stones larger than 6 mm in diameter, stones in the common hepatic duct, a cystic duct smaller than 4 mm, a CBD smaller than 6 mm, and a posterior or distal cystic duct entrance. Laparoscopic choledochotomy should not be performed if there is marked inflammation or if the tissue is too weak to hold sutures (36). The exploration is conducted in a similar fashion to the open technique. A T-tube is left in place for drainage of the CBD.

The postoperative ERCP is a valuable option if the surgeon is reluctant to perform a laparoscopic exploration and if the institution has good endoscopists. A transcystic catheter can be passed into the duodenum through the cystic duct at the time of surgery to facilitate the retrograde approach to the ampulla (35).

How is an open CBD exploration conducted?
Through a small longitudinal incision on the anterior wall of the CBD, calculi are removed directly with forceps or scoops, extracted with tools such as Fogarty balloon-tipped catheters, or irrigated out. In this manner, the distal CBD, the proximal bile ducts, and right and left hepatic ducts are explored in that order. After all of the calculi are removed, a Bakes dilator is passed through the ampulla into the duodenum, confirming the patency of the sphincter. The tip of the T-tube is placed in the CBD through the incision to drain the bile postoperatively. The incision is closed with interrupted sutures, assuring no leakage of bile around the T-tube. Postexploration cholangiography is performed to confirm the absence of retained stones in the CBD and passage of dye into the duodenum.

Following open CBD exploration as described here, how often do retained CBD stones occur?
Retained CBD stones occur in approximately 10% of cases (37).

What technique can reduce the incidence of retained stones following CBD exploration?
Use of choledochoscopy for direct visualization of the biliary ducts during stone extraction can reduce the likelihood of a missed or retained stone. Although the reported rates vary greatly, choledochoscopy can decrease the rate from approximately 10% to less than 2% (37).

What can be done to remove an impacted stone?
The Kocher maneuver can be used to remove an impacted stone. It is done by incising the lateral peritoneal reflection of the second portion of the duodenum for exposure. Afterward, a longitudinal incision on the anterior duodenum is made to expose the sphincter from within the lumen. The impacted stone may be removed directly, and if there is fibrosis at the orifice, a limited sphincterotomy may facilitate the extraction.

Before the abdomen is closed after open CBD exploration, should the gallbladder fossa be drained?
Routine drainage of the gallbladder fossae after any form of cholecystectomy is not warranted. In elective cholecystectomies, use of drains actually may increase the incidence of postoperative fever and wound infection. However, in cases of CBD exploration or excessive fluid accumulation, drainage may be employed. Drainage-related complications may be decreased by using a closed-suction drain, separating the drain exit wound from the incisional wound, and removing the drain within 48 hours.

Mrs. Rodriguez undergoes a successful transcystic laparoscopic CBD exploration. After closure of the cystic duct and control of the cystic artery, the surgeon dissects the gallbladder off the liver bed. During this procedure, the gallbladder is punctured and bile and stones are spilled. The young scrub nurse and the medical students are aghast.

What is the significance of this incident?
A study of 52 patients who underwent laparoscopic cholecystectomy for acute cholecystitis did not show any increase in early complications after intraoperative spillage of bile and stones. Other studies have had similar results (31). However, case reports of late complications after spillage of stones during laparoscopic cholecystectomy include intraabdominal abscesses, chronic suppuration of the umbilical incision secondary to entrapped infected stones, persistent abdominal wall sinuses, tracks from the port site abscesses, subhepatic inflammatory masses, cholelithoptysis, liver abscesses, and empyema. These complications present weeks or months after the original procedure. Most of them necessitate exploratory laparotomy. A recent experimental study suggests that infected bile in combination with multiple stones increases the chances of formation of intraabdominal abscesses as opposed to the spillage of stones in the absence of infected bile (38). It is recommended that if infected bile is spilled, attempts should be made to close the defect either by placing laparoscopic clips or by stitching the defect to avoid spillage of infected stones. The abdominal cavity should be thoroughly irrigated, and if the stones cannot be recovered, conversion to an open cholecystectomy should be considered.

Are there any other options for the treatment of acute cholecystitis?
In critically ill patients and those with a very high risk of developing complications due to significant associated conditions, a simple drainage of the gallbladder without removal (i.e., cholecystostomy) can be performed. With the recent advances in interventional radiology, this procedure is done under local anesthesia, percutaneously, with ultrasound guidance. Both the transhepatic and the transperitoneal approaches are safe. The response rates vary from 59 to 93%, with the morbidity rates of 0 to 18% and mortality rates of 0 to 12% (39, 40). Complications include misplacement in the colon, exacerbation of sepsis, bile leakage, and bleeding (39–41). The overall recurrence of cholecystitis is 15% (42). The procedure is thought to be definitive in patients with acalculous cholecystitis (40, 41, 43). Factors determining a good response include the presence of cholelithiasis, wall thickening, distension of the gallbladder, pericholecystic fluid, and absence of gangrene, indicating that the procedure is beneficial when the gallbladder is the source of sepsis (39, 44, 45). In patients who have a high operative risk and whose cardiorespiratory status prevents elective surgery, the procedure can be combined with contact dissolution with MTBE or with percutaneous extraction of the stones (40, 46).

The defect in the wall of the gallbladder is repaired with laparoscopic clips, and the peritoneal cavity is copiously irrigated after the cholecystectomy is completed. No stones are left in the abdomen. Approximately 36 hours after completion of the laparoscopic cholecystectomy, Mrs. Rodriguez is still complaining of significant abdominal pain and nausea. The abdomen is moderately distended and somewhat tender. She has a low-grade fever, her white blood cell count is 12,000/mm^3, and her bilirubin level is 1.9 mg/dL.

What is the differential diagnosis of these findings?
The differential diagnosis includes postoperative pancreatitis, retained CBD stone, cystic duct leak, accessory duct leak, and injury to the bile ducts. Bile leaks usually present 5.3 plus or minus 4.2 days after laparoscopic cholecystectomy. Manifestations, which are nonspecific, include unusual pain, nausea, vomiting, fever, and tenderness (47). Most bile leaks are from the cystic duct (77% of cases); 31% of patients with a cystic duct leak have a retained stone (47). Leaks from accessory bile ducts after cholecystectomy are also well known (discussed earlier).

The amylase and the lipase levels are normal. What should be the next step in management of Mrs. Rodriguez?
The HIDA scan has a very good sensitivity and specificity for the diagnosis of bile leakage after laparoscopic cholecystectomy (48, 49). Both ultrasound and CT are very good in diagnosing intraabdominal collections. The relative roles of these three tests have not been well defined in the literature. If any of these tests are positive, ERCP should be performed to confirm the leak, identify the site and the cause, and plan the management. Minor leaks usually respond to sphincterotomy, bile duct stenting, or nasobiliary drainage. Percutaneous drainage of a biloma or of peritoneal bile is also indicated in these situations. In more severe injuries with intact ducts, endoscopic dilation and stenting may be useful in closing the leaks or preventing strictures.

For more severe injuries involving the CBD, a multidisciplinary approach that includes the interventional radiologist, the endoscopist, and the surgeon is always necessary (50–54). The best results are obtained when the injury is recognized early during surgery and is immediately repaired. For a surgical approach to CBD injury, hepaticojejunostomy seems to have a better outcome than primary end-to-end repair (54).

A HIDA scan raised suspicion of a bile leak. Mrs. Rodriguez underwent ERCP and sphincterotomy with stent placement combined with percutaneous drainage of a large biloma. She was found to have a leak from a patent cystic duct. The drainage decreased 5 days later, and a repeat HIDA scan showed no leakage. She was discharged.

What should be done if the pathology report reveals cancer of the gallbladder?
There are numerous reports of implantation of the cancer in the trocar sites and of peritoneal dissemination with manipulation of the gallbladder during laparoscopic cholecystectomy. It has been suggested that the risk is higher than with open cholecystectomy (52, 55, 56). If the cancer is confined to the mucosa of the organ and the gallbladder was removed intact, laparoscopic cholecystectomy may be sufficient. If the malignancy invades the wall or if the gallbladder was torn during the procedure, the patient should undergo laparotomy, local reexcision, and excision of the trocar sites (52). However, gallbladder cancer is found among the elderly, and the prognosis is extremely poor. An honest and open discussion of the value of additional surgery should be held with the patient.

Is laparoscopic cholecystectomy safe during pregnancy?
Recent reports of small numbers of patients suggest that laparoscopic cholecystectomy may be safe during pregnancy (57–59). Only a recent study of a small number of patients suggests otherwise (60). This study reports four fetal deaths among seven pregnant women who underwent laparoscopic procedures. Of the seven patients, three had acute appendicitis, three had gallstone pancreatitis, and one had acute cholecystitis. Postulated risks include trocar injury to the uterus, decreased uterine blood flow, premature labor from the increased intraabdominal pressure, and increased fetal acidosis (61). The Society of American Gastrointestinal and Endoscopic Surgeons recommends the following maneuvers to enhance safety of the procedure: defer the intervention until the second trimester of pregnancy; use pneumatic compression devices to prevent deep venous thrombosis; continuously monitor the fetal heart rate and maternal end-tidal carbon dioxide level; protect the fetus with a lead shield over the lower abdomen if intraoperative cholangiogram is planned; use the open technique for access to the abdomen; use the partial (15 to 30°) left decubitus position to shift the uterus off the vena cava; maintain the intraabdominal pressure at 8 to 12 mm Hg; and always obtain an obstetric consultation before operating (61).

Giles Sampson is a 73-year-old man who goes to the emergency department complaining of abdominal pain that started 3 days ago. It is now in the right upper quadrant. It is not associated with meals and does not respond to antacids. He states that he had a temperature of 38.3°C and that he has felt chills intermittently. He reports dark urine during the past 2 days. The patient had a laparoscopic cholecystectomy 2 years ago for acute cholecystitis.

What do the symptoms and history suggest?
These symptoms suggest acute cholangitis. With the history of a laparoscopic cholecystectomy, the patient may have a retained stone or an iatrogenic bile duct stricture.

What is Charcot's triad?
Charcot's triad is fever, right upper quadrant abdominal pain, and jaundice. It was described in 1987 by Jean M. Charcot, a French neurologist. Approximately 70% of patients describe three symptoms: 80 to 95% have fever; 80 to 86%, jaundice; and 67 to 80%, pain (62–64). Pain has become less common because of the increased incidence of cholangitis with obstruction of percutaneous draining biliary catheters and internal biliary stents. Pain is usually seen with cholangitis because of stones (65).

Physical examination reveals a well-developed and well-nourished man in no apparent distress. He is mildly tachycardic. His temperature is 38°C. The patient has jaundiced sclerae. Examination of the abdomen reveals a soft, nondistended abdomen that is mildly tender in the right upper quadrant. There are no peritoneal signs or palpable masses. Rectal examination shows guaiac-negative stools. Laboratory data show a total bilirubin level of 13.8 mg/dL, alkaline phosphatase level of 381 mIU/mL, SGPT of 126 mIU/mL, SGOT of 101 mIU/mL, and a lactate dehydrogenase level of 122 mIU/mL. The white blood cell count is 20,800/mm³.

What is the pathophysiology of acute cholangitis?
Three key elements are necessary for the development of acute cholangitis: bacteriobilia, biliary stasis, and obstruction. The bile can be contaminated during percutaneous procedures, endoscopy, and biliary bypass procedures. Reflux through the ampulla of Vater has also been postulated. Bacteria also can reach the bile through lymphatics, arterial circulation, and the portal venous circulation.

What causes the sepsis in acute cholangitis?
The biliary obstruction increases the intraluminal pressure in the bile ducts. With the increased pressure, bacteria regurgitate into the lymphatics and the portal system. From there, the infection enters the systemic circulation. With obstruction, the pressure is higher than 200 mm Hg. These pressures can easily be increased during percutaneous or endoscopic cholangiography (65).

How frequently is bacteriobilia present?
Bile has been found to be colonized in 20 to 40% of cases of cholelithiasis, 90% of cases of choledocholithiasis, and 12 to 20% of cases of malignant obstruction (65).

What is the most common cause of bile duct obstruction?
The most common cause is secondary stones from the gallbladder. Other causes
of obstruction are primary bile duct stones; benign strictures caused by surgical procedures, congenital pathologies, or rare conditions such as sclerosing
cholangitis; malignant strictures; pancreatitis, both acute and chronic; extrinsic
compression such as in Mirizzi's syndrome; parasites; and obstructed biliary
stents or percutaneous catheters.

What is the most common malignant obstruction?
Carcinoma of the head of the pancreas is the most common malignant obstruction. Other malignant causes are ampullary carcinoma, bile duct adenocarcinoma, duodenal carcinoma, and gallbladder carcinoma.

How are the CBD stones classified?
They are generally classified as primary or secondary. Primary stones are formed
de novo in the bile duct. They are usually soft, smooth, yellowish tan, and not
formed of cholesterol. They often conform to the shape of the bile duct. They
are usually formed in the presence of biliary stasis and bacterial contamination.
Production of β-glucuronidase by the organisms catalyzes the hydrolysis of
bilirubin diglucuronide to unconjugated bilirubin, which binds to calcium to
form insoluble calcium bilirubinate. Secondary stones are formed in the gallbladder and pass to the CBD through the cystic duct or via a fistulous communication (66).

What organisms are most commonly found in the bile of patients with acute cholangitis?
Most patients are infected with gut organisms, the most common being *Escherichia coli* and Klebsiella. *Streptococcus faecalis* have been common in the past,
but Enterococcus is now the most common gram-positive organism seen in biliary tract infections. Increasing numbers of cultures show Enterobacter,
Pseudomonas, and Serratia. The most common anaerobes are the Bacteroides.
Approximately 50% of patients have more than one organism. Fungal infections are rare, but fungi are occasionally found in diabetics and in patients with
enterobiliary stents. More patients have recently had recurrent cholangitis related to occluded stents and percutaneous drainage catheters. This has caused a
shift toward resistant organisms (65).

What are the characteristic laboratory findings in patients with acute cholangitis?
There is elevation of the total bilirubin, direct bilirubin, alkaline phosphatase,
SGOT, and SGPT. These enzymes begin to rise within an hour of the onset
of obstruction and continue to rise for weeks. The increase in serum bilirubin
results from blockage of excretion, and alkaline phosphatase rises because of increased synthesis of the enzyme by the canalicular epithelium. Consequently,
serum alkaline phosphatase may be elevated, but bilirubin may be normal or

slightly elevated in partial obstruction. The elevation of alkaline phosphatase is out of proportion to that of SGOT and SGPT. Blood cultures are positive in 25% of patients.

What is Courvoisier's law?
Courvoisier's law states that when the CBD is obstructed by a stone, dilation of the gallbladder is rare, but when it is obstructed in another way, dilation is common. For example, obstructive jaundice due to a CBD stone is not associated with a palpable mass in the right upper quadrant (i.e., a distended gallbladder) because the organ is either scarred from chronic inflammation or surgically removed. However, in patients with periampullary cancer, the jaundice is associated with a palpable mass because the gallbladder is dilated without scarring.

A diagnosis of acute cholangitis is made according to the history, physical examination, and laboratory tests.

What additional test may be useful at this point?
An ultrasound of the upper abdomen can differentiate obstructive from nonobstructive lesions with an accuracy of 99% for showing dilated bile ducts (64). Cholescintigraphy is not generally useful for cholangitis because the degree of anatomic precision needed to plan the treatment of this condition is not attainable with this technique (65).

What other tests are useful for this condition?
CT is complementary to ultrasound. It is excellent for the detection of dilated ducts, and it is very useful in cholangitis caused by malignancy because it may detect pancreatic masses, adenopathy, or liver metastases. Direct cholangiography via percutaneous technique or endoscopy provides essential diagnostic and anatomic information for determining the source of cholangitis and for treating the cause of obstruction (65).

An ultrasound of the right upper quadrant reveals a dilated CBD. This is followed by CT of the abdomen. There are no pancreatic masses, and there are no abscesses or metastases in the liver. Both the extrahepatic and intrahepatic bile ducts are dilated. The patient is admitted to a general surgical floor.

What is the initial approach to the management of a patient with cholangitis?
First and foremost is to support the patient hemodynamically and treat the infection. Intravenous administration of fluids and ascertainment of adequate urine output are essential. Antibiotics that are effective on the biliary tract organisms are started immediately. The secondary aspect of management is to find the underlying cause of obstruction.

**Upon admission to the ward, Mr. Sampson's fever rises to 39.1°C. In-
travenous fluids and antibiotics are started immediately.**

What is the likelihood that the infection will be controlled by hydration and antibiotics?
Approximately 70 to 85% of patients with cholangitis respond to antibiotics and
hydration. However, 15% progress to a more severe form of cholangitis with
continued sepsis, shock, and central nervous system depression (64). Patients
with malignancy respond to antibiotics alone in fewer than 50% of cases (65).

What is Reynolds' pentad?
Reynolds' pentad is mental status deterioration and severe shock in addition to
the right upper quadrant pain, jaundice, and fever traditionally seen in patients
with cholangitis.

What are the different types of cholangitis?
Ascending cholangitis has a wide spectrum of clinical manifestations depending on the location and the type of obstruction. Acute nonsuppurative cholangitis generally is the milder clinical presentation, which is commonly caused by
partial obstruction of the biliary tract. Usually responsive to antibiotics, nonsuppurative cholangitis is most often seen with benign strictures, sclerosing
cholangitis, extrinsic compression of the CBD, and CBD stones.

Acute toxic cholangitis ("suppurative" cholangitis) is a more aggressive process,
usually caused by complete or nearly complete obstruction of the biliary tract,
resulting in pus under pressure. Even when treated with systemic antibiotics,
patients with suppurative cholangitis manifest a rapidly deteriorating condition,
leading to high fever, hyperbilirubinemia greater than 4 mg/dL, septic shock,
and eventual death if not treated (62). Reynolds' pentad of symptoms is associated with this form of the disease. Cholangiohepatitis, also known as recurrent pyogenic cholangitis, is endemic to the Orient. It is a chronic, recurrent
form of the disease characterized by intrahepatic stones, strictures, and infection. These patients also develop hepatic abscesses. The principles of management include delineation of ductal anatomy, extraction of stones, drainage of
strictured segments, and resection of badly damaged liver parenchyma (66).

Sclerosing cholangitis is a progressive disease that causes inflammation and fibrosis of the bile ducts. It can involve the intrahepatic and extrahepatic segments of the biliary tract. It is thought to be immune related, and it is well documented in the setting of ulcerative colitis.

AIDS-related cholangiopathy is characterized by right upper quadrant and epigastric pain, cholestasis and dilated bile ducts, diffuse abnormalities on imaging
of the biliary tree, papillary stenosis, and abnormal liver function tests. In 75%

of cases, an opportunistic infection can be identified. In patients with biliary disease, pain is often relieved by endoscopic sphincterotomy, whereas cholecystectomy provides pain relief in patients with acalculous cholecystitis (67, 68).

What is the appropriate treatment of progressively worsening ascending cholangitis?
Acute toxic cholangitis is treated with intravenous antibiotics and aggressive fluid therapy guided by monitoring of central pressures and cardiopulmonary indices to attain good tissue perfusion. Vasopressor medication may be necessary to achieve this goal. However, aggressive intensive care management should not delay the mainstay of treatment, which is the emergency decompression of the biliary obstruction.

On the morning after admission, the patient's fever spiked to 39.4°C, and his blood pressure fell to 70/30 mm Hg. The patient was transferred to the intensive care unit and was resuscitated aggressively. The blood pressure returned to 110/60 mm Hg, and preparations were made for emergency decompression of the biliary tract.

What are the modalities of emergency biliary duct decompression?
The three modalities are percutaneous transhepatic cholangiography (PTC), ERCP, and surgical decompression. The choice of modality depends on the level of expertise of the operator, the degree of dilation of the bile ducts, the location and cause of the obstruction, and any previous surgical procedures (e.g., biliary enteric bypasses and gastric resections).

ERCP is the preferred method for emergency decompression for impacted CBD stones, for suspected proximal malignancies, and for nondilated bile ducts. A prospective randomized study comparing ERCP with surgical emergency decompression showed a lower mortality rate for ERCP (10 versus 32%; $P < 0.03$). Fewer patients in the ERCP group needed ventilatory support (12 versus 26 patients; $P < 0.005$), and residual stones were significantly less frequent (3 versus 12, $P = 0.03$) (69). A stent or a nasobiliary drainage tube can be left until definitive treatment is carried out.

Complications include bleeding (2%), pancreatitis (5%), and perforation. The rate of complications after sphincterotomy is related to the indications for the procedure (e.g., dysfunction of sphincter of Oddi and cirrhosis) and to the endoscopic technique (e.g., difficulty in cannulating the bile duct, achievement of access to the bile duct by precut sphincterotomy, and use of combined percutaneous-endoscopic procedure) (69, 70).

PTC is preferred in cases of proximal obstruction with dilated ducts and in patients whose anatomy has been disrupted by previous biliary enteric bypass or gastric resections. Advantages include simplicity and safety, no need for general anesthesia, and a high rate of success. Possible complications include bacteremia, bile leak, formation of cholangiovenous communications, and blockage of the drainage catheter. The incidence of immediate complications is approximately 2 to 5% (65).

Surgical decompression in the presence of severe cholangitis with sepsis and coagulopathy carries reported mortality rates of 20 to 60% (69). It is now reserved for patients for whom ERCP and PTC are unavailable or were unsuccessful. A CBD exploration is carried out initially, and a T-tube is left in the CBD to allow drainage of the infected bile and to have a port of access for later study of the biliary tract. The role of laparoscopic CBD exploration in acute cholangitis has not been defined. Laparoscopic cholecystectomy after endoscopic clearance of CBD stones is recommended in the presence of cholelithiasis and if the patient has no significant operative risks.

The surgical options for formal decompression of the biliary tract are transduodenal sphincteroplasty, choledochoduodenostomy, and choledochojejunostomy. A formal surgical decompression is absolutely indicated in patients with primary CBD stones because stasis plays a significant role in the pathogenesis of these stones (66, 71). These procedures also have been recommended for recurrent stones after a second CBD exploration, multiple large stones, and stones in the hepatic ducts. A recent randomized study showed no difference in morbidity, mortality, and long-term results between choledochoduodenostomy and choledochojejunostomy. Choledochoduodenostomy may be preferable because it is technically easier and permits easy access for further endoscopic exploration or treatment if necessary (72).

What are the treatment options for benign strictures and for intrahepatic stones with recurrent cholangitis?
These conditions require a close interaction between surgeons, interventional radiologists, and endoscopists. ERCP can be used to define the anatomy and to stent distal lesions in the biliary tract. This modality has been particularly useful for the treatment of strictures after repairs of laparoscopic injuries of the bile ducts. PTC is used for definition of the anatomy and for definitive or adjunctive treatment. Radiologic treatment options include dilation of strictures, stent placement, and transhepatic cholangioscopy with lithotripsy or lithotomy (73, 74). The interventional radiologist can place transhepatic catheters through strictures that surgeons can use as guides for locating the lesion and stenting biliary enteric bypasses. The principles of successful repair of biliary strictures are exposure of healthy proximal bile ducts that provide drainage to the entire liver; preparation of a suitable segment of intestine that can be brought to the area of the stricture without tension, most frequently a Roux-en-Y jejunal

Management Algorithm for Presumed Acute Cholecystitis

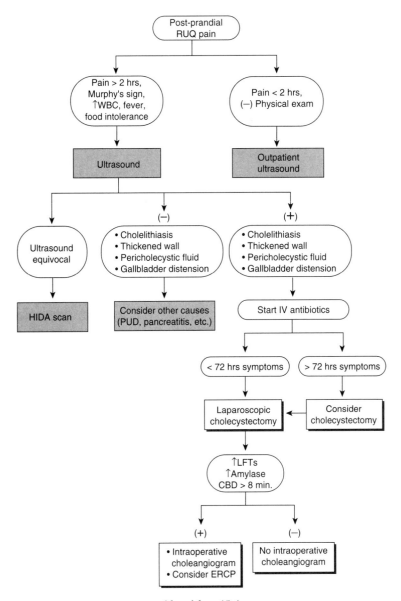

Algorithm 15.1.

limb; and creation of a direct biliary enteric mucosal-to-mucosal anastomosis. Excellent long-term results can be achieved in 70 to 90% of cases. Approximately two-thirds of restrictures are evident within 2 years, and 90% are seen within 7 years (75).

Mr. Sampson had a successful ERCP and sphincteroplasty. He was found to have a retained stone from his previous laparoscopic cholecystectomy. No abnormalities of the bile ducts were identified. His overall condition improved with the antibiotics, and he was discharged a week after admission.

REFERENCES

1. Gieugiu DIN, Roslyn JJ. Calculous biliary disease. In: Greenfield LJ et al., ed. Surgery: Scientific Principles and Practice. 2nd ed. Philadelphia: Lippincott-Raven, 1997.
2. Cuschieri A. Acute and chronic cholecystitis. In: Cameron JL. Current Surgical Therapy. 5th ed. St. Louis: Mosby, 1995.
3. Jazrawi RP, Pazzi P, Petroni ML, et al. Post prandial gallbladder motor function: refilling and turnover of bile in health and in cholelithiasis. Gastroenterology 1995;109:582.
4. Soper NJ. Biliary anatomy and physiology. In: Greenfield LJ et al. Surgery: Scientific Principles and Practice. 2nd ed. Philadelphia: Lippincott-Raven, Philadelphia, 1997.
5. Janowitz P, Klatzer W, Zemnler T, et al. Gallbladder sludge: spontaneous course and incidence of complications in patients without stones. Hepatology 1994;20:291.
6. McSherry CK, Ferstenberg H, Calhoun WF, et al. The natural history of diagnosed gallstone disease in symptomatic and asymptomatic patients. Ann Surg 1985;202:59.
7. Friedman GD, Raviola CA, Fireman B, et al. Prognosis of gallstones with mild or no symptoms: 25 years of follow up in a health maintenance organization. J Clin Epidemiol 1989;42:127.
8. Gracie WA, Ransohoff DF. The natural history of silent gallstones. Gastroenterology 1981;80:1161.
9. Del Favero G, Caroli A, Meggiato T, et al. Natural history of gallstones in non-insulin dependent diabetes mellitus: a prospective 5-year follow up. Dig Dis Sci 1994;39:1704.
10. Aucott JN, Cooper GS, Bloom AD, et al. Management of gallstones in diabetic patients. Arch Intern Med 1993;153:1053.
11. Adamek HE, Jorg S, Bachor OA, et al. Symptoms of post-extracorporeal shock wave lithotripsy: long-term analysis of gallstone patients before and after successful shock wave lithotripsy. Am J Gastroenterol 1995;90:1125.
12. Sackmann M, Niller H, Klueppelberg U, et al. Gallstone recurrence after shock-wave therapy. Gastroenterology 1994;106:225.
13. Pauletzki J, Althaus R, Holl J, et al. Gallbladder emptying and gallstone formation: a prospective study on gallstone recurrence. Gastroenterology 1996;111:765.
14. Pauletzki J. Gallstone recurrence after direct contact dissolution with methyl tert-butyl ether. Dig Dis Sci 1995;40:1775.
15. Nahrwold DL. Gallstone lithotripsy. Am J Surg 1993;165:431.
16. Russell JC, Walsh SJ, Maltie AS, et al. Bile duct injuries 1989–93: a state-wide experience. Connecticut Laparoscopic Cholecystectomy Registry. Arch Surg 1996;131:382.

17. Kullman E, Borch K, Lindstrom E, et al. Value of routinely intraoperative cholangiography in detecting aberrant bile ducts and bile duct injuries during laparoscopic cholecystectomy. Br J Surg 1996;83:171.
18. Singer AJ, McCracken G, Henry MC, et al. Correlation among clinical, laboratory, and hepatobiliary scanning findings in patients with suspected acute cholecystitis. Ann Emerg Med 1996;28:267.
19. Gruber PJ, Silverman RA, Gottesfeld S, et al. Presence of fever and leukocytosis in acute cholecystitis. Ann Emerg Med 1996;28:273.
20. Cooperberg PL, Gibney RG. Imaging of the gallbladder. Radiology 1987;163:605.
21. Fink-Bennett D, Freitas JE, Ripley SD, et al. The sensitivity of hepatobiliary imaging and real-time ultrasonography in the detection of acute cholecystitis. Arch Surg 1985;120:904.
22. Ferrucci J. The radiological diagnosis of gallbladder disease. Radiology 1980;141:49.
23. Kim CK. Pharmacologic intervention for the diagnosis of acute cholecystitis: cholecystokinin pretreatment or morphine, or both? J Nucl Med 1997;38:647.
24. Chen CC, Holder LE, Maunoury C, et al. Morphine augmentation increases gallbladder visualization in patients pre treated with cholecystokinin. J Nucl Med 1997;38:644.
25. Nahrwold DL. The biliary system. In: Sabiston DC, ed. Textbook of Surgery. 13th ed. Philadelphia: WB Saunders, 1986.
26. Hakala T. Microangiopathy in acute acalculous cholecystitis. Br J Surg 1997;84:1249.
27. Eldar S. Laparoscopic cholecystectomy for acute cholecystitis: prospective trial. World J Surg 1997;21:540.
28. Garber SM. Early laparoscopic cholecystectomy for acute cholecystitis. Surg Endosc 1997;11:347.
29. Coo KP, Thirlby RC. Laparoscopic cholecystectomy in acute cholecystitis: what is the optimal timing for operation? Arch Surg 1996;131:540.
30. Unger SW, Rosenbaum G, Unger HM, et al. A comparison of laparoscopic and open treatment of acute cholecystitis. Surg Endosc 1993;7:408.
31. Rattner DW, Ferguson C, Warshaw AL. Factors associated with successful laparoscopic cholecystectomy for acute cholecystitis. Ann Surg 1993;217:233.
32. Diez J, Arozamena CJ, Ferraina P, et al. Relation between postoperative infections and gallbladder bile leakage during laparoscopic cholecystectomy. Surg Endosc 1996;10:529.
33. MacFadyen BV, Passi RB. The role of endoscopic retrograde cholangiopancreatography in the area of laparoscopic cholecystectomy. Semin Laparosc Cholecystect Semin Laparosc Surg 1997;4:18.
34. Schwartz SI. Gallbladder and exerbiliary system. In: Schwartz SI et al., ed. Principles of Surgery. 4th ed. New York: McGraw-Hill, 1984.
35. Johnson AB, Hunter JG. Future treatment of common bile duct stones. Semin Laparosc Surg 1997;4:45.
36. Petelin JB. Techniques and cost of common bile duct exploration. Semin Laparosc Surg 1997;4:23.
37. King ML, String ST. Extent of choledoscopic utilization in common bile duct exploration. Am J Surg 1983;146:322.
38. Zorluoglu A, Ozguc H, Yilmazlar T, et al. Is it necessary to retrieve dropped gallstones during laparoscopic cholecystectomy? Surg Endosc 1997;11:64.
39. England RE, McDermott VG, Smith TP, et al. Percutaneous cholecystostomy: who responds? AJR Am J Roentgenol 1997;168:1247.

40. Vauthey JN, Lerur J, Martini M, et al. Indications and limitations of percutaneous cholecystostomy for acute cholecystitis. Surg Obstet Gynecol 1993;176:49.

41. Boland GW, Lee MJ, Leung J, et al. Percutaneous cholecystostomy in critically ill patients: early response and final outcome in 82 patients. AJR Am J Roentgenol 1994; 163:339.

42. Hamy A, Visset J, Likholatnikov D, et al. Percutaneous cholecystostomy for acute cholecystitis in critically ill patients. Surgery 1997;121:398.

43. van Overhagen H, Meyers H, Tylanus HW, et al. Percutaneous cholecystostomy for patients with acute cholecystitis and an increased surgical risk. Cardiovasc Intervent Radiol 1996;19:72.

44. Hultman CS, Hergst CA, McCall JM, et al. The efficacy of percutaneous cholecystostomy in critically ill patients. Am Surg 1996;62:263.

45. Lo LD, Vogelzang RL, Braun MA, et al. Percutaneous cholecystostomy for the diagnosis and treatment of acute calculous and acalculous cholecystitis. J Vasc Intervent Radiol 1995;6:629.

46. Hamy A, Visset J, Likholatnikov D, et al. Percutaneous cholecystostomy for acute cholecystitis in critically ill patients. Surgery 1997;121:398.

47. Barkun AN, Rezieg M, Mehta SN, et al. Postcholecystectomy biliary leaks in the laparoscopic era: risk factors, presentation, and management. McGill Gallstones Treatment Group. Gastrointest Endosc 1997;45:277.

48. Mirza DF, Narsimhan KL, Ferraznet BH, et al. Bile duct injury following laparoscopic cholecystectomy: referral pattern and management. Br J Surg 1997;84:786.

49. Sandoval BA, Goettler CE, Robinson AV, et al. Cholescintigraphy in the diagnosis of bile leak after laparoscopic cholecystectomy. Am Surg 1997;63:611.

50. Ponsky JL. Endoscopic approaches to common bile duct injuries. Surg Clin North Am 1996;76:505.

51. Barton JR, Russell RC, Hatfield AR, et al. Management of bile leaks after laparoscopic cholecystectomy. Br J Surg 1995;82:780.

52. Barthel J, Scheider D. Advantages of sphincterotomy and nasal biliary tube drainage in the treatment of cystic duct stump leak complicating laparoscopic cholecystectomy. Am J Gastroenterol 1995;90:1322.

53. Raijman I, Catalano MF, Hirsch GS, et al. Endoscopic treatment of biliary leakage after laparoscopic cholecystectomy. Endoscopy 1994;26:741.

54. Gough D, Donohue JH. Characteristics of biliary tract complications during laparoscopic cholecystectomy: a multi-institutional study. Am J Surg 1994;167:27.

55. Jacobi CA, Keller H, Monig S, et al. Implantation of metastases of unsuspected gallbladder carcinoma after laparoscopy. Surg Endosc 1995;9:351.

56. Copher JC, Rogers JJ, Dalton ML. Trocar-site metastasis following laparoscopic cholecystectomy for unsuspected carcinoma of the gallbladder: case report and review of the literature. Surg Endosc 1995;9:348.

57. Eichenberg BJ, Vanderlinden J, Miguel C, et al. Laparoscopic cholecystectomy in the third trimester of pregnancy. Am Surg 1996;62:874.

58. Martin IJ, Dexter SP, McMahon MJ. Laparoscopic cholecystectomy in pregnancy: a safe option during the second trimester? Surg Endosc 1996;10:508.

59. Wishner JD, Zolfaghari D, Wohlgemuth SD, et al. Laparoscopic cholecystectomy in pregnancy: a report of six cases and review of literature. Surg Endosc 1996;10:314.

60. Amos JD, Schorr SJ, Norman PF, et al. Laparoscopic surgery during pregnancy. Am J Surg 1996;171:435.
61. Guidelines for laparoscopic surgery during pregnancy. Society of American Gastrointestinal Endoscopic Surgeons. Surg Endosc 1998;12:189–190.
62. Boey HA, Way LW. Acute Cholangitis. Ann Surg 1980;191:264.
63. O'Connor MJ, Schwartz ML, McQuarrie DG, et al. Acute bacterial cholangitis. Arch Surg 1982;117:437.
64. Sievert W, Vakil N. Emergencies of the biliary tract. Gastroenterol Clin North Am 1988;17:247.
65. Sharp KW. Acute cholangitis. In: Cameron JL. Current Surgical Therapy. 5th ed. St. Louis: Mosby, 1995.
66. Roslyn JJ, Zinner MJ. Gallbladder and extrahepatic biliary system. In: Schwartz SI, et al. Principles of Surgery. 6th ed. New York: McGraw-Hill, 1994.
67. Nash JA, Cohen SA. Gallbladder and biliary tract disease in AIDS. Gastroenterol Clin North Am 1997;26:323.
68. Ducreux M, Buffet C, Lamy P, et al. Diagnosis and prognosis of AIDS-related cholangitis. AIDS 1995;9:875.
69. Lai EC, Mok FP, Tan ES, et al. Endoscopic biliary drainage for severe acute cholangitis. N Engl J Med 1992;326:1582.
70. Freeman ML, Nelson DB, Sherman S, et al. Complications of endoscopic biliary sphincterotomy. N Engl J Med 1996;335:909.
71. Giurgiu DIN, Roslyn JJ. Calculous biliary disease. In: Greenfield LJ et al., ed. Surgery: Scientific Principles and Practice. 2nd ed. Philadelphia: Lippincott-Raven, 1997.
72. Panis Y, Faguiez PL, Brisser D, et al. Long term results of choledochoduodenostomy versus choledochojejunostomy for choledocholithiasis. French Association for Surgical Research. Surg Gynecol Obstet 1993;177:33.
73. Yeh YH, Huang MH, Yang JC, et al. Percutaneous trans-hepatic cholangioscopy and lithotripsy in the treatment of intrahepatic stones: a study with 5 years follow-up. Gastrointest Endosc 1995;42:13.
74. Jan YY, Chen MF. Percutaneous trans-hepatic cholangioscopic lithotomy for hepatolithiasis: long-term results. Gastrointest Endosc 1995;42:1.
75. Lillemoe KD. Biliary strictures and sclerosing cholangitis. In: Greenfield LJ et al., ed. Surgery: Scientific Principles and Practice. 2nd ed. Philadelphia: Lippincott-Raven, 1997.

Liver Disease: Portal Hypertension

Jeffrey L. Kaufman

Henry Norman is a 60-year-old man who goes to the emergency department because of intermittent vomiting of bright red blood over the previous 4 hours. Until the bleeding started, he felt normal. His bowel movements are normal in consistency, and both stool and urine have normal color. He felt weak and slightly dizzy when moving around his house before the vomiting started. After vomiting, he laid down and could not get up to go to the bathroom to vomit again. He has no history of peptic ulcer disease. He has smoked 1 to 1.5 packs per day for years and, for most of his working life, has drunk a fifth of vodka every 2 days or consumed two six-packs of beer after work. He had jaundice once in his youth; a physician attributed it to hepatitis. He is a metal fabricator and has not missed work because of accidents or binge drinking; he has never had a drunk driving violation. His father was said to be alcoholic and died of liver failure at age 57. His siblings are alive and well, and none of them use alcohol.

Mr. Norman is a thin man who appears chronically ill. His vital signs are as follows: respiratory rate, 24 breaths per minute; supine pulse rate, 142 beats per minute; supine blood pressure, 80/45 mm Hg; and body temperature, normal. The muscles of his arms and temporal fossae appear wasted, his sclerae are mildly icteric, and there are prominent telangiectases over the nose and cheeks. The chest and cardiac examination are normal, but the abdominal examination reveals mild tympany. The liver edge is firm and is at the right costal margin. There is no visceral tenderness to palpation. The stool is dark, tarry, and guaiac positive. The genitalia are those of a normal man, but the testes are atrophic. His femoral pulses are 2+, but popliteal and pedal pulses are absent. His fingers reveal yellow staining of the right index and middle fingernails, and he is right-handed. He has no asterixis. He is unable to produce a urine sample.

What are the key findings of the initial evaluation and treatment of Mr. Norman?
Mr. Norman's history indicates a recent and perhaps ongoing hemorrhage. Acute blood loss is indicated by the history and vital signs, which are best explained by severe hypovolemia. A priority is to resuscitate by placing large-bore intravenous lines and rapidly infusing isotonic saline solution. Blood should be drawn for typing and cross-matching. Additional tests include a complete blood count, platelet count, clotting studies (prothrombin time and partial thromboplastin time), and determination of electrolyte, blood urea nitrogen, and creatinine levels. Because of his history, liver function should be studied, including determination of albumin, total protein, bilirubin, alkaline phosphatase, aspartate transaminase, and alanine transaminase. The amylase level should also be checked.

What are the end points for volume infusion?
The pulse rate, blood pressure, and urine formation should be evaluated. If the ability to urinate is in doubt, a Foley catheter should be placed to guide resuscitation.

What is the role of vasopressors in this patient?
Mr. Norman should not be treated with vasopressors because the hypovolemia is caused by hemorrhage; the shock is therefore treated with volume resuscitation, including blood transfusion when cross-matched blood is available.

Mr. Norman responds to infusion of 1.5 L saline: his pulse decreases to 115 beats per minute, and his blood pressure increases to 122/75 mm Hg. A nasogastric tube is passed, and lavage with warm saline partially clears clots and liquid blood with repeated rinses. Some of the rinses appear stained with bile.

What is the differential diagnosis for this patient?
The most likely diagnosis is gastric or duodenal ulceration with bleeding. Other possibilities include gastritis with bleeding, portal hypertension with esophageal varices that have hemorrhaged, gastric variceal bleeding from portal hypertension, bleeding from gastric varices as a result of splenic vein thrombosis, gastric or duodenal neoplasm with extrahepatic portal obstruction, Mallory-Weiss tear with hemorrhage, esophagitis with bleeding, and a myeloproliferative disorder with sclerosis of the portal system (1).

Despite the patient's history of alcohol consumption, peptic ulcer disease remains highest on the list, because it accounts for half to two-thirds of cases of upper gastrointestinal (GI) bleeding. Gastritis accounts for another 15% of cases (2).

Mr. Norman's initial laboratory tests show the following results: hematocrit, 21%; platelet count, 55,000/mL; sodium, 147 mEq/L; potassium,

3.7 mEq/L; chloride, 101 mEq/L; CO_2, normal; blood urea nitrogen, 35 mg/dL; creatinine, 1.8 mg/dL; prothrombin time, 16 seconds (international normalized ratio, 1.4); partial thromboplastin time, 44 seconds. The chest radiograph is normal. He continues to retch and vomit blood.

What diagnostic study should be performed next?
Upper GI endoscopy should be performed as soon as possible.

Mr. Norman is given 3 U of blood. His blood pressure stabilizes at 120/75 mm Hg, his pulse is maintained at 75 to 85 beats per minute, and he begins voiding urine. He undergoes upper GI endoscopy, which reveals active bleeding from large esophageal varices.

What therapeutic options should the endoscopist consider?
Endoscopic sclerotherapy should be performed if possible. The technique of sclerotherapy is to visualize the varices directly and to inject a sclerosant in and around them. As early as 1939, Crafoord considered using specially modified rigid esophagoscopes to inject esophageal varices with material that would cause them to scar and thrombose (3). The procedure did not become prominent because of its technical difficulty in comparison with shunting, but when fiberoptic endoscopes became clinically available in the 1970s, it was revived. Because of its ease, most centers used sclerotherapy as the main procedure for early control of bleeding varices, especially in poor-risk patients (4).

Agents available for sclerotherapy in the United States include sodium morrhuate and ethanolamine oleate. The procedure is successful in the initial control of bleeding varices in 80 to 90% of patients, in combination with other measures for medical management. In patients with acute bleeding, such as Mr. Norman, technical success depends on a clear view of the site of hemorrhage without interference from bleeding sites or persistent blood in the gastroesophageal lumen. Bleeding from gastric varices is more difficult to control with sclerotherapy because the stomach cannot be fixated for injection and because there are more veins that can bleed. Gastropathy from portal hypertension, including submucosal hyperemia, cannot be treated with sclerotherapy (5). The outcome is influenced by the Child classification of the patient at the time of sclerotherapy (6). An alternative surgical procedure, early portacaval shunting, has produced better results in the short- and long-term management of people with bleeding varices than has sclerotherapy (7). Additional studies favorably compare esophageal transection with sclerotherapy for control of acute bleeding (8).

What causes esophageal varices?
In normal conditions, blood flows through the portal veins under low pressure (less than 10 mm Hg), which is consistent with the low resistance in the portal

circulation of the liver. Significant increases in portal venous blood flow can be accommodated (e.g., during digestion) without an increase in portal venous pressure. In a diseased liver, with alteration of the microscopic portal architecture, obstruction to portal venous flow leads to elevation of portal venous pressure. The physiologic response to this rise in pressure is the formation of alternative channels for blood flow from the intestine to the central venous system, which bypass the liver altogether. These varices occur in the retroperitoneum, along the esophagus and stomach, around the anal canal, and around the umbilicus. Patients with symptoms of portal hypertension have portal venous pressures typically higher than 20 mm Hg, sometimes higher than 40 mm Hg.

What causes portal hypertension?
The causation of portal hypertension is complex. Fibrosis of the liver, regeneration of liver nodules, and hepatocyte swelling all lead to distortion of portal architecture. The cause of rapid swings in portal pressure is uncertain. In North America and Europe, the most common cause of portal hypertension is alcoholic liver disease, or Laennec's cirrhosis. Worldwide, extrahepatic obstruction and fibrosis from schistosomiasis (bilharzia) are the leading causes. Other causes of portal hypertension include portal or splenic vein thrombosis, which can be spontaneous or iatrogenic (e.g., use of umbilical vein catheters in neonatal intensive care units was a significant cause in the past); hepatic vein or vena cava obstruction (Budd-Chiari syndrome); hypersplenism with secondary portal hypertension caused by massive increases in portal vein blood flow (the liver architecture is normal but overwhelmed).

Which findings on initial history and physical examination suggest that portal hypertension with cirrhosis is the cause of bleeding?
Alcohol abuse is common in the general population, and practitioners should therefore check for warning signs by asking each patient about the quantity of alcohol used, binge drinking if any, and any societal adverse events such as being away from work or being arrested for drunk driving (9). The physical examination often shows a general loss of muscle mass, and wasting can be severe in the end-stage patient. The liver feels firm and is often enlarged below the costal margin. Spider angiomata over the chest and upper back can occur, as can gynecomastia. Testicular atrophy is common. There are no direct signs of portal engorgement other than the rare appearance of a caput medusae from periumbilical collateral venous channels.

How are patients with portal hypertension classified in terms of prognosis?
Child classified patients with alcoholic cirrhosis in terms of the expected morbidity and mortality from surgery for portal hypertension (2). The original intent was to stratify outcomes on the basis of a worst-case analysis. This classification was later modified by Pugh (2) to provide a general classification of the

severity of disease. It describes the degree of liver damage in terms of protein synthetic function and ability to process digestive products (Table 16.1). A patient's classification is based on the worst criterion. For example, a patient who has fixed ascites but all other factors in the B group range is still placed in group C. No single test assesses liver function overall in a manner analogous to the creatinine clearance for renal function or ejection fraction for cardiac function. Other tests that describe liver function include prothrombin time as a measure of synthetic function and the bromsulphalein clearance test for ability to process products of digestion (10). A cofactor in the prognosis of these patients is alcoholic hepatitis as established by liver biopsy. Biopsy is not routinely performed for patients with portal hypertension, but when tissue is obtained, the architectural changes in the liver and the prominence of Mallory bodies correlate with the outcome of surgery (11).

Why do varices bleed?
The specific reason a patient with varices who has been stable for years suddenly hemorrhages is unknown. Portal pressure varies significantly over the day, especially with changes in the degree of inflammation of the liver. Other factors include esophageal or gastric erosion over varices. A prospective study of the predictors of bleeding from extant varices indicated that dominant risk factors are Child class, size of varices, and any abnormal markings over the varices (red wale markings) (12). Other factors that correlated with bleeding in other studies include the location of varices, other markings over the varices (cherry-red spots and hematocystic spots), color of varices, esophagitis, ascites, and prothrombin time.

Mr. Norman is admitted to the intensive care unit for stabilization. An hour later, his blood pressure falls to 90/60 mm Hg, and his heart rate increases to 120 beats per minute. He continues to pass melanotic

Table 16.1.   CHILD CLASSIFICATION OF
PATIENTS WITH CIRRHOSIS

Liver Function Patient's Status	Group A	Group B	Group C
Bilirubin (mg/dL)	<2	2–3	>3
Albumin (g/dL)	>3.5	3–3.5	<3
Ascites	None	Some (easily controlled)	Fixed
Encephalopathy	None	Minimal	Significant
Nutritional status	Normal	Adequate	Poor (muscle wasting prominent)

stools that are more copious and more liquid. He receives a bolus of crystalloid, which normalizes the blood pressure, but he continues to have tachycardia.

How should a patient such as Mr. Norman be stabilized?
Recurrence of bleeding is very common, even after technically satisfactory sclerotherapy. The patient must be resuscitated with fluids and blood products. Any coagulopathy must be corrected. Fresh frozen plasma must be administered, as must vitamin K. If the platelet count is severely depressed, platelet transfusion may be needed. If there is the slightest suspicion that alcoholism is the cause of bleeding varices, precautions against acute alcohol withdrawal syndrome must be taken. The patient should be treated with prophylactic doses of a sedative-hypnotic drug, commonly lorazepam, and be closely observed for signs of agitation or delirium. In addition, thiamine should be given to prevent Wernicke's encephalopathy.

What is the role of drugs in the control of bleeding?
For many years, vasopressin was used to control acute bleeding from esophageal varices. Octreotide is now the favored drug, because vasopressin at high doses causes coronary vasoconstriction, which may induce clinically significant myocardial ischemia, especially when there is underlying coronary artery disease. Both drugs cause vasoconstriction on the arterial side of splanchnic blood flow, which leads to reduction in portal pressure. All vasoconstrictors should be considered stopgap measures that allow control of bleeding; no drug has long-term effectiveness. Studies with systemic vasopressin show that after the drug is withdrawn, hemorrhage recurs in more than 50% of patients (13). In several controlled trials, administration of propranolol reduced long-term bleeding from esophageal varices (14–16). Some clinicians are concerned about the potential for accentuation of shock by β-blocking agents if significant rebleeding occurs in patients with esophageal varices; however, European studies have not confirmed this complication.

What are the mechanical techniques for stopping acute variceal bleeding?
A Sengstaken-Blakemore (SB) tube can be placed in the stomach and esophagus. This large-bore nasogastric tube has a 300-mL gastric balloon, a long esophageal balloon, and two aspiration ports. The tube is guided into place by fluoroscopy to ensure that the gastric balloon is safely in the stomach before it is inflated; blind placement carries risk of esophageal rupture. Traction is placed on the tube initially, with only the gastric balloon inflated to determine whether pressure on the varices at the gastroesophageal junction will lead to hemostasis. If this fails, the esophageal balloon can be inflated to put direct pressure on the varices. SB tubes are fixed to a helmet or over pulleys to gentle traction with weights. The airway must be controlled with intubation. Because the tube

completely obstructs the esophagus functionally, aspiration of blood or saliva is a major risk. In addition, the tube is so uncomfortable that sedation may be needed. Also, encephalopathy may further compromise the patient's ability to protect the airway. For these reasons, the patient should be intubated when SB tubes are employed.

SB tubes can quickly lead to esophageal erosion and thus recurrent bleeding from varices. In general, the SB tube is used as a temporary measure after initial failure to control bleeding; endoscopic sclerotherapy should be repeated in 12 to 18 hours. If this is not possible, the esophageal balloon, if inflated initially, should be deflated as a trial within the first 24 hours, and the gastric balloon should be taken off traction thereafter. If hemostasis is maintained, the tube is left in place for 12 to 24 hours of observation and sedation; it can then be removed and further sclerotherapy can be performed. If bleeding recurs, the tube is available for reinflation in preparation for further intervention.

Mr. Norman is given octreotide and he has another sclerotherapy session. His condition stabilizes, and no further bleeding is noted for the next 48 hours. He is allowed small amounts of fluid by mouth, and his loose melenotic stools decrease in frequency. His hematocrit stabilizes, and the octreotide is successfully tapered off. He is sent to the general medical floor. His total protein level is 3.1 mg/dL and the prothrombin time is 14 seconds (international normalized ratio, 1.3); he has mild tenderness to deep palpation of the liver edge under the right costal margin. On the sixth day in hospital, he has another sclerotherapy session and is found to have some distal esophagitis, but the varices are still prominent halfway up the esophagus. Sclerotherapy is repeated. He is prescribed an H_2-antagonist and antacids by mouth and discharged home. A month later, he returns to the emergency department with nearly identical symptoms of bleeding, hematemesis, and melenotic stools. His family confirms that he consumed a pint of vodka on the day bleeding recurred. He receives a blood transfusion, and endoscopy reveals bleeding esophageal varices. He is readmitted to the intensive care unit, where he is given octreotide again. The bleeding slows but it does not stop completely. He is now noted to have mild encephalopathy and jaundice, with a total bilirubin level of 4 mg/dL.

What are the options for treatment?
The options include more sclerotherapy, portasystemic decompression surgery, esophagogastric transection surgery (Sugiura procedure), transjugular intrahepatic portal shunt procedure, and liver transplantation. The condition of the patient guides treatment decisions. The Child class must be determined, because it is an important prognosticator of surgical outcome, although it has been

modified over the years to provide a more general estimate of liver function. In addition, the liver disease should be evaluated in the context of any other organ system that has failed, because patients with multiple organ system failure have a poor prognosis. In most patients, the decision at this point is to intervene to decrease portal pressure or directly remove varices from the esophagus or stomach. In the case of patients with a particularly poor prognosis because of underlying liver disease, the clinician should discuss end-of-life issues with the family.

What is a portasystemic shunt, and what are some common shunting techniques?
Portasystemic shunting consists of diverting high-pressure portal blood into the systemic circulation. It is the oldest treatment (Figure 16.1). The earliest model of this shunt was used by Eck in dogs in 1877. Pavlov followed these experiments and determined that shunting was complicated by hepatic encephalopathy. The operation was unused until the 1930s, when Whipple and others revived the concept of portacaval shunting. The operation was modified after it was recognized that the development of encephalopathy depended on whether liver blood flow was completely or partially diverted and whether the patient used a low-protein diet after surgery. Because the liver normally receives 70% of its blood supply through the portal vein, total diversion of portal blood flow results in complete bypass of the liver's ability to metabolize various body metabolites. This leads to accumulation of harmful metabolites that cause encephalopathy. Ingestion of a protein-rich diet aggravates this condition.

These are the main shunt procedures:

End-to-side portacaval shunt was one of the two main operations used through the 1960s. The portal vein is totally diverted into the vena cava, leaving the liver to survive on hepatic artery flow.

Side-to-side shunt was the other commonly used procedure, in which the technique of Eck was applied to create a partial diversion of portal flow.

Mesocaval shunt, a modification of the partial diversion technique, was popularized by Drapanas. A graft is used to connect the side of the superior mesenteric vein to the vena cava (17).

Linton central splenorenal shunt is the procedure in which the splenic vein distally is turned into the left renal vein.

Distal splenorenal shunt was devised by Warren and Zeppa in the late 1960s in an attempt to reduce the rate of encephalopathy. The portal system is divided into two parts by dividing the splenic vein off the portal vein at its junction with the superior mesenteric vein and turning the splenic vein into an anastomosis with the left renal vein (18, 19). This shunt diverts portal flow from the stomach, spleen, and esophageal varices but leaves portal flow from the small and large intestine intact.

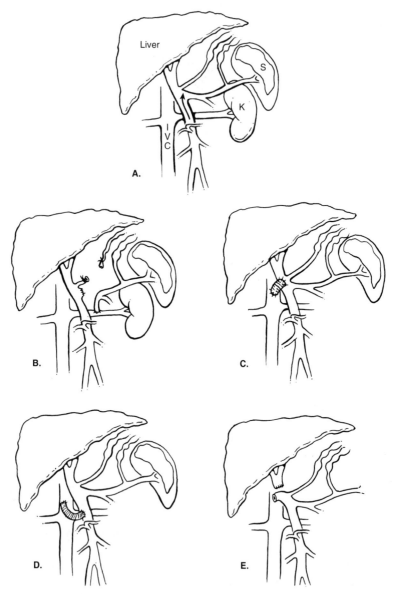

Figure 16.1.   Portal anatomy and major shunt types. **A.** Baseline condition with varices.
B. Distal splenorenal shunt. **C.** H-graft interposition portocaval shunt. **D.** Mesocaval shunt.
E. End-to-side portocaval shunt. *IVC*, Inferior vena cava; *K*, kidney; *S*, spleen.

H-graft bridge, used by Sarfeh to create a more facile central partial shunt that was in effect a side-to side-shunt, is a 10-mm H-graft to bridge the portal vein and vena cava (20).

All shunt procedures have complications in common: all are major abdominal or retroperitoneal operations and carry significant risk for chronically ill patients. The main concerns in the immediate postoperative period are worsening of liver failure, worsening of ascites, exacerbation of hepatic encephalopathy, and shunt failure with recurrent hemorrhage.

What is the prognosis after shunt surgery?
Shunt surgery does not alter the long-term prognosis for survival, which is based on the Child class of the patient at the time of surgery. Shunt surgery is intended to stop variceal hemorrhage, which in the short term causes significant mortality—approximately 25% per major bleeding episode, even in recent studies (2). The operation chosen should stop the hemorrhage and have a low risk of short-term encephalopathy. Shunt surgery does not cure the liver disease, which remains a significant cause of death. Because the Child classification can be used easily with bedside criteria and tests that have been available for decades, it is possible to compare current survival with that in the 1940s and earlier. For patients with bleeding esophageal varices, 1-year survival has remained constant at 30 to 40%. This poor prognosis applies predominantly to alcoholic cirrhosis and to diseases in which hepatocellular functional reserve is destroyed. The prognosis is better for patients with a disease such as primary splenic vein thrombosis or schistosomiasis, in which hepatic reserve can be maintained.

What is the Sugiura procedure?
Dissatisfaction with the results of shunting, even in the 1960s and 1970s, led to a search for an alternative approach that preserved blood flow to the liver. Transesophageal open ligation of varices was attempted, but the mortality and morbidity from this procedure were high. Sugiura modified this approach by defining a multiple-stage devascularization of esophageal and gastric varices in a large cohort of Japanese patients. This procedure has been modified in the United States and Europe, with use of a transabdominal approach and stapling. The Sugiura procedure is rarely used now in North America and Europe, except for patients in whom shunting or sclerotherapy is not possible, but it remains popular in Japan (21, 22).

What is the role of transjugular shunting?
In the late 1980s, interventional radiology gained importance in the treatment of portal hypertension. Images of the portal architecture are required before any shunt operation can be planned. Imaging was originally performed by di-

rect puncture of the spleen and injection of radiopaque contrast medium. As aortography developed, it became easy to obtain selective angiograms of the celiac and superior mesenteric circulation by tracking the contrast through to the portal venous phase. These techniques became easier with computed angiography, which produces high-quality digital subtraction images. Angiographers attempted transhepatic puncture into the portal system, with direct injection of sclerosing material, thrombogenic agents, or even emboli into the largest varices, but these techniques generally failed to achieve long-term benefit. Finally, after the development of endovascular stents, it became possible to create an artificial channel between the hepatic veins and the portal vein, dilate the channel, and maintain it with a metal stent. This procedure, transjugular intrahepatic portasystemic shunting (TIPS), has been moderately successful in recent years as an alternative to surgery in the highest-risk patients (23–25). Nevertheless, TIPS has been associated with a problematic rate of recurrent portal hypertension because of stent thrombosis or fibrosis.

What is the role of hepatic transplantation?
The only curative procedure for primary liver disease is transplantation, which was introduced in the 1970s and has progressed to be an option today (26). Transplantation is the only procedure that treats portal hypertension and restores hepatic metabolic function, but it remains a problem for several reasons:

1. Livers remain in short supply, and therefore only a few thousand procedures can be performed each year in the United States.
2. The procedure is very expensive because of the cost of surgery and the ongoing cost of immunosuppression, and many potential recipients do not have the needed insurance or personal finances.
3. Ethical concerns have been raised about the propriety of allowing transplantation for alcoholic cirrhosis, with opponents noting that the significant medical resources used for a transplant would be more properly distributed to people who have not abused alcohol.

Nevertheless, liver transplantation has generally been performed in centers that treat relatively large numbers of patients, and a high success rate has been achieved in the 1990s for this technically demanding operation (27).

When should surgery be considered in the management of liver failure and portal hypertension?
Surgery has a smaller role today than it did 20 years ago (28). Most medical consultants consider surgical portal decompression after bleeding has not been controlled by other means. A shunt operation is uncommon, and in general the patients at the time of operation have significant risk factors and are in Child class

B or C. In such situations, early surgical consultation is encouraged so that the surgeon is familiar with the patient in case a shunt is necessary, and the surgeon should encourage early portal system angiography for the patient in whom medical management seems to be failing.

Management Algorithm for Portal Hypotension/Bleeding Esophageal Varices

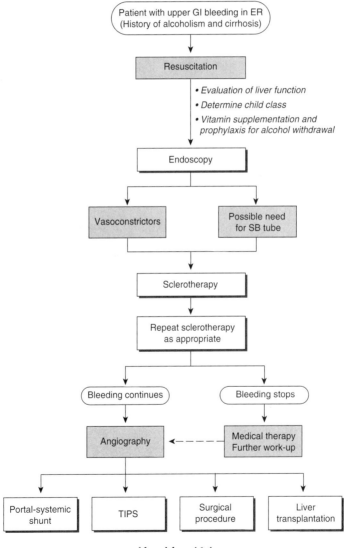

Algorithm 16.1.

Patients with severe hemorrhage should be aggressively treated with medical therapy and sclerotherapy. Repeated endoscopic sclerotherapy should be performed at short intervals to obliterate varices as quickly as possible (29). Failure to follow this procedure is likely to cause rebleeding. A problem for the surgeon is that the longer a patient with marginal liver function remains without proper nutrition and the greater the number of hemorrhagic episodes, the more likely that the patient's Child classification will deteriorate and the higher the mortality will be after surgery (30, 31). Because some centers have obtained results with surgery that are equivalent to those with sclerotherapy, some authors strongly advocate early surgery, before the patient's status deteriorates (5, 32).

Should patients with varices that have not yet hemorrhaged have surgery?
Approximately 30% of patients with asymptomatic esophageal varices bleed (1). The outcome of a prospective study performed more than 20 years ago did not favor preemptive surgery for nonhemorrhaging varices. Intervention with prophylactic medical therapy may be cost-effective (33). Most patients who have incidental esophageal varices from portal hypertension should be evaluated to establish the cause of the liver dysfunction if alcoholism is not the apparent cause. Measures to restore liver function include avoidance of the noxious stimulus, use of vitamins, and perhaps medication with a β-blocker. A low-protein diet should be used to avoid encephalopathy, and patients with ascites should be treated with diuretics and/or repeated paracentesis (34). Those with refractory ascites should be considered for TIPS or for hepatic transplantation but rarely for a portacaval shunt.

REFERENCES

1. Collini FJ, Brener B. Portal hypertension. Surg Gynecol Obstet 1990;170:177–192.
2. Resnick RH. Portal hypertension. Med Clin North Am 1975;59:945–953.
3. Terblanche J, Kahn D, Bornman P. Long-term injection sclerotherapy treatment for esophageal varices. Ann Surg 1989;210:725–731.
4. Cello JP, Grendell JH, Crass RA, et al. Endoscopic sclerotherapy versus portacaval shunt in patients with severe cirrhosis and acute variceal hemorrhage. N Engl J Med 1987;316: 11–15.
5. Orloff MJ, Orloff MS, Orloff SL, Hanes KS. Treatment of bleeding from portal hypertensive gastropathy by portacaval shunt. Hepatology 1995;21:1011–1017.
6. Garrett KO, Reilly JJ, Schade RR, van Thiel DH. Sclerotherapy of esophageal varices: long-term results and determinants of survival. Surgery 1988;104:813–818.
7. Orloff MJ, Orloff MS, Rambotti M, Girard B. Is portal-systemic shunt worthwhile in Child's class C cirrhosis? Ann Surg 1992;216:256–268.
8. Burroughs AK, Hamilton G, Phillips A, et al. A comparison of sclerotherapy with staple transection of the esophagus for the emergency control of bleeding from esophageal varices. N Engl J Med 1989;321:857–862.
9. Adams WL, Barry KL, Fleming MF. Screening for problem drinking in older primary care patients. JAMA 1996;276:1964–1967.

10. Galambos J. Evaluation of patients with portal hypertension. Am J Surg 1990;160: 14–18.

11. Andreoni B, Chiara O, Maggioni D, et al. Role of hepatic histologic findings in the prognosis and treatment of bleeding esophageal varices. Am J Surg 1989;157: 220–224.

12. North Italian Endoscopic Club for the study and treatment of esophageal varices. Prediction of the first variceal hemorrhage in patients with cirrhosis of the liver and esophageal varices. N Engl J Med 1988;319:983–989.

13. Burnett DA, Rikkers LF. Nonoperative emergency treatment of variceal hemorrhage. Surg Clin North Am 1990;70:291.

14. Teran JC, Imperiale TF, Mullen KD, et al. Primary prophylaxis of variceal bleeding in cirrhosis: a cost-effectiveness analysis. Gastroenterology 1997;112:473–482.

15. Bernard B, Lebrec D, Mathurin P, et al. Propranolol and sclerotherapy in the prevention of gastrointestinal rebleeding in patients with cirrhosis: a meta-analysis. J Hepatol 1997;26:312–324.

16. Burroughs AK, Pangou E. Pharmacological therapy for portal hypertension: rationale and results. Sem Gastrointest Dis 1995;6:148–164.

17. Lillemoe KD, Cameron JL. The interposition mesocaval shunt. Surg Clin North Am 1990;70:379–394.

18. Warren WD, Zeppa R, Fomon JJ. Selective trans-splenic decompression of gastroesophageal varices by distal splenorenal shunt. Arch Surg 1967;168:437–455.

19. Millikan WJ Jr, Warren WD, Henderson JM, et al. The Emory prospective randomized trial: selective versus nonselective shunt to control variceal bleeding: ten-year follow-up. Ann Surg 1985;201:712–722.

20. Sarfeh IJ, Rypins EB, Mason GR. A systematic appraisal of portacaval H-graft diameters. Ann Surg 1986;204:356–394.

21. Abouna GM, Baissony H, Al-Nakib BM, et al. The place of Sugiura operation for portal hypertension and bleeding esophageal varices. Surgery 1987;101:91–98.

22. Takenaka H, Nakao K, Miyata M, et al. Hemodynamic study after devascularization procedure in patients with esophageal varices. Surgery 1990;107:55–62.

23. Zemel G, Katzen BT, Becker GJ, et al. Percutaneous transjugular portasystemic shunt. JAMA 1991;266:390–393.

24. Pursnani KG, Sillin LF, Kaplan DS. Effect of transjugular intrahepatic portasystemic shunt on secondary hypersplenism. Am J Surg 1997;173:169–173.

25. LaBerge JM, Ring EJ, Gordon RL, et al. Creation of transjugular intrahepatic portasystemic shunts with the Wallstent endoprosthesis: results in 100 patients. Radiology 1993;187:413–420.

26. Garrett KO, Reilly JJ, Schade RR, van Thiel DH. Bleeding esophageal varices: treatment by sclerotherapy and liver transplantation. Surgery 1988;104:819–823.

27. Henderson JM, Gilmore GT, Hooks MA, et al. Selective shunt in the management of variceal bleeding in the era of liver transplantation. Ann Surg 1992;216:248–254.

28. Conn HO, Lebrec D, Terblanche J. The treatment of oesophageal varices: a debate and a discussion. J Inter Med 1997;241:103–108.

29. Chung RS, Dearlove J. The sources of recurrent hemorrhage during long-term sclerotherapy. Surgery 1988;104:687–696.

30. Grossman MD, McGreevy JM. Effect of delayed operation for bleeding esophageal varices on Child's class and indices of liver function. Am J Surg 1988;156:502–505.

31. Pomerantz RA, Eckhauser FE, Knol JA, et al. Operative timing and patient survival following distal splenorenal shunt. Am Surg 1989;55:333–337.
32. Rikkers LF, Jin G, Burnett DA, et al. Shunt surgery versus endoscopic sclerotherapy for variceal hemorrhage: late results of a randomized trial. Am J Surg 1993;165:27–33.
33. Greig JD, Garden OJ, Carter DC. Prophylactic treatment of patients with esophageal varices: is it ever indicated? World J Surg 1994;18:176–184.
34. Runyon BA. Care of patients with ascites. N Engl J Med 1994;330:337–342.

17

Pancreatitis

Jeannie F. Savas

Anne Ryan is a 29-year-old woman who visits the emergency department with severe epigastric abdominal pain, nausea, and vomiting during the previous 2 to 3 days. She has a history of pancreatitis. She denies having fever, chills, or any other associated
complaints. She denies the use of alcohol. Her medical history is significant for familial hypertriglyceridemia for which she is prescribed
medication; she has a history of noncompliance. She has had no
surgery. She is very thin and in moderate distress during physical
examination. She has poor capillary refill; her blood pressure is
90/60 mm Hg; her heart rate, 120 beats per minute; her temperature, 38.3°C; her respiratory rate, 30 breaths per minute. The midepigastrium is quite tender, but there is no peritonitis or palpable
mass.

What diagnosis is most likely?
Given Ms. Ryan's history of pancreatitis and her epigastric pain associated with
nausea and vomiting, acute pancreatitis is the likely culprit. The differential diagnosis includes gastritis, peptic ulcer disease, biliary disease, pneumonia, and
myocardial infarction.

What are the symptoms and signs of pancreatitis?
The classic history is epigastric pain radiating to the back. The pain is described
as a constant boring or knifelike pain often associated with anorexia, nausea,
vomiting, and occasionally fever. The patient may give a history of pancreatitis. The abdominal findings may range from mild epigastric tenderness to diffuse peritonitis. A mass or ascites may be found with complicated pancreatitis
(e.g., pseudocyst, abscess, pancreatic duct leak, severe acute pancreatitis). Any
ecchymosis in the flank (Grey-Turner's sign) or periumbilical area (Cullen's
sign) should be noted. Though very rare, they are both signs of retroperitoneal
hemorrhage, which may accompany severe acute pancreatitis (1).

What laboratory or radiologic tests support this diagnosis?
Elevated serum amylase, lipase, or urinary amylase is expected. However, many other conditions may result in hyperamylasemia. Abdominal film may show pancreatic calcification if the patient has chronic pancreatitis. The abdominal film often shows an ileus pattern of some dilated loops of small bowel with a few air-fluid levels. The ileus pattern may be diffuse or local, as with the sentinel loop, a single dilated jejunal loop in the upper abdomen, or colon cutoff signs. Here the colon is dilated to the mid–transverse colon, and little gas is seen distally. An upright chest film rules out pneumonia and free intraabdominal air. A left pleural effusion is visible. Ultrasound may show an edematous pancreas and, more important, the presence or absence of gallstones or a dilated common bile duct (CBD). Abdominal computed tomography (CT) may show pancreatic edema, fluid collections, soft tissue stranding, necrosis, or associated complications of pancreatitis. However, CT generally is not recommended as a primary diagnostic tool in patients with simple acute pancreatitis.

What causes pancreatitis?
Pancreatitis is most frequently caused by gallstones or alcohol ingestion (Table 17.1). Other causes include congenital abnormalities of the pancreas and its ductal system, hypertriglyceridemia, trauma, drugs (e.g., thiazides, azathioprine) (Table 17.2), and iatrogenic causes (e.g., surgery, endoscopic retrograde cholangiopancreatography [ERCP]).

What is the treatment for acute pancreatitis?
Because oral intake stimulates the pancreas, the patient should be given nothing by mouth (NPO). If the patient is vomiting or has gastric distension, nasogastric decompression alleviates these symptoms and prevents aspiration. Intravenous fluids should be given, and parenteral nutrition should be considered if enteral nutrition for a long time is not possible. Histamine (H_2) blockers may help suppress pancreatic secretion (2).

The patient receives a fluid bolus of 1 L normal saline (NS), after which her vital signs stabilize. A Foley catheter is placed and laboratory tests performed, yielding the following results: calcium, 5.9 mg/dL; carbon dioxide, 18 mEq/L; creatinine, 1.4 mg/dL; glucose, 250 mg/dL; amylase, 1200 U/L; lipase, 9200 IU/L; triglycerides, 31,000 mg/dL; liver function tests, normal; hemoglobin, 10 g/dL; white blood cell count, 12,000/mm³. She is administered intravenous calcium 2 g and transferred to her room, where she is kept NPO and receives pain medication and maintenance intravenous fluids. She receives furosemide for oliguria. The next morning, she is in respiratory distress and has the following values: calcium, 4.2 mg/dL; creatinine, 4.9 g/dL; hemoglobin, 8 g/dL. She is transferred

Table 17.1.   CAUSES OF ACUTE PANCREATITIS AND
HYPERAMYLASEMIA

Acute Pancreatitis	Hyperamylasemia
Alcohol	Renal insufficiency
Biliary tract disease	Mumps
Hyperlipidemia	Macroamylasemia
Hypercalcemia	Mesentric thrombosis
Familial tendency	Perforated peptic ulcer
Trauma	Cardiopulmonary bypass
External disease	Tumors
Operative	Head trauma
Retrograde pancreatography	Peritonitis
Ischemia	Salivary hyperamylasemia
Hypotension	Drugs
Cardiopulmonary bypass	Small-bowel obstruction
Atheroembolism	
Vasculitis	
Pancreatic duct obstruction	
Tumor	
Pancreatic divisum	
Ampullary stenosis	
Ascaris infestation	
Duodenal obstruction	
Viral infection	
Scorpion venom	
Drugs	
Idiopathy	

to the intensive care unit, intubated, and given more intravenous calcium and fluid boluses.

Why did Ms. Ryan deteriorate?
She was severely dehydrated and hypocalcemic. Although attempts were made to correct these deficiencies in the emergency department, she should have had more frequent monitoring of her vital signs and laboratory values to be sure she was adequately resuscitated.

What are Ranson's criteria?
Ranson (3) described a series of signs that help determine the severity of acute pancreatitis. They have recently been modified and are now known as the Glasgow criteria (4). One group of signs are assessed at the time of admission and the others are assessed within 48 hours (Table 17.3). At the time of Ranson's

**Table 17.2.   DRUGS IMPLICATED IN THE INITIATION OF
ACUTE PANCREATITIS**

Definite Association	Probable Association
Azathioprine	Thiazide diuretics
Estrogens	Furosemide
	Ethacrynic acid
	Sulfonamides
	Tetracycline
	L-Asparaginase
	Corticosteroids
	Phenformin
	Procainamide
	Valproic acid
	Clonidine
	Pentamidine
	Dideoxyinosine

Reprinted with permission from Sabiston. Textbook of Surgery. 15th ed. Philadelphia: Saunders, 1997.

Table 17.3.   RANSON'S CRITERIA FOR PANCREATITIS

At Admission	During Initial 48 Hours
Age above 55 yr[a]	Hematocrit falling >10%
WBC >16,000 cells/mm^3	BUN >5 mg/100 mL[a]
Blood glucose >200 mg/100 mL[a]	Serum calcium <8 mg/100 mL[a]
Serum lactate dehydrogenase >350 IU/L[a]	Arterial PO_2 <60 torr[a]
AST >2250 U/100 mL	Base deficit >4 mEq/L
	Estimated fluid sequestration >6 L

Reprinted with permission from Sabiston. Textbook of Surgery. 15th ed. Philadelphia: Saunders, 1997.

study, patients with fewer than two criteria had 1% mortality; those with three or four signs, 15%; those with five or six signs, 40%; and those with more than six signs, 100%. With the advances in monitoring and treatment, the mortality for each subgroup has probably decreased, but it has not been studied recently. The usefulness of these criteria is to help one identify severe pancreatitis and treat it aggressively. Because only five signs are assessed on admission, however, one should consider the possibility of severe pancreatitis if more than two or three signs are seen initially or if there are signs of hemodynamic instability or respiratory distress. Treatment should not wait until all criteria are met, which takes 48 hours.

Was this patient treated appropriately?
Ms. Ryan did not have all appropriate tests to determine how many Ranson's or Glasgow signs she had. With her hemodynamic compromise, severe hypocalcemia, tachypnea, and oliguria, Ms. Ryan required more aggressive monitoring and resuscitation, even without accurate assessment of her pancreatitis.

During the next 48 hours in the intensive care unit, Ms. Ryan requires 15 L crystalloid, 6 units blood, 8 g calcium, and emergency plasmapheresis to manage her severe hypertriglyceridemia. With this treatment, her hemoglobin and calcium levels return to normal, and her creatinine decreases to 2.9 after reaching a high of 9. As her pancreatitis improves, she requires less respiratory support as well. Antibacterial treatment with imipenem is started. A week later, although hemodynamically improved, Ms. Ryan continues to require ventilatory support and begins to spike fevers to 39.4°C. Her white blood cell count rises to 22,000/mm³. She is now receiving total parenteral nutrition.

Is there a role for prophylactic antibiotics in patients with acute pancreatitis?
In a recent study, patients with severe acute pancreatitis who received prophylactic treatment with imipenem had fewer infectious complications (5). Imipenem is the only drug that has been studied for this indication, although other broad-spectrum antibiotics may be as effective.

What are the infectious complications of pancreatitis?
Pancreatic abscess, infected pancreatic necrosis, infected pancreatic pseudocyst, line sepsis, pneumonia, infected pleural effusion, catheter-related urinary tract infection, and pancreatic or enteric fistulas may result from severe acute pancreatitis.

How is the cause of infection diagnosed?
All indwelling catheters, urinary or vascular, should be changed, and a thorough physical examination should be performed in search of factors such as cellulitis, abdominal mass, and increased abdominal tenderness. A chest radiograph helps assess for pneumonia and large pleural effusion. Often, the abdominal examination is difficult in a patient with pancreatitis either because of preexisting tenderness or because the patient is sedated or receiving pain medication. Therefore, when infection is suspected, abdominal CT is often required. If available, dynamic or spiral CT with contrast is best because it demonstrates any abscess, pseudocyst, or pancreatic necrosis.

What is the treatment for pancreatic abscess or infected pseudocyst?
If possible, radiology-guided percutaneous drainage is best, especially in already compromised patients (6). If this cannot be done, surgical drainage is required.

What is the treatment for pancreatic necrosis?
Although it is controversial, most studies advocate nonoperative therapy for patients with only small areas of necrosis (less than 20 to 30%) or when no infection is suspected (7). However, when infection is suspected—because of fever, leukocytosis, bacteremia, failure to improve clinically, or positive Gram stain on aspirated necrosis—surgical management is indicated. Intraoperative findings are thick necrotic tissue surrounding the pancreas, sometimes extending into the transverse mesocolon, small-bowel mesentery, or retroperitoneum. Extensive debridement is performed. Most often, this requires multiple visits to the operating room with the abdomen packed between visits. When no further debridement is necessary, drains are placed and the abdomen is closed. A sample of the necrotic tissue is sent to the laboratory for Gram stain and culture to guide antimicrobial therapy. It is prudent to place a feeding jejunostomy so that an elemental diet may be given when tolerated.

What is the treatment for gallstone pancreatitis?
If a patient with pancreatitis has gallstones, even if there are other possible causes of pancreatitis, the gallbladder should be removed after the pancreatitis has resolved. This is usually done before the patient is discharged from the hospital to prevent another attack of pancreatitis, which may be more severe than the initial attack. Some literature supports early ERCP to remove the stone or a sphincterotomy if there is suspicion of a persistent, obstructing distal CBD stone in a patient whose pancreatitis fails to improve (8, 9). However, ERCP itself may worsen pancreatitis (10). Some centers use magnetic resonance cholangiopancreatography (MRCP) as a diagnostic maneuver prior to ERCP because it is noninvasive (11). This technique is new, so its accuracy and usefulness, although promising, are not yet fully elucidated.

Ms. Ryan underwent 6 to 8 surgical debridements for her infected pancreatic necrosis, which was diagnosed with dynamic abdominal CT. She also had a surgical jejunostomy feeding tube. Her enteral elemental diet was advanced over several weeks, and TPN was discontinued. She required a tracheostomy because of prolonged ventilator dependence. After long stays in the intensive care unit and hospital, she was able to tolerate a low-fat oral diet and be discharged home.

See Algorithm 17.1A and B at the end of this chapter.

Gerald Stevens is a 45-year-old man who visits the hospital with acute onset of epigastric pain, hematemesis, and dizziness. He has a history of alcoholic pancreatitis. The patient has mild epigastric tenderness. A nasogastric tube confirms fresh blood clots in his stomach. His vital signs are stable, although his hemoglobin is 8 g/dL. Intravenous access is obtained. Esophagoduodenoscopy reveals a large opening in

the posterior gastric wall that is filled with clotted blood. No active bleeding is seen. Abdominal CT shows evidence of chronic pancreatitis and a large pseudocyst adherent to the posterior gastric wall.

What are the most common causes of gastrointestinal bleeding in a patient with pancreatitis?
The most common causes are not related to pancreatitis; they include alcoholic gastritis, peptic ulcer disease, varices, Mallory-Weiss tear, and tumor. Rarely, as in this patient, a large untreated pseudocyst may erode into an adjacent organ and cause bleeding.

What causes a pseudocyst?
A pancreatic pseudocyst forms as a result of a contained pancreatic duct leak, often the result of a proximal ductal obstruction. This usually occurs during a bout of acute pancreatitis, and the surrounding inflammatory reaction forms a wall and thus a pseudocyst.

What is the surgical treatment for a pseudocyst?
A pseudocyst may be treated with internal or external drainage. The pseudocyst is opened and sewn to an adjacent structure, usually the stomach (cystgastrostomy) or jejunum (cystojejunostomy). This is the preferred method of drainage if no infection is present. External drainage, which is the best option for an infected pseudocyst, may be percutaneous with radiologic guidance or surgical. The risk of external drainage is that the patient may develop a pancreatic-cutaneous fistula if there is still a connection between the pseudocyst and the pancreatic duct. It is customary to send a portion of the wall of a suspected pseudocyst to the pathologist to rule out cystic tumor of the pancreas, in which case there is a true epithelial-lined cyst wall. Another option is resection of the pseudocyst. This is usually reserved for pseudocysts in the tail of the pancreas when no proximal strictures are present.

When is surgery indicated for a pseudocyst?
Surgery or percutaneous drainage is indicated for all infected pseudocysts. Uninfected pseudocysts should undergo surgical drainage if they are very large (more than 6 cm) or persist after the pancreatitis has resolved, to avoid further complications, such as rupture or bleeding. Unless they are very large, most pseudocysts spontaneously resolve within 4 to 6 weeks after a bout of acute pancreatitis (12). Large pseudocysts may cause abdominal discomfort, bloating, and early satiety because of compression of adjacent organs. They also may erode into vascular structures, resulting in bleeding into the intestine, as in this patient, or rupture free into the peritoneal cavity, causing pancreatic ascites if the pseudocyst communicates with the pancreatic duct.

How is a pseudocyst diagnosed?
A pseudocyst should be suspected in a patient with a history of pancreatitis who has early satiety, abdominal distention, or an abdominal mass. Abdominal ultrasound or CT confirms the diagnosis and rules out tumor. Infection is suspected if the patient has a high fever, marked abdominal tenderness, leukocytosis, or typical radiologic features. MRCP or ERCP may be useful to document ductal strictures or connection to the pseudocyst if therapy is contemplated. ERCP, if performed, should be done within 24 hours of surgery to avoid infecting the pseudocyst.

Mr. Stevens underwent operative exploration for his gastrointestinal bleeding. An anterior gastrotomy revealed that the pseudocyst had spontaneously ruptured into the posterior gastric wall. The edges of gastric mucosa, adjacent to the cystgastrostomy, were bleeding and therefore were oversewn. The clot was evacuated from the pseudocyst, and no further bleeding was noted. The gastrotomy was closed. Mr. Stevens recovered uneventfully.

Dennis Keith is a 35-year-old man who visits the emergency department with abdominal pain and weakness of acute onset. During physical examination, he is notably pale, tachycardiac, and hypotensive, and he has a distended abdomen. After initial intravenous fluid boluses of 2 L lactated Ringer's solution, he remains unstable and is immediately taken to the operating room. A midline abdominal incision reveals 2 to 3 L of blood in his abdomen. The abdomen is packed in four quadrants while the anesthesiologist transfuses him and achieves normal blood pressure. As the packs are removed, bleeding is noted to be coming from the left upper quadrant, and a splenectomy is performed. The bleeding continues and is found to originate from the splenic artery proximal to the site of its division. The bleeding artery is controlled, and the patient recovers uneventfully. The spleen appears grossly normal when inspected in the operating room after its removal. The physician later learns that Mr. Keith had a recent episode of gallstone pancreatitis.

What is the diagnosis?
This patient ruptured a splenic artery pseudoaneurysm that developed during pancreatitis. With no history of trauma, other possibilities include a perforated viscus; spontaneous splenic rupture; and rupture of an abdominal aortic, iliac, or visceral artery aneurysm.

What are the vascular complications of pancreatitis?
The most common complication is splenic artery pseudoaneurysm because of inflammation of the pancreas in proximity to the vessel. Other causes of bleeding include rupture of a pseudocyst, erosion of a pseudocyst into vascular struc-

tures or bowel, and varices arising from splenic vein thrombosis. Splenectomy is curative for management of bleeding varices in this situation, which is called sinistral hypertension.

While intoxicated, John Roberts, a 27-year-old man, sustains a stab wound to his midepigastrium and complains of severe abdominal pain. On exploration, he is found to have two gastrotomies, one anterior and one posterior, which are repaired. A thorough exploration reveals no other evidence of injury. He recovers well, except that on postoperative day 5 he still has a significant amount of abdominal pain, anorexia, and nausea. Mr. Roberts has no fever or leukocytosis, but his amylase level is elevated. The physician suspects that he has either alcoholic pancreatitis or some degree of injury to his pancreas not recognized at surgery. Two days later, Mr. Roberts has sudden onset of severe abdominal pain and massive distention that causes respiratory distress. After initial resuscitation, abdominal CT demonstrates ascites, a left pleural effusion, and possibly a pancreatic laceration. Analysis of ascitic and pleural fluid demonstrates an amylase level above 50,000 U/L.

What is the diagnosis?
This patient had an acute free rupture of his pancreatic duct. Probably some injury to the pancreas from the stab wound ruptured the duct. This led to his pancreatic ascites and pancreaticopleural fistula.

What is the treatment for pancreatic ascites?
Initial management is resuscitation of the patient: respiratory support if needed, fluids, nasogastric decompression, and pancreatic rest. Next, one must determine whether there is an ongoing pancreatic leak and, if so, its cause. When a leak is caused by a major disruption of the duct or gland, surgery is indicated to resect, repair, or drain the injury (13). When no major disruption is noted, ERCP with stenting or external drainage may be sufficient. MRCP or ERCP is usually necessary to diagnose the cause of the pancreatic ascites and determine whether there is an ongoing leak.

Is pancreatic juice corrosive to the peritoneal cavity and its organs?
Pancreatic enzymes are secreted in their inactive form into the duodenum, where they are activated. Therefore, when the ascites results from a pancreatic leak, no direct injury results. The major symptoms are pain from acute pancreatitis and discomfort or respiratory compromise due to massive abdominal distention.

How do pancreatic fistulas develop?
The pancreas is a retroperitoneal structure, so if the leak does not rupture through the peritoneum, it can track along the retroperitoneum into the pleural cavities,

mediastinum, or pericardium. When there is any open connection to the skin, such as a surgical incision or drain, a pancreatic-cutaneous fistula may develop.

How are pancreatic fistulas treated?
The treatment is similar to that of pancreatic ascites (Table 17.4). Any major ductal disruption requires surgery, whereas minor leaks may be treated with ERCP and stenting. Treatment also includes avoiding pancreatic stimulation; the patient should take nothing by mouth, instead receiving parenteral nutrition or alternatively, an elemental diet administered via a jejunal feeding tube. The use of somatostatin analogs is controversial (14). Although somatostatin diminishes the volume of pancreatic fluid secretion, its use has not yet been correlated with quicker or higher rates of closure of pancreatic fistulas; furthermore, it is very expensive.

Mr. Roberts required no further intervention, since the splenic artery pseudoaneurysm was repaired during surgery. He should have no future bouts of pancreatitis, since his gallbladder was removed at the time of his initial attack.

Janet Morgan is a 13-year-old girl referred for a second opinion. She has a history of chronic relapsing pancreatitis, and a brother and two cousins have the same problem. She is not taking any medications and

Table 17.4.   MANAGEMENT OF PATIENTS WITH
INTERNAL PANCREATIC FISTULA

Nonoperative treatment
  Prohibition of oral intake
  Nasogastric tube suction
  Paracentesis for pancreatic ascites
  Thoracentesis or chest tube for pancreatic pleural effusion
  Hyperalimentation
  Somatistatin (octreotide)
Operative treatment
  Direct duct leak
    Roux-en-Y drainage of duct leak
    Pancreatic resection for distal duct leak with Roux-en-Y drainage of proximal
      pancreatic remnant for any proximal duct disease
  Leaking pseudocyst
    Roux-en-Y drainage of pseudocyst to jejunum
    Small distal pseudocyst: possible resection with Roux-en-Y drainage of proximal
      pancreatic remnant for any proximal duct disease
    External drainage

---

denies any drug or alcohol use. She gives no history of abdominal trauma.

How will the physician diagnose and treat Janet's pancreatitis?
With a young patient, one must consider familial pancreatitis and congenital anomalies such as pancreas division and cystic fibrosis. Abdominal CT, ERCP, or MRCP may help to define the anatomy and rule out complications of pancreatitis such as pseudocysts and stricture. Again, MRCP is a new technology not available in many centers, and its accuracy is not yet known. Ultrasound should be performed to rule out cholelithiasis. Treatment is conservative (i.e., NPO, pancreatic rest, analgesia) during the acute phase and in the long term may entail chronic dietary modifications—that is, low-fat diet with or without pancreatic enzyme supplementation.

Janet's ultrasound reveals no gallstones or dilated ducts. No masses or pseudocysts are seen on abdominal CT. MRCP demonstrates normal pancreatic ductal anatomy without dilation or stricture. It is determined that she has familial pancreatitis and is treated medically as described earlier.

Rhys Williams is a 45-year-old man who is a frequent visitor to the emergency department. He is a recalcitrant alcoholic who has repeated bouts of pancreatitis. His abdominal pain is exacerbated by a recent binge. He says this pain feels just the same as every time he has pancreatitis—a gradually worsening midepigastric pain that radiates to his back. He has been vomiting for 2 days, and furthermore, he has no desire for any food or alcohol. He denies any other symptoms but demands pain medication. During physical examination, he appears thin, has mild tachycardia at 105 beats per minute, and has rebound tenderness in the upper abdomen. No masses are palpated, and he is heme negative on rectal examination. His laboratory tests are all within normal limits except for an elevated urinary amylase level and a white blood cell count of 12,000/mm³. The abdominal radiograph demonstrates pancreatic calcification. Last year, Mr. Williams had an ultrasound that showed no gallstones.

What is the diagnosis?
Mr. Williams has the classic presentation of chronic relapsing pancreatitis caused by alcohol use. The history and physical examination were performed to rule out other causes of pain, such as gastritis, gallstone pancreatitis, and peptic ulcer disease. The serum amylase level often is normal in patients with a history of chronic pancreatitis, but an elevated urinary amylase level confirms that there is an acute exacerbation.

What is the treatment for chronic relapsing pancreatitis?
In the acute setting, the treatment is pancreatic rest, nasogastric decompression
if vomiting persists, analgesia, and fluid resuscitation. Serial abdominal examinations determine when the patient is improved. This usually requires 1 or 2
days, at which time the diet is advanced as tolerated and pain medicines are
tapered.

**After 2 days, Mr. Williams is tolerating a low-fat diet and requires only
occasional acetaminophen with codeine (Tylenol 3) for pain. He is
discharged and given a follow-up appointment in 2 weeks. He misses
this appointment but comes back in 2 months complaining of foul-
smelling diarrhea, especially after eating greasy foods. He has no pain
or nausea but continues to drink excessively.**

What is the cause of his current symptoms?
Mr. Williams has steatorrhea, which is confirmed by finding fat in the stool.
This is a result of pancreatic insufficiency.

What advice and treatment should this patient receive?
Mr. Williams needs counseling about his alcohol abuse. Pancreatic enzyme supplementation, to be taken with meals, will help the steatorrhea, as will avoidance of greasy foods.

*Does Mr. Williams need insulin or oral hypoglycemics because of his pancreatic insuffi-
ciency?*
Endocrine insufficiency may result from pancreatitis, although exocrine deficiency is much more common. Diabetes mellitus may develop in up to 38% of
patients with chronic pancreatitis (15).

**The nutritionist speaks with Mr. Williams at length about a proper
low-fat diet. He understands her recommendations and promises to
try to modify his diet. He is shocked when the physician tells him that
his problem is a result of his alcohol use and says no one ever told
him that. The physician explains that his pancreatitis will likely continue to get worse unless he abstains, and Mr. Williams agrees to quit.
Six months later, Mr. Williams returns because he ran out of pills. He
states they helped him with the diarrhea. He tried to quit drinking but
says it was just too hard. He now has pain every day, although it has
not been severe enough to get admitted to the hospital. He is angry
at the physicians in the emergency department because they refuse to
give him any more intravenous pain medication. He says he had some
pain medication left over from a tooth extraction that took care of**

his pain, so he wants a prescription for more. The physician again counsels him about his need to abstain from alcohol and gives him information on several detoxification centers. His physical examination is significant only for a 10-pound weight loss, and there is no evidence of acute pancreatitis.

What is the cause of his chronic pain?
Mr. Williams suffers from chronic pancreatitis and will likely have progressive worsening of his pain if he continues to drink.

The physician prescribes Mr. Williams oxycodone hydrochloride with acetaminophen (Percocet), which controls his pain if he takes 4 or 5 per day. He goes to an alcohol detoxification center and stops drinking. He continues to require pancreatic enzyme replacement with meals and has no further problems. He gets a job as a construction worker and works 40 to 60 hours per week. He keeps his appointments at 2-month intervals to get his medicine refilled and shows no progression of disease. Approximately 1 year later, still sober, Mr. Williams calls his physician to say he is out of pain medicine, although his last refill was just 2 weeks earlier. He says he now requires 10 to 15 pills per day to control his pain, but they just do not seem to be working anymore. He denies nausea, vomiting, steatorrhea, or any other problems. He comes to the office for a physical examination, which is unremarkable.

Is this patient getting addicted to the pain medicine?
Although this is a definite possibility, the physician must first search for a pathologic reason for the increased pain. This patient has remained abstinent for more than 1 year and was managed for a long period on a stable dose of pain medication; now he has a relatively sudden increase in his analgesic requirement. One possibility is that he has begun drinking again. This information may be sought by speaking with family members or friends or with random toxicology screening. If there is nothing to suggest a relapse, further diagnostic tests should be done.

How should Mr. Williams be worked up at this point?
As always, it is prudent to begin with a thorough history and physical examination. Are the character and location of this pain the same as with his previous pancreatitis? Does he have an abdominal mass or unexplained weight loss? Is there any evidence to suggest other diagnoses, such as peptic ulcer disease, reflux esophagitis, biliary disease, or tumor? If the findings suggest progressive pancreatitis, further evaluation of the pancreas is indicated. Abdominal CT is

helpful to assess the size of the gland and the main pancreatic duct, the CBD, any pseudocyst or abscess, and any intrinsic or extrinsic mass or adenopathy. ERCP is helpful to image the pancreatic duct for strictures. MRCP may also be helpful but is still considered experimental. Its role and accuracy have not been proved.

Mr. Williams's laboratory tests are normal. Abdominal CT shows pancreatic calcifications and a dilated pancreatic duct. The CBD is normal. No gallstones are seen. No masses or adenopathy is seen, and there is no edema of the pancreas. There is no ascites or fluid around the pancreas. ERCP shows multiple pancreatic duct strictures with dilation of the intervening segments of the duct, the so-called chain of lakes.

What causes strictures of the pancreatic duct?
They may be caused by tumor or more commonly by recurrent bouts of pancreatitis with resultant scarring. If only a single stricture is seen, especially with no history of pancreatitis, brush cytology of the duct should be done during ERCP, and CT should be performed to search for a mass.

What is the treatment for a stricture of the pancreatic duct?
If a tumor is suspected, surgical resection is indicated when technically feasible. For benign strictures, management depends on symptoms. If the patient has minimal or no pain, expectant management is preferred. If, as in this case, the patient has progressive pain while abstinent and compliant with medical therapy, surgery should be considered.

What is the surgery for benign strictures?
Therapy is aimed at relieving the obstruction of the duct. If there is a single stricture in the body or tail of the gland, a distal pancreatectomy is curative. A Puestow procedure is performed for multiple strictures. The pancreatic duct is identified, then opened along its length to obliterate all strictures. Some advocate the removal of any pancreatic duct stones. A Roux-en-Y pancreatojejunostomy is then formed to drain the pancreas. This relieves pain in selected patients; however, those who continue to imbibe or who have idiopathic pancreatitis do not have such good results. Surgery is therefore reserved for compliant, good-risk patients who understand that the procedure may or may not result in permanent or even temporary pain relief (Table 17.5).

Are there any other options?
Pancreatic duct stents may be placed via ERCP and may provide temporary relief for patients who are not candidates for surgery. These stents oc-

Table 17.5. PAIN RELIEF AFTER SURGERY
FOR CHRONIC PANCREATITIS

Procedure	Good + Fair (%)	Poor (%)	Average Follow-up (yr)
Longitudinal pancreaticojejunostomy	81.0	19.0	5.7
Short pancreaticojejunostomy	35.0	65.0	8.0
Short pancreaticogastrostomy	83.0	17.0	4.0
Caudal pancreaticojejunostomy	34.0	66.0	5.7
Total pancreatectomy	72.5	27.5	5.8
Pancreaticoduodenectomy	82.0	18.0	4.7
Duodenal preservation and local resection	88.0	12.0	2.7
Distal pancreatectomy			
Less 80%	85.0	15.0	5.8
Greater 80%	65.0	35.0	6.5

Reprinted with permission from Cameron J. Current Surgical Therapy. 5th ed. St. Louis: Mosby–Year Book, 1995:443.

clude and thus require repeated ERCP for stent changes, usually at 2-month intervals. Another option for patients who have persistent pain or who are not candidates for surgery is celiac ganglionectomy, or percutaneous nerve blocks. Results with this are variable as well. The only other option is to prescribe stronger analgesics, but one should be aware of potential for abuse.

The patient undergoes a successful Puestow procedure (pancreatojejunostomy) and recovers uneventfully. Within 2 weeks, he no longer requires any pain medication, although he still takes enzyme replacement. He has a friend who was recently diagnosed with unresectable pancreatic cancer after being told for years he had pancreatitis. He wants to be sure he does not have cancer too.

How can this patient be reassured that he does not have cancer?
There is a higher incidence of pancreatic cancer in patients with previous pancreatitis than in the general population, but this risk is still very low. The physician can explain that no evidence of tumor is seen, but frequent follow-up may help detect a mass if it develops. Most masses seen on CT in patients with pancreatitis are acute inflammation, but a new mass discovered without acute increase in pain should be evaluated for possible tumor.

Management Algorithm for Acute Pancreatitis

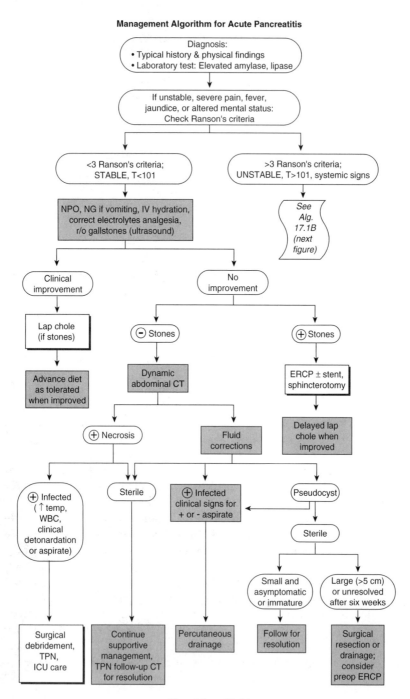

Algorithm 17.1A.

Management Algorithm for Acute Pancreatitis

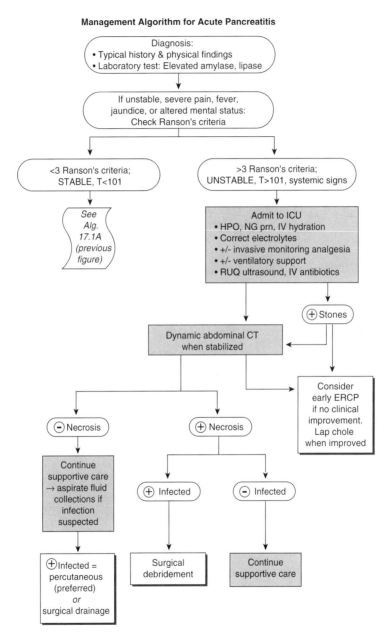

Algorithm 17.1B.

Management Algorithm for Chronic Pancreatitis

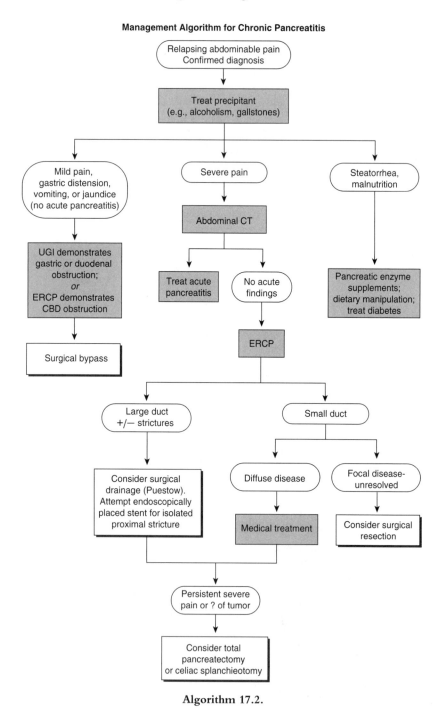

Algorithm 17.2.

REFERENCES

1. Beger HG, Rau B, Mayer J, Pralle U. Natural course of acute pancreatitis. World J Surg 1997;21:130–135.
2. Steinberg W, Tenner S. Acute pancreatitis. N Engl J Med 1994;330:1198.
3. Ranson JHC, Rifkind KM, Roses DF, et al. Prognostic signs and the role of operative management in acute pancreatitis. Surg Gynecol Obstet 1974;139:69.
4. Wassef W, Zfass A. Gallstone pancreatitis: an update. Gastroenterologist 1996;4:70–75.
5. Pederzoli P, Bassi C, Vesentini S, et al. A randomized multicenter clinical trial of antibiotic prophylaxis of septic complications in acute necrotizing pancreatitis with imipenem. Surg Gynecol Obstet 1993;176:480.
6. Lang EK, Paolini RM, Pittmeyer A. The efficacy of palliative and definitive percutaneous versus surgical drainage of pancreatic abscesses and pseudocysts: a prospective study of 85 patients. South Med J 1991;84:55.
7. Bradley EL III. Fifteen year experience with open drainage for infected pancreatic necrosis. Surg Gynecol Obstet 1993;177:215–222.
8. Sheung-Taf F. Early treatment of acute biliary pancreatitis by endoscopic papillotomy. N Engl J Med 1993;328:228–232.
9. Neoptolemos JP, Carr-Locke DL, London NJ, et al. Controlled trial of urgent endoscopic retrograde cholangiography and endoscopic sphincterotomy versus conservative treatment for acute pancreatitis due to gallstones. Lancet 1988;2:979.
10. Sherman S, Lehman GA. ERCP- and endoscopic sphincterotomy-induced pancreatitis. Pancreas 1991;6:350.
11. Soto JA. Magnetic resonance cholangiography: comparison with ERCP. Gastroenterology 1996;110:589–597.
12. Yeo CJ, Bastidas JA, Lynch-Nyhan A, et al. The natural history of pancreatic pseudocysts documented by computed tomography. Surg Gynecol Obstet 1990;170:411.
13. Ridgeway MG, Stabile BE. Surgical management and treatment of pancreatic fistulas. Surg Clin North Am 1996;76:1159–1173.
14. Parekh D, Segal I. Pancreatic ascites and effusion: risk factors for failure of conservative therapy and the role of octreotide. Arch Surg 1992;127:707.
15. Steer ML, Waxman I, Freedman S. Chronic pancreatitis. N Engl J Med 1995;332:1482.

Pancreatic Cancer

James L. Frank

Edwin Snood is a 77-year-old man with a 3-week history of painless jaundice and pruritus. He thinks he had the flu about 2 months ago and since then has felt quite run down. Although he has lost 15 pounds, he ascribes this to a loss of interest in eating rather than inability to eat. Recently, he has noticed that his urine is much darker and his stools are lighter. A yellowing of the eyes that he noticed the previous day has progressed. His medical history is significant for a cholecystectomy for symptomatic cholelithiasis 2 years ago. He drinks one to two cans of beer per night and smokes one pack of cigarettes a day.

What is the significance of the absence of pain in this patient?
Patients with obstructive jaundice without associated abdominal pain are likely to have a neoplasm. In a patient such as Mr. Snood, who has a history of gallstones and biliary surgery, the possibility of choledocholithiasis or a benign postoperative biliary stricture should also be entertained. Pain in a patient with malignant biliary obstruction may be related to cholangitis or tumor invasion of retroperitoneal neural structures. The latter finding suggests that the tumor is likely to be incurable.

Why is a recent change in food intake important?
Alterations in dietary patterns may be secondary to tumor-related anorexia or gastric outlet obstruction. The latter finding is serious because it suggests that an advanced, bulky tumor is invading or compressing the foregut, and it mandates immediate operative exploration for gastrointestinal bypass, minimally. Although biliary decompression can be percutaneous or endoscopic, reestablishment of foregut continuity requires surgery. Laparoscopic gastrojejunostomy has been described and may be increasingly available as more surgeons acquire expertise in advanced laparoscopic techniques (1). Neither radiation therapy nor chemotherapy will dependably relieve gastric outlet obstruction.

Which other systems must be assessed by history for optimal management of patients suspected of having pancreatic cancer?
Many patients with pancreatic cancer have comorbid diseases that may affect their outcomes. Many patients, like Mr. Snood, are heavy tobacco users, and such persons may have concomitant cardiac or pulmonary disease. Cirrhosis or signs of irreversible hepatocellular dysfunction are precautions to resection. A history of significant weight loss may indicate malnutrition. Assessment of these systems reveals any inherent risks in a patient's ability to tolerate surgery (e.g., radical pancreaticoduodenectomy) and any potential for complications.

What causes pancreatic cancer?
Although many factors have been implicated in pancreatic cancer, most of these associations are weak and have not been borne out. Among environmental influences, epidemiologic studies have linked cigarette smoking to pancreatic cancer (2). A genetic component has also been suggested because patients with pancreatic cancer have a high incidence of mutations in the K-*ras* oncogene (3).

On physical examination, Mr. Snood is noted to be somewhat ill at ease, and he is obvious jaundiced. There are several skin excoriations. He has a well-healed right subcostal incision. Palpation reveals no abdominal masses or tenderness. His liver percusses to 6 cm below the right costal margin and is smooth. The remainder of his examination produces normal findings.

What findings from a physical examination indicate unresectable tumor?
Signs of disseminated disease or advanced comorbid conditions lessen the likelihood of a successful pancreaticoduodenectomy. A palpable Virchow's lymph node (left supraclavicular node), nodular liver, multiple intraabdominal masses, and rectal cul-de-sac shelf are all signs of incurability because of distant metastases. Signs of advanced cardiac or pulmonary disease and stigmata of portal hypertension or cirrhosis, including spider angiomata, ascites, varices, and periumbilical veins (caput medusae), raise concerns about a patient's ability to tolerate major intraabdominal surgery. Some patients with pancreatic cancer have a palpable enlarged gallbladder. This finding, Courvoisier's sign, is not an indication of unresectability. It suggests that the biliary obstruction is inferior to the level of the cystic duct and is probably not caused by stone disease, in which the gallbladder tends to be chronically inflamed and contracted.

Which laboratory evaluations should be performed?
The patient should have a complete blood count and liver function panel, including coagulation studies. If pancreatic malignancy is suspected, a nutritional profile (total protein, albumin, and prealbumin) should also be ordered. Evaluation of tumor markers, such as carcinoembryonic antigen and Ca 19–9, is

not particularly useful in pancreatic cancer, and these tests should not be ordered routinely. In patients with advanced unresectable disease, a high Ca 19–9 level may lend sufficient support to the diagnosis to initiate nonoperative management (i.e., chemotherapy and radiation therapy) without further histologic confirmation. After potentially curative resection of pancreatic exocrine tumors, routine monitoring with tumor markers has no established role because recurrent pancreatic cancer is incurable.

Laboratory data show a white blood cell count of 10.1; hemoglobin, 12.4; and platelet count, 114,000. Liver function tests show serum glutamic-oxaloacetic transaminase (SGOT), 55; serum glutamate pyruvate transaminase (SGPT), 62; lactate dehydrogenase (LDH), 150; alkaline phosphatase, 412; and total bilirubin, 6.1. Coagulation studies show prothrombin time (PT), 20 (international normalized ratio, or INR, 1.8); and partial thromboplastin time (PTT), 31. Mr. Snood's nutritional profile is normal, with a serum albumin of 3.6.

What is the significance of increased PT? How should this abnormality be managed?
The coagulation defect is the result of vitamin K deficiency or hepatocellular dysfunction. Malabsorption of vitamin K resulting from biliary obstruction is readily reversible either by relieving the obstruction and returning bile to the gastrointestinal tract or by parenteral supplementation of vitamin K. In rare instances, the clotting abnormality is caused by hepatocellular dysfunction stemming from long-standing biliary obstruction or preexisting liver disease, and the potential for postoperative hepatic failure is substantial. This coagulopathy is not corrected by vitamin K administration, and the patient requires clotting factor transfusions. In such cases, pancreatic resection should be undertaken only with extreme caution or should be omitted.

Mr. Snood is having trouble sleeping because of itching. He is told that itching is a result of bile duct obstruction and high bilirubin levels in his blood. Unable to find relief with antihistamines alone, he inquires about other ways to relieve this problem.

Should a patient who may be operated on for tumor resection undergo preoperative biliary decompression?
Randomized clinical trials in the 1980s failed to show a survival benefit from preoperative biliary drainage. However, those studies were performed with percutaneous transhepatic drainage, which carries a risk of significant complications, before the widespread availability of endoscopic decompression. Because most patients with pancreatic cancer are best treated nonoperatively, preoperative endoscopic retrograde cholangiopancreatography (ERCP) with drainage can assess the efficacy of nonoperative biliary drainage in patients who will require no further surgical intervention if they are found to have unre-

sectable tumors. Surgeons skilled in advanced laparoscopic biliary surgery may omit ERCP and perform a palliative bypass if the tumor is found to be unresectable at the time of diagnostic laparoscopy. If preoperative chemotherapy and radiation therapy are to be given, biliary decompression should be performed first.

Mr. Snood is told that his jaundice may stem from any of a number of causes, including cancer. He asks how the cause will be determined.

What are the imaging modalities employed to characterize a condition such as Mr. Snood's?

Spiral computed tomography (CT) with oral and intravenous contrast is the best radiologic evaluation, because it is unlikely that choledocholithiasis, for which ultrasonography is the best initial imaging modality, is responsible for this patient's presentation. This test permits evaluation of the suspected periampullary tumor, including local extension, relation to the mesenteric vessels, and signs of significant nodal or hepatic dissemination. Although ultrasonography, visceral angiography, positron emission tomography, and magnetic resonance imaging (MRI) may be useful in individual patients for highly specific reasons, CT is still the preferred imaging modality because it yields considerable accurate information with limited cost and morbidity.

MRI with fat suppression technique is sensitive to hepatic metastases and may be preferred for patients allergic to intravenous contrast. If the level of biliary obstruction is indeterminate, an MRI cholangiogram may also be of use, although this test is available only in selected referral centers.

Angiography to assess for anomalous vessels and vascular invasion by tumor used to be performed often. However, the expense and potential for morbidity of this test are no longer justifiable. Spiral CT with intravenous contrast gives sufficient information about vessel involvement, which in some instances is no longer considered a contraindication to resection. Also, vascular anomalies are fairly common and should be readily apparent to the exploring surgeon.

CT portography is extremely sensitive in detecting hepatic metastases and portraying the tumor–mesenteric vasculature relation. However, as with angiography, CT portography is expensive and requires arterial catheterization.

Mr. Snood's CT demonstrates a 3-cm mass in the head of the pancreas and dilation of the common bile duct and pancreatic ducts. There are no signs of hepatic or nodal metastases, and there appears to be a fat plane between the tumor and the superior mesenteric vessels. A chest radiograph is normal. He returns with his family for a discussion of management options and is informed that the result from the CT strongly suggests cancer. They have several questions.

What is the long-term outlook for cure in patients with pancreatic cancer?
Ductal adenocarcinoma of the pancreas, which accounts for 75% of periampullary neoplasms, is a biologically virulent disease with a poor prognosis.
The overall survival rate for all patients is less than 1% (4). The resectability rate
is only 10 to 20% because most patients have disseminated or locally advanced
disease at diagnosis. Of patients who undergo resection, 7 to 30% can expect
to survive beyond several years (5). Part of the difficulty in interpreting survival
analyses in pancreatic cancer stems from lack of uniformity in reporting results
and the occasional inclusion of patients with periampullary cancers that exhibit
a more indolent behavior (e.g., distal bile duct, duodenal, and islet cell tumors).

*Why should pancreaticoduodenectomy be considered if the probability of long-term sur-
vival after resection is so low?*
Occasionally a patient with ductal adenocarcinoma survives for the long term.
In addition, some authors think the Whipple operation provides excellent palliation even for patients with a poor prognosis (6). Finally, 20 to 25% of patients with periampullary tumors have a histologic tumor type other than ductal adenocarcinoma, and the 5-year survival for such patients can be as high as
50%, depending on lymph node status. Exploration should not be denied these
patients, because resection offers the only chance for cure.

What is the Whipple procedure?
The classic Whipple procedure is pancreaticoduodenectomy with resection of
gastric antrum, gallbladder, duodenum, head of pancreas, and common bile duct,
with anastomoses to stomach, common hepatic duct, and pancreatic duct (Figure
18.1). Many surgeons prefer a pylorus-preserving pancreaticoduodenectomy
(Figure 18.2).

*How can a pancreatic mass observed on CT be confirmed to be cancer? If no tissue diag-
nosis has been made, is it necessary to perform a preoperative or intraoperative biopsy?*
After periampullary malignancy is suspected, the tumor should be staged and
explored for resectability. A preoperative percutaneous biopsy should be
avoided because of risk of seeding the peritoneal cavity or biopsy tract with tumor cells. Intraoperative biopsy is often not diagnostic and wastes significant
time in an already lengthy procedure. Once the lesion is deemed resectable,
pancreaticoduodenectomy should be performed, with the acceptance that occasionally the pathology report demonstrates benign disease.

What are the morbidity and mortality for this operation?
This operation has a perioperative mortality of 1 to 5% when performed by experienced pancreatic surgeons. In part, this is because of the centralization of
subspecialty expertise in tertiary referral centers, at which the procedure is done
frequently with appropriate backup from specialized ancillary support services
(7). Notwithstanding such coordination of specialized services, significant

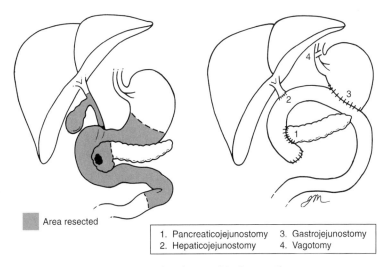

Area resected

1. Pancreaticojejunostomy	3. Gastrojejunostomy
2. Hepaticojejunostomy	4. Vagotomy

Figure 18.1.   The classic Whipple procedure.

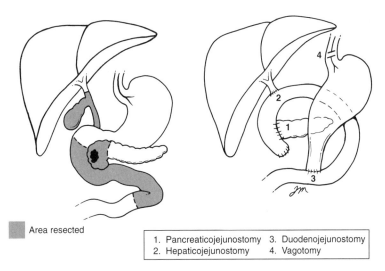

Area resected

1. Pancreaticojejunostomy	3. Duodenojejunostomy
2. Hepaticojejunostomy	4. Vagotomy

Figure 18.2.   Pylorus-preserving Whipple procedure.

complications occur in as many as 46% of patients (8). The most common complications are pancreatic fistula, gastrointestinal bleeding, delayed gastric emptying, postgastrectomy syndromes, weight loss, intraabdominal abscess, and wound infection. Common postoperative complications are thromboembolism, pneumonia, and urinary tract infections.

How can complications be prevented?
In addition to meticulous surgical technique and careful perioperative care, recent randomized clinical trials suggest that perioperative use of octreotide (somatostatin analog) and erythromycin may be appropriate for patients undergoing elective pancreatic surgery. Erythromycin, a motilin agonist, decreases the
extent of delayed gastric emptying and the need for reinstitution of nasogastric decompression after pancreaticoduodenectomy (9). This may be particularly advantageous after pylorus-preserving pancreaticoduodenectomy, a procedure in which delayed gastric emptying is a common postoperative problem.
Two studies have also shown that parenteral somatostatin decreases the risk of
pancreatic fistula after pancreatic resection (10, 11).

What factors contribute to pancreatic fistula formation after the Whipple procedure?
Discussion on this topic has been extensive for 3 decades, but as yet there is no consensus as to the optimal method of managing the pancreatic remnant after pancreaticoduodenectomy. Factors that may promote leakage include large remnant size,
friable parenchymal texture, and absence of pancreatic ductal dilation. Management options include ligation and drainage of the pancreatic stump, pancreaticojejunostomy, and pancreaticogastrostomy, with or without duct-to-mucosa anastomosis. Many variations of pancreaticojejunostomy, the most common
reconstruction, have been tried in attempts to improve its outcome. Proponents of
pancreaticogastrostomy cite the proximity of the stomach to the remnant and absence of an alkaline pancreatic enzyme–activating environment as factors favoring
this reconstruction (12). For the normal, unobstructed pancreatic remnant, stapling
and drainage of the remnant to create a controlled fistula has also been advocated
(13). Pancreatic surgeons should be familiar with the full spectrum of techniques
so that management can be based on the specific operative findings in each patient.

What are the advantages of a pylorus-sparing pancreaticoduodenectomy?
Sparing the pylorus presumably provides the patient with a more nearly normal digestive tract. Patients undergoing pylorus-preserving pancreaticoduodenectomy exhibit more postoperative weight gain and better nutritional status than those undergoing the standard Whipple procedure (14). There is no
survival difference between the two procedures.

**Mr. Snood is still concerned about the poor survival rate after the
Whipple procedure.**

*Should patients with pancreatic cancer routinely receive chemotherapy and radiation after
"curative" resection because surgical management is relatively ineffective in improving
long-term survival?*
A randomized clinical trial by the GI Tumor Study Group demonstrated a small
but statistically significant survival benefit for patients receiving adjuvant 5-

fluorouracil and external beam radiation therapy after potentially curative resection (15). Although the results of this small study have not been duplicated, many medical oncologists cite these data when advocating treatment. Because the issue remains unresolved, participation in randomized clinical trials should be encouraged.

Preoperative chemotherapy with radiation therapy has recently been advocated as possibly improving survival (16). Proponents of neoadjuvant therapy cite as possible advantages the improved drug delivery to the undisturbed tumor and regional lymph nodes and earlier treatment of disseminated disease. This approach is investigational at present and should be undertaken only in clinical trials. Responses to neoadjuvant therapy in patients with unresectable disease have been modest, and patients with resectable tumors should be offered resection as the standard of care. Also, progression to unresectability has been reported in patients with potentially resectable tumors who receive preoperative chemotherapy.

Mr. Snood's preoperative evaluation does not reveal any prohibitive comorbid medical condition or signs of disseminated cancer. After a detailed discussion about all aspects of his disease, Mr. Snood and his family elect surgery and an attempt at curative resection. He is operated on 1 week later. Equipment and supplies for laparoscopic surgery are also kept available.

What operative plan does a surgeon follow to determine resectability? What is the role of minimally invasive surgery in pancreatic cancer?
All patients with pancreatic cancer should undergo diagnostic laparoscopy as the initial step of their operation. This permits detection of peritoneal or small hepatic metastases that have eluded preoperative identification. In addition, laparoscopic ultrasonography may yield critical information about the relation of the tumor to the mesenteric vessels. Such an approach may increase resectability to 75 to 80% in patients undergoing celiotomy (17). If diagnostic laparoscopy does not show evidence of unresectability, the abdomen should be opened for further inspection and palpation, and particular attention should be directed to areas and conditions that are difficult to evaluate laparoscopically (e.g., regional lymph nodes, relation between tumor and mesenteric vessels, involvement of the mesocolon). If curative resection is contraindicated, the patient should be managed with minimally invasive (endoscopic or laparoscopic) bypass procedures.

Diagnostic laparoscopy on Mr. Snood does not show any evidence of tumor on the liver or the peritoneum. Laparoscopic ultrasound

shows the tumor to be invading the lateral wall of the superior
mesenteric vein.

How should the surgeon proceed?
Although experience with major vascular resections, including regional pancreatectomy, in pancreatic cancer has not shown the efficacy of extended resection, recent reports suggest that mesenteric or portal vein involvement
should no longer be considered a contraindication to resection (18). In many
instances, a primary anastomosis can be readily performed; should an interposition graft be required, autogenous vein (internal jugular) is the reconstructive
conduit of choice.

**When the abdomen is explored further laparoscopically, large celiac
nodes are palpated, biopsied and examination of frozen sections
shows tumor metastases.**

How should patients with incurable pancreatic cancer be managed?
Patients and family members should be questioned before the surgery about
their concerns and goals for palliation and improved quality of life. Endoscopic
stenting can easily relieve biliary obstruction and pruritus with minimal cost and
low morbidity. Should this approach fail, percutaneous transhepatic stenting
may be undertaken, with subsequent conversion to internal drainage. Patients
undergoing laparotomy for attempted resection or relief of foregut obstruction
should be managed with gastrojejunostomy and choledochojejunostomy (19).
If peritoneoscopy has determined incurability and the surgeon has mastered advanced gastrointestinal laparoscopic techniques, laparoscopic biliary and gastrointestinal bypasses should be performed.

*Should all patients with incurable disease undergo gastric bypass as part of their pallia-
tion?*
Of patients with unresected periampullary tumors, 15 to 25% develop gastric
outlet obstruction during the course of their disease. It may be appropriate to
omit gastric bypass in patients with systemic metastases who do not have gastric outlet obstruction (20). These patients are unlikely to live long enough to
require gastric decompression and may benefit from avoidance of the additional
morbidity imposed by gastrojejunostomy.

**Before surgery, Mr. Snood considered the benefits and risks of gastric
and biliary decompression, and he decided if possible to seek relief
from pruritus, jaundice, and future gastric outlet obstruction. Therefore, laparoscopic gastrojejunostomy and cholecystojejunostomy are
performed. His recovery is uneventful, and he is discharged on the
eighth postoperative day. Two months later, he develops progressive**

Management Algorithm for Periampullary Neoplasm

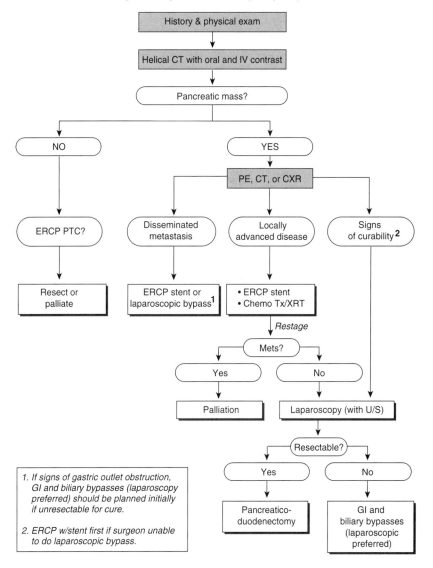

Algorithm 18.1.

gnawing upper abdominal and back pain. His workup demonstrates local progression of the pancreatic tumor.

How is the pain of pancreatic cancer palliated?
Most patients can be kept comfortable with oral opioids. These should be made readily available, and the dosage should be escalated at the patient's request. Pain arising from splanchnic nerve invasion may be controlled by celiac plexus neurolysis. This may be done at the time of laparotomy or by a percutaneous technique during the postoperative period.

Should patients with incurable pancreatic cancer receive chemotherapy?
In a comparison study with historical controls who received no further therapy, 5-fluorouracil in conjunction with external beam radiation therapy was shown to provide a modest survival benefit to patients with unresected pancreatic cancer (21). The treatments, commonly associated with significant side effects, offer no hope of cure and should be administered only after a thorough discussion of risks and potential benefits. Octreotide, tamoxifen, and gemcitabine also have considerable activity in pancreatic cancer. These agents are well tolerated and may significantly improve a patient's quality of life.

Mr. Snood decides against receiving any adjunctive therapy. His gastric and biliary bypass functions well. His bilirubin concentration decreases to a normal level, and he continues to tolerate an oral diet despite poor appetite and progressive malaise. Six months after surgery, he enters a hospice for terminal care.

REFERENCES

1. Wilson RG, Varma JS. Laparoscopic gastroenterostomy for malignant duodenal obstruction. Br J Surg 1992;79:1348.
2. Silverman DT, Dunn JA, Hoover RN, et al. Cigarette smoking and pancreas cancer: a case-control study based on direct interviews. J Natl Cancer Inst 1994;86:1510–1516.
3. Hahn SA, Kern SE. Molecular genetics of exocrine pancreatic neoplasms. Surg Clin North Am 1995;75:857–869.
4. Gudjonsson B. Carcinoma of the pancreas: critical analysis of costs, results of resections and the need for standardized reporting. J Am Coll Surg 1995;181:483–503.
5. Nitecki SS, Sarr MG, Colby TV, van Heerden JA. Long-term survival after resection for ductal adenocarcinoma of the pancreas. Ann Surg 1995;221:59–66.
6. Watanapa P, Williamson RCN. Surgical palliation for pancreatic cancer: developments during the past two decades. Br J Surg 1992;1992:8–20.
7. Lieberman MD, Kilburn H, Lindsey M, Brennan MF. Relation of perioperative deaths to hospital volume among patients undergoing pancreatic resection for malignancy. 1995;222:638–645.

8. Miedema BW, Sarr MG, van Heerden JA, et al. Complications following pancreatico-duodenectomy. Arch Surg 1992;127:945–950.

9. Yeo CJ, Barry MK, Sauter PK, et al. Erythromycin accelerates gastric emptying after pancreaticoduodenectomy. Ann Surg 1993;218:229–238.

10. Montorsi M, Zago M, Mosca F, et al. Efficacy of octreotide in the prevention of pancreatic fistula after elective pancreatic resection: a prospective, controlled, randomized clinical trial. Surgery 1995;117:26–31.

11. Buchler M, Friess H, Klempa I, et al. Role of octreotide in the prevention of postoperative complications following pancreatic resection. Am J Surg 1992;163:125–131.

12. Mason G R, Freeark RJ. Current experience with pancreatogastrostomy. Am J Surg 1995;169:217–219.

13. Reissman P, Perry Y, Cuenca A, et al. Pancreaticojejunostomy versus controlled pancreaticocutaneous fistula in pancreaticoduodenectomy for periampullary carcinoma. Am J Surg 1995;169:217–219.

14. Zerbi A, Balzano G, Patuzzo R, et al. Comparison between pylorus-preserving and Whipple pancreaticoduodenectomy. Br J Surg 1995;82:975–979.

15. Douglass HO, Nav HR, Panahon A, et al. Further evidence of effective adjuvant combined radiation and chemotherapy following curative resection of pancreatic cancer. Cancer 1987;59:2006–2010.

16. Coia L, Hoffman J, Scher R, et al. Preoperative chemoradiation for adenocarcinoma of the pancreas and duodenum. Int J Radiat Oncol Biol Phys 1994;30:16–167.

17. Warshaw AL, Gu ZY, Wittenberg J, Waltham AC. Preoperative staging and assessment of resectability of pancreatic cancer. Arch Surg 1990;125:230–233.

18. Roder JD, Stein HJ. Carcinoma of the periampullary region: who benefits from portal vein resection? Am J Surg 1996;171:170–175.

19. Sarfeh IJ, Rypins EB, Jakowatz JG, Juler GL. A prospective, randomized clinical investigation of cholecystoenterostomy and choledochoenterostomy. Am J Surg 1988; 155:411–414.

20. Wade TP, Neuberger TJ, Swope TJ, et al. Pancreatic cancer palliation: using tumor stage to select appropriate operation. Am J Surg 1994;167:208–213.

21. Moertel CG, Frytak S, Hahn RG, et al. Therapy of locally unresectable pancreatic carcinoma: a randomized comparison of high dose (6000 rads) radiation alone, moderated dose radiation (4000 rads + 5-fluorouracil) and high dose radiation + 5-fluorouracil. Cancer 1981;48:1705–1710.

Inguinal Hernia

Timothy Emhoff

John Jones is a 72-year-old man who visits the emergency room with a complaint of abdominal pain, nausea, vomiting, and poor appetite during the preceding 2 days. His last bowel movement was 3 days ago. His medical history is significant for recently diagnosed hypertension, myocardial infarction 4 years ago, and a stab wound to the abdomen. When questioned about the stab wound, he indicates that exploratory surgery was performed but no significant findings were detected. He smoked one to two packs of cigaretes a day for 50 years but quit just this year. His medications include occasional nifedipine, nitroglycerin (which he has not used for months), and on occasion, antibiotics for his seasonal bronchitis. A physical examination reveals the following vital signs: temperature, 37.2°C; blood pressure, 140/85 mm Hg; pulse, 100 beats per minute; and respiratory rate, 24 breaths per minute. The head and neck examination produces normal findings, the chest examination reveals mild wheezes in both lower lung fields, and the heart examination shows mild tachycardia. Mr. Jones is moderately obese, and his abdomen is distended (larger than normal) and diffusely tender. There is no guarding. A few high-pitched bowel sounds are discernible. The prostate gland is slightly enlarged and firm and has no irregularities. The stool examination reveals traces of occult blood. Pedal pulses are intact.

What is the working diagnosis on the basis of these findings?
Bowel obstruction is the likely diagnosis.

What further tests confirm the diagnosis?
Tests that can confirm this diagnosis are discussed in Chapter 9.

A radiographic series for diagnosis of acute abdominal pain is ordered along with blood tests. Radiographs of the abdomen reveal multiple loops of small bowel with air and fluid levels; the colon is free of gas.

The chest radiograph does not show free air under the diaphragm but does indicate some mild streaking in both lower lung fields. The following are results of laboratory tests: sodium, 145 mEq/L; chloride, 95 mEq/L; potassium, 3.2 mEq/L; bicarbonate, 17 mEq/L; hematocrit, 48%; amylase, 50 mIU/mL; and white blood cell count, 14,000/mL with 10% bands. Urinalysis is unremarkable except for a specific gravity of 1.035. The electrocardiogram shows sinus tachycardia without signs of ischemia.

Mr. Jones is admitted to the surgical service. A nasogastric tube is inserted, and normal saline with potassium replacement is administered intravenously after the urine output is confirmed. He is allowed nothing by mouth. Repeat radiographs are ordered for the next day. The admitting diagnosis is small-bowel obstruction, most likely the result of adhesions arising from the previous abdominal exploration. During the admitting physical examination, a firm, painful swelling is noted in Mr. Jones's right groin, midway between the testicle and the symphysis pubis. The penis, testicles, and scrotum are otherwise normal, as is the skin over the mass.

What is the diagnosis?
The patient has an incarcerated inguinal hernia that is causing small-bowel obstruction. There is a possibility of a strangulated bowel.

What are the most common causes of small-bowel obstruction?
In patients of all ages, the most common cause of small-bowel obstruction is adhesive bands, followed by groin hernias and small-bowel tumors. These three conditions account for 80% of bowel obstructions. Groin hernia is the leading cause in children, and diverticulitis and colorectal carcinoma are the common causes in the elderly. Incisional and groin hernias are easily detected during a physical examination and must be sought in all cases of bowel obstruction.

What are other significant history and laboratory findings?
Smoking and chronic bronchitis may predispose patients to development of groin hernias because of frequent coughing and straining. Smokers may actually develop a defect in collagen that increases the risk of both new and recurrent herniation. Occult blood in the stool may indicate a problem with the bowel mucosa. The occult blood may be explained by a tumor or ischemic necrosis from strangulation (1). Although in the past all patients with hernias were evaluated for large-bowel tumors because hernia was believed to result from increased intraabdominal pressure from the narrowed bowel lumen, the association between hernia and large-bowel tumors has never been proven.

What is a hernia?
A hernia is a defect in a wall through which contents normally contained by that wall may protrude. In a groin hernia, abdominal contents may protrude through a congenital defect. This is best exemplified by an indirect hernia, in which abdominal contents protrude through an enlarged internal ring and a patent processus vaginalis. Groin hernias may also develop over time because of thinning of the abdominal wall itself. For example, a direct inguinal hernia results when the transversalis fascia (the inguinal floor in the region of Hesselbach's triangle) has thinned, allowing abdominal contents to protrude.

What are the symptoms of a hernia?
A hernia is often asymptomatic and can be found only on physical examination when the patient is asked to strain or cough, actions that force abdominal contents through the defect. Patients who have large defects may have abdominal contents in the sac at all times but may have no symptoms. Some patients complain of a dull ache or intermittent pain and notice periodic bulging. Small defects can produce a constricting ring around protruding contents and when swelling increases, can become very painful and lead to ischemia. The hernia contents occasionally become necrotic.

How should a patient with a hernia be examined?
The patient should be standing if possible, facing the seated examiner. Often the protruding bulge can be seen above or below the inguinal ligament, which passes between the anterior superior iliac spine and the symphysis pubis. The internal ring lies midway along this line. Femoral hernias are usually felt below this line, but a large bulge may appear to be above the line. If the hernia is not readily apparent, the examiner should ask the patient to indicate where the bulge was. Palpation of the inguinal canal while the patient strains may reproduce the bulge. The physician can best produce a Valsalva effect by asking the patient to bear down as during a bowel movement. Using the index finger of the gloved hand, the physician should invaginate the upper scrotal skin and follow the testicular cord (vessels and vas deferens) up into the canal. Attention must be directed at palpating the inguinal floor and the external inguinal ring. Indirect hernias may be felt protruding through this ring, and a weak floor can sometimes be palpated lateral to this ring. When both protrusions are felt simultaneously, the hernia is called a pantaloon type.

Can the three types of hernia (direct, indirect, and femoral) be accurately differentiated during a physical examination?
Femoral hernias are differentiated from inguinal hernias on physical examination because the bulge of femoral hernia is below the inguinal ligament and medial to the femoral pulsation. However, reliable differentiation between a direct and an indirect inguinal hernia can be done only at surgery because the distinction

is based on the relation of the epigastric vessels to the defect. Direct hernias lie medial to these vessels, whereas indirect hernias originate lateral to the vessels. The location of the hernia in relation to the epigastric vessels and the size of the opening are important determinants of the type of repair needed and the propensity for recurrence. The size of the hernia orifice is classified as follows: grade I, less than 1.5 cm; grade II, 1.5 to 3 cm; and grade III, more than 3 cm. The average size of the examining fingertip is approximately 1.5 cm (2, 3).

Where are the most common sites of hernias?
The sites of the different types of hernia are as follows (1):

Direct and indirect inguinal hernias and femoral hernias are in the groin, the most common site of hernia (Figure 19.1).
Umbilical hernias are ventral, occurring in the anterior abdominal wall excluding the groin.

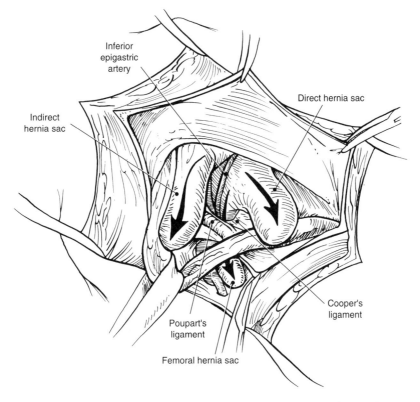

Figure 19.1. Locations of groin hernias. (Reprinted with permission from Nyhus LM, Baker RJ. *Mastery of Surgery*. Vol 2. Philadelphia: JB Lippincott, 1992.)

Epigastric hernias occur in the midline of the abdomen, above the umbilicus. **Spigelian hernias,** which are unusual, occur along the lateral border of the rectus muscle below the umbilicus, at its junction with the linea semilunaris.

What is the incidence of hernias?
Half of hernias are inguinal, followed by femoral, incisional, and umbilical types. Hernias are five times as prevalent in men as in women, and 5% of men have at least one. Inguinal hernias are more common than femoral hernias in women, although women are more likely than men to have a femoral hernia. Indirect inguinal hernias are the most common in both men and women.

What is an incarcerated hernia?
A hernia is considered incarcerated when the sac contents cannot be pushed back through the hernia ring into the cavity from which it protruded. Strangulation occurs when the incarcerated contents lose their blood supply and tissue necrosis sets in. A hernia is considered reducible if its contents can be pushed back into the abdominal cavity, in which case there is no risk of strangulation.

Which intraabdominal organ is incarcerated most frequently within the inguinal canal?
The omentum is the most frequently incarcerated structure. The large or small bowel or a woman's ovary may also be involved. Herniation of ovaries is especially common in newborn girls. In rare cases, the appendix protrudes into the inguinal canal, which leads to obstruction of the appendix and acute appendicitis within the hernia sac. Treatment consists of appendectomy and hernia repair (1). In a sliding hernia, the bowel wall or bladder forms one wall of the hernia.

What are the complications of incarceration?
Incarceration may lead to swelling of the sac contents against a tight hernia ring. A loop of bowel that has been incarcerated can present as an acute bowel obstruction. Strangulation occurs when a reduction in blood flow to the incarcerated contents leads to tissue ischemia and ultimately to necrosis. A strangulated bowel may rupture and cause peritonitis, sepsis, and even death.

When should an incarcerated hernia be repaired?
An incarcerated hernia is a surgical emergency and should be repaired as soon as the diagnosis is made. Delaying surgery can result in strangulation, tissue necrosis, infection, and sepsis. These complications are associated with high morbidity and mortality. Tissue necrosis not only makes hernia repair more difficult because of swelling but is also associated with higher rates of infection and recurrence. In addition, ischemic tissue may preclude the use of prosthetic materials to repair the hernia defect, which can further increase the recurrence rate.

When should a reducible hernia be repaired?
All hernias are susceptible to incarceration and strangulation and should therefore be repaired when discovered. Hernias do not disappear, and over time

they almost always enlarge. The rates of complications and recurrence are higher after surgical repair of incarcerated or strangulated hernias than after elective repair.

Are small hernias less likely to incarcerate than large ones?
Contents that have herniated through a small ring are more prone to constriction, swelling, and strangulation than if the ring is large.

Mr. Jones is taken to the operating room for exploration of the groin, reduction of the hernia, and repair of the defect. At surgery, a loop of small bowel is found in a large indirect hernia sac. The bowel is thickened and hyperemic, but it softens and assumes its normal color when the constricting ring is cut.

Which body layers must be traversed for entry into the inguinal canal?
The skin, subcutaneous tissue, Scarpa's fascia, external oblique fascia (which makes up the external inguinal ring), and external oblique aponeurosis (which is contiguous with the inguinal ligament) are anatomic layers that must be crossed. The spermatic cord lies over the transversalis fascia, beneath the external oblique aponeurosis. The cord enters the abdomen laterally through the transversalis fascia (internal ring), forming the floor of the inguinal canal.

What are the surgical options if the bowel is strangulated and nonviable?
The strangulated loop of bowel must be resected if it appears nonviable. A primary anastomosis can be performed for small-bowel involvement, and both resection and anastomosis can be carried out through the original incision. If the colon is to be resected, a proximal diverting colostomy must be performed. These procedures require a separate incision, and the floor of the inguinal canal may have to be opened to obtain proper exposure.

What is the intraoperative procedure if the hernia's contents cannot be reduced?
The hernia opening is made larger by incising the floor of the inguinal canal through the constricting internal ring.

Mr. Jones's hernia is reduced with high ligation of the hernia sac. When palpated through the sac before closure, the floor of the inguinal canal feels lax, and there is a grade II opening (1.5 to 3 cm).

How can a direct hernia defect such as Mr. Jones's be repaired?
Several options are available for repair of a defect in the floor of the inguinal canal. Mr. Jones has a pantaloon hernia; that is, his hernia has both direct and indirect components. The direct portion is defined by the lax fascia found

medial to the epigastric vessels. The indirect component is indicated by the ligated sac, which is lateral to the epigastric vessels. Tension-free repair is the guiding principle in any hernia operation. Because of the dual nature of Mr. Jones's hernia, an appropriate repair can include a mesh plug inserted into the indirect defect (Figure 19.2) and an onlay mesh that covers the inguinal floor for repair of the direct defect. This mesh can be sutured circumferentially and without tension. Mesh such as Marlex sticks to the tissues. Ultimately, tissue grows into the patch and permanently secures it in place. Most surgeons sew at least one edge of the mesh to the inguinal ligament or to the iliopubic tract, the fascia which appears as a yellow layer of tissue lying just below and medially to the inguinal ligament. Some surgeons also tack the mesh to the aponeurotic layer just under the external oblique. This type of repair, in which a mesh onlay is used, is known as Lichtenstein repair (4–6).

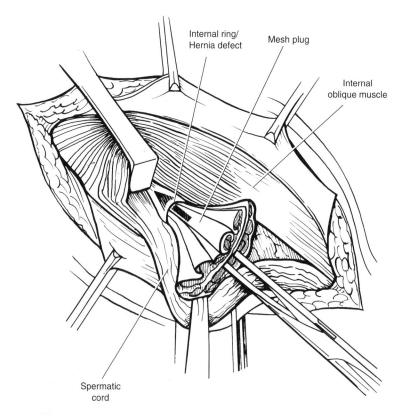

Figure 19.2.   Mesh plug inserted into indirect defect. (Reprinted with permission from Soper NJ, Bendavid R, Arregui ME, eds. Problems in General Surgery. Problems in the Management of Inguinal Hernias. Part 1. Philadelphia: Lippincott-Raven, 1995:123.)

Which other procedures can be used to repair hernias?
Three other repair procedures can be used for hernias (7, 8).

Shouldice repair, in which the patient's own tissues are used. The transversalis fascia is opened from the pubic bone into the internal ring; any thinned redundant tissue (the direct hernia) is removed; and the tissues are sewn, imbricating in four layers, to form a new floor for the inguinal canal.
McVay repair, in which the transversalis fascia and conjoint tendon are used. The tendon is sewn to the deeper Cooper's ligament medially, with a transition area over the femoral vessels as the repair progresses laterally onto Poupart's ligament. Interrupted sutures are used in the McVay repair, and care must be taken not to injure the femoral vein or artery. This procedure can also be used to close the femoral canal for treatment of femoral hernias.
Bassini repair, in which the transversalis fascia and conjoint tendon are used as in the McVay procedure, but sewn to Poupart's ligament (inguinal ligament) from the pubic tubercle medially to the internal ring laterally.

If a bowel resection with or without an anastomosis is required, repair with a foreign body mesh plug or patch should be avoided. A Shouldice, McVay, or Bassini repair should be undertaken. Unlike repairs that use mesh plugs or patches, hernia repairs performed with only native tissue are more likely to develop tension, hence recurrence.

Can hernias be repaired laparoscopically?
Although some surgeons repair groin hernias exclusively with laparoscopic techniques, Mr. Jones's situation is not one in which the laparoscope would be an advantage. Laparoscopic herniorrhaphy may be advantageous for uncomplicated recurrent hernia or bilateral hernias. Further studies on laparoscopic repair are under way.

Should antibiotics be given to patients undergoing hernia repair?
High infection rates are associated with the following conditions:

1. Patient more than 70 years old
2. Use of a drain
3. Repair of incarcerated hernia
4. Repair of recurrent hernia
5. Surgery lasting longer than 90 minutes

Use of a foreign body such as mesh in a repair is believed to increase the risk of infection because significantly fewer bacteria can cause infection when a foreign body is present. A topical antibiotic such as bacitracin or iodine solution is therefore applied to the mesh itself. Parenteral antibiotics have no advantage unless they are administered preoperatively, and if used, they should target only skin organisms. With a patient such as Mr. Jones, both parenteral and topical antibiotics are necessary because he is over age 70, he has incarcerated bowel in the hernia, and mesh is used for the repair.

Mr. Jones has an uncomplicated hernia repair. No bowel is resected, and a mesh plug with onlay patch is used to repair the defects. His small-bowel obstruction rapidly resolves, and he is eating on the third postoperative day.

What is the most serious postoperative complication of hernia repair?
The use of a foreign body in the wound makes infection a serious potential complication. Infection prolongs treatment and may require removal of the mesh.

How is an infection in a groin incision treated?
The wound must be opened and antibiotics administered intravenously if mesh was used and not initially removed. Otherwise, simple drainage of the infection is the most important treatment. After the wound is opened, care includes removing necrotic tissue, providing a moist, occlusive wound environment, and allowing secondary closure (granulation and wound contraction). Use of a calcium alginate wound packing after removal of necrotic tissue is a good way to allow moist wound healing with dressing changes only daily every other day. The alginate absorbs wound exudate and prevents wound maceration while providing a moist healing environment. After it is hydrated, the alginate dressing can easily be removed because it does not adhere to tissue.

What is the recurrence rate after inguinal herniorrhaphy, and what are the risk factors?
Recurrences within 2 to 3 years of operation are the result of poor technique. Examples of technical error include inadequate dissection of an indirect sac, poor choice of suture (using braided absorbable suture), excessive tissue tension in the repair, and infection (1). Late recurrences are usually caused by collagen or fascial degradation, producing a new hernia. This type of recurrence is found around an old hernia in patients in whom a localized herniorrhaphy was used to repair a direct floor defect. Recurrence rates after the classic Shouldice herniorrhaphy have been reported to be less than 1.% when the surgery is performed by experienced surgeons. The McVay (Cooper's ligament) repair is reported to have a recurrence rate of 3.5%. Comparable recurrence rates are claimed with the mesh plug onlay techniques. Advocates of the tension-free mesh technique report low recurrence rates even in inexperienced hands (4–8).

A week after his operation, Mr. Jones is examined and is found to have a swollen, painful right scrotum, with the testicle high in the scrotal sac. His hernia incision has healed and is not painful or swollen.

Management Algorithm for Hernia

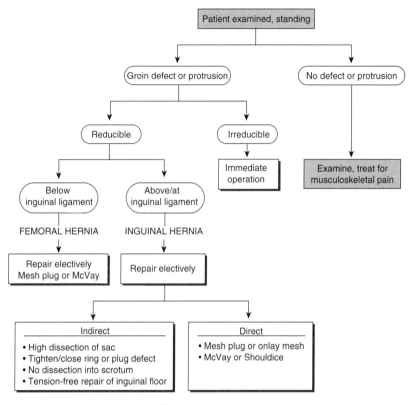

Algorithm 19.1.

What is the problem and how can it be treated?
Mr. Jones has ischemic orchitis, a condition that may ultimately result in testicular atrophy. Ischemic orchitis can be prevented by limiting the dissection around the spermatic cord. Limited dissection prevents injury to the delicate testicular veins and the pampiniform plexus. Therapy consists of symptomatic care. Analgesics and anti-inflammatory medications can alleviate the symptoms.

REFERENCES

1. Nyhus LM, Condon RE, eds. Hernia. 4th ed. Philadelphia: Lippincott, 1995.
2. Soper NJ, Bendavid R, Arregui ME, eds. Problems in General Surgery: Problems in the Management of Inguinal Hernias. Part 1, vol 12, no 1. Philadelphia: Lippincott-Raven, 1995.
3. Soper NJ, Bendavid R, Arregui ME, eds. Problems in General Surgery: Problems in the Management of Inguinal Hernias. Part 2, vol 12, no 2. Philadelphia: Lippincott-Raven, 1995.

4. Lichtenstein, IL, Shulman, AG, Amid PK, Montilor MM. The tension-free hernioplasty. Am J Surg 1989;157:188–193.
5. Amid PK, Shulman AG, Lichtenstein IL. Critical scrutiny of the open "tension free" hernioplasty. Am J Surg 1993;165:369–375.
6. Amid PK, Shulman AG, Lichtenstein IL. Open, tension-free repair of inguinal hernias: the Lichtenstein technique. Eur J Surg 1996;162:447–453.
7. Contemporary Surgery. Symposium: Operative Repair of Inguinal Hernias. Part 1. Torrence, CA: Bobit Publishing, 1997:387–397.
8. Contemporary Surgery. Symposium: Operative Repair of Inguinal Hernia. Part 2. Torrence, CA: Bobit Publishing, 1998:61–72.

Carotid Artery Disease

Jeffrey H. Widmeyer

Matthew Hooper is a 72-year-old man with no significant medical history. He presents with expressive aphasia that occurred 2 hours before his arrival at the hospital. He also has slight weakness in his right arm and leg. His symptoms resolve over 4 hours, leaving him able to speak but at times unable to find the word he is searching for.

What is a transient ischemic attack (TIA)?
A TIA is a temporary focal neurologic deficit that lasts less than 24 hours. The most common cause of TIA is carotid occlusive disease; however, embolization from the heart must be considered. TIAs resulting from extracranial occlusive disease tend to be the same each time, whereas those caused by cardiac emboli tend to produce varying symptoms (1).

What is amaurosis fugax?
Amaurosis fugax is transient loss of vision or blurring in the eye ipsilateral to a carotid plaque. Often, it is described as if a shade were coming down over the affected eye or as a quadrant visual field defect.

This is the first time the patient has had this type of episode, and he has no headache, seizure, aura, or changes in vision. Physical examination findings are normal except for a left-side carotid bruit. Vital signs are normal, and electrocardiogram (ECG) shows normal sinus rhythm.

What is the significance of a carotid bruit?
A bruit indicates turbulent flow in a vessel that causes vibration and therefore noise. The extreme manifestation of this vibration is a palpable thrill. It may be caused by plaque in or narrowing of the common, internal, or external carotid artery. In the absence of symptoms, a carotid bruit should not cause alarm. Even in the presence of cerebrovascular symptoms, a bruit alone is insufficient to predict a high-grade stenosis (2). Because noninvasive vascular technology is read-

ily accessible, a carotid bruit is best evaluated by carotid Doppler (duplex) study to evaluate for significant stenosis.

What if a bruit is found on physical examination before an elective general surgical procedure or before vascular or cardiac surgery?
Prospective studies show no significant increase in stroke rate for elective general surgery (3). Symptomatic carotid stenosis is shown to increase the risk of stroke in vascular and coronary surgery, but asymptomatic carotid stenosis is not (4).

Mr. Hooper undergoes a carotid duplex study, which is normal on the right and shows a 90% stenosis of the left internal carotid artery just above the bifurcation.

How does a carotid duplex study identify carotid lesions, and how accurate is it?
Imaging ultrasound identifies atherosclerotic plaques as an echogenic area in an otherwise homogeneous vessel. The Doppler mode measures relative blood velocity. Areas of turbulent flow and increased velocity occur at points of stenosis. Stenoses may be quantified as a range (e.g., 50 to 75% stenosis) when compared with the adjacent "normal" vessel. Carotid duplex is operator dependent, but in experienced hands it is very accurate. Studies comparing carotid duplex with angiography (the gold standard) show good correlation (5).

Mr. Hooper has an arch angiogram with injection of both carotid arteries and shows a 90% stenosis of the left internal carotid artery. These findings correlate well with the findings on carotid duplex study. In accordance with his presentation, the angiogram and carotid duplex study findings, and his lack of cardiac history or evidence of arrhythmia, Mr. Hooper is diagnosed with symptomatic 90% stenosis of the left internal carotid. Carotid endarterectomy is recommended.

What are the indications for carotid endarterectomy, and what prospective randomized trials support those indications?
Symptomatic patients with high-grade stenosis (70 to 99%), such as Mr. Hooper, derive more benefit from carotid endarterectomy than from medical treatment (aspirin). The North American Symptomatic Carotid Endarterectomy Trial (NASCET), a multicenter prospective randomized trial, demonstrated a significant reduction in stroke in patients randomized to carotid endarterectomy compared with those treated medically. Data on patients with intermediate stenosis (30 to 69%) are still being collected (6). In the Asymptomatic Carotid Atherosclerosis Study (ACAS), another multicenter prospective randomized trial, asymptomatic patients with 60% or greater carotid stenosis show a significant reduction in risk of stroke when carotid endarterectomy instead of medical therapy is used (7). Both studies required surgeons experienced

in carotid endarterectomy with documented histories of morbidity and mortality rates below 3%. Many older multicenter trials show a benefit of surgery in stroke reduction for severe carotid stenosis, but the study design of NASCET and ACAS is believed to be the most reliable to date (8).

How soon after a TIA can carotid endarterectomy be performed? How soon after a completed stroke can it be performed?
Endarterectomy can be performed immediately after TIA. Traditionally, a 6-week waiting period following a cerebrovascular accident (CVA) was advocated because of the risk of converting an ischemic, or dry, infarct into a hemorrhagic, or wet, infarct. Today, the trend is toward waiting until the patient's recovery from the stroke has reached a plateau. An emergency endarterectomy should be carefully considered if the stroke is in evolution or if the patient has crescendo TIAs (i.e., frequent, repeated attacks of a neurologic deficit without full recovery between attacks) (9). In these cases, endarterectomy is unusual and risky, and it requires an experienced surgeon and careful consideration.

Mr. Hooper is under general anesthesia; his head is turned to the right and slightly extended. His neck is gently prepped and draped, and an incision is made along the anterior border of the sternocleidomastoid muscle, through the platysma. The anterior, or crossing, facial vein is identified, ligated, and divided. The internal jugular vein is retracted laterally, and the carotid artery is identified.

What arterial, venous, muscular, and nervous system structures are identified during this dissection?

Arteries. The common, internal, and external arteries are identified and controlled with vessel loops or umbilical tapes. The superior thyroid artery is the first branch of the external carotid artery and is usually controlled separately. There are no extracranial branches of the internal carotid artery.
Veins. The internal jugular vein and the facial vein are the important venous structures; the facial vein is a landmark for the carotid bifurcation.
Muscles and nervous system structures. The **omohyoid muscle inferiorly** usually marks the larger aspect of the dissection of the common carotid; it may be retracted or divided if further exposure is needed. The **digastric muscle superiorly is a good landmark** for the hypoglossal nerve, which crosses the internal carotid at this level. The hypoglossal nerve should be identified and preserved. Injury to this nerve is commonly a result of retraction and causes deviation of the tongue toward the side of injury. The ansa hypoglossi branches from the hypoglossal nerve as it crosses the internal carotid and then courses inferiorly. It innervates the strap muscles, and it may be divided with minimal consequence if exposure is needed. The vagus nerve lies

in a posterolateral position in the carotid sheath, and injury causes vocal cord paralysis. The carotid body is located in the carotid bifurcation, and manipulation in this area can cause hypotension and bradycardia. Local injection with 1% lidocaine blocks these effects; this is done routinely by some surgeons and selectively by others. The marginal mandibular branch of the facial nerve at the superior aspect of the incision is also at risk; injury of this branch can paralyze the lower lip. Finally, the greater auricular nerve, which provides sensation to the earlobe, is in the same region and should be preserved if exposure is not compromised.

The common, internal, and external carotid arteries are dissected and controlled with vessel loops. The surgeon takes great care to handle the vessels gently so as not to dislodge and embolize plaque material. Heparin is administered systemically. The internal carotid artery is clamped first, followed by the external and then the common carotid artery. The artery is opened longitudinally, starting in the common below the plaque, extending up through the plaque, and into the internal. A shunt is placed into the common carotid first; blood is allowed to flush through the shunt, and the shunt is clamped. The distal end is carefully placed in the internal carotid and opened. Both ends of the shunt are secured in the artery with clamps that seal the artery around the shunt.

What is a shunt, and why is it used in this patient? Do all surgeons use them? What are the risks associated with shunts? Are there alternatives to using a shunt?
A shunt is a soft plastic (Silastic) tube inserted proximally and distally through the endarterectomy incision to maintain cerebral blood flow during a carotid endarterectomy. It is used in this patient because the surgeon is a routine shunter (as opposed to a nonshunter or a selective shunter). Those who shunt routinely prefer the comfort of nearly continuous cerebral perfusion during the endarterectomy and note that shunt placement is easily performed and takes some of the time pressure off the surgeon, allowing a meticulous endarterectomy without concern for cerebral hypoperfusion or the need for expensive cerebral monitoring. Nonshunters prefer an unobstructed operative field and note that shunt placement carries its own (albeit low) risk of embolization and stroke. They correctly note that nearly all patients tolerate 20 to 30 minutes of carotid occlusion. Selective shunters agree that shunt placement is not benign and that most patients do not need it for a safe endarterectomy but recognize that some patients are at relatively high risk for complications of cerebral hypoperfusion. They rely on some form of cerebral monitoring to identify patients who need a shunt. Routine shunting, nonshunting, and selective shunting have all been demonstrated to yield excellent results.

How do surgeons monitor for cerebral hypoperfusion during carotid endarterectomy? Common techniques for monitoring of cerebral perfusion during carotid endarterectomy include monitoring the patient's mental status under local or regional anesthesia, measurement of distal stump pressure, monitoring electroencephalography (EEG) intraoperatively, and more recently, near-infrared spectroscopy.

Mental status. A change in mental status in a patient with carotid occlusion whose endarterectomy is being performed under local anesthesia is a very sensitive and specific indicator of cerebral hypoperfusion and is the most clinically relevant. However, significant cooperation is required of the patient, and anesthetic techniques are critical.

Distal stump pressure. The carotid stump pressure is the pressure in the distal internal carotid artery measured after clamping the common and external carotid arteries. It reflects the collateral circulation within the brain via the circle of Willis. This stump pressure correlates roughly with the perfusion pressure seen in that clamped hemisphere. What constitutes an acceptable stump pressure above which no shunt is necessary is controversial, but many surgeons use a minimum stump pressure of 35 mm Hg as the cutoff point below which a shunt is placed (10). Patients with stump pressure below this level may tolerate clamping without problems, and conversely, a stump pressure above 50 mm Hg does not rule out a postoperative neurologic deficit.

EEG. EEG monitors electrical activity of both cerebral cortices, but it does not monitor brainstem or subcortical tissue (10, 11). It is a sensitive index of ischemia, perhaps too sensitive, since up to 15% of patients have EEG changes during endarterectomy. EEG changes occur well before permanent ischemic damage. EEG does require extensive monitoring and expertise for interpretation.

Near-infrared spectroscopy. Near-infrared spectroscopy is a new technique that directly measures cerebral tissue oxygenation by emitting and sensing a near-infrared light source that penetrates bone. After placement of the leads on the skin, changes in cerebral tissue oxygenation are recorded noninvasively (analogous to pulse oximetry). Measurements are regional, recorded only in areas immediately below the sensor. Changes in cerebral oxygenation mandating shunting are not as yet clear-cut. Neuroprotective agents, such as thiopental, have been used without shunting with excellent results (12). As the understanding and monitoring of cerebral ischemia continue to improve, the use of neuroprotective agents is likely to increase.

The endarterectomy continues, with blunt dissection in a plane in the mid- to outer media. The dissection begins in the distal common carotid and continues distally. The external and then the internal carotid portion of the plaque are then removed. Great care is taken at the distal end of the internal carotid dissection to leave a smooth

feathered edge of transition between the endarterectomized and normal vessel, so that no abrupt edge can serve as a lead point for a dissection. If this type of flap is left, it is tacked down with a 7–0 prolene suture. The remaining luminal surface is carefully inspected for
loose fragments, which are removed. The arteriotomy is then closed
with a preclotted polyester (Dacron) patch and secured in place with
a 6–0 prolene suture. The wound is irrigated and closed in layers after hemostasis is adequate. The heparin is not reversed.

What is the purpose of the patch closure?
By necessity, primary closure of the arteriotomy causes a small amount of luminal narrowing. Patch closure not only eliminates narrowing but actually widens
the lumen. Intuitively, this widening of the lumen leads to less restenosis; whether
this is clinically significant is difficult to demonstrate. Comparisons of both saphenous vein patch and prosthetic patch with primary closure have not demonstrated
an advantage of either approach (13, 14). Many surgeons use patches routinely,
knowing that this type of closure leaves a widely patent vessel.

**Mr. Hooper awakes from surgery neurologically intact and recovers
uneventfully. He is discharged home on postoperative day 2. He remains asymptomatic, and his wound heals well. He returns for yearly
carotid Doppler studies, which at 5 years reveal a 60% restenosis of
his left internal carotid artery.**

Should all postendarterectomy patients have routine follow-up Doppler examinations?
Follow-up duplex studies are valuable to track progression of contralateral
carotid disease and to look for the relatively uncommon recurrence of stenosis on the operated side (15).

How should Mr. Hooper's recurrent left internal carotid artery stenosis be managed?
Most surgeons observe an asymptomatic 60% lesion. Current data support repeat carotid endarterectomy for symptomatic as well as high–grade (more than
75%) asymptomatic stenoses (16). As with any reoperative surgery, morbidity
is slightly higher for repeat carotid endarterectomy; however, in experienced
hands it can be performed safely (17). Some groups are looking at angioplasty
and stenting as a treatment for recurrent carotid stenosis with some success, but
long term follow-up is not yet available (18).

*If Mr. Hooper has coronary artery disease requiring bypass surgery as well as carotid dis-
ease, what should be done?*
Since atherosclerosis is a systemic disease, patients with carotid artery stenosis
often have coronary artery disease (symptomatic or not) and vice versa. Up to
50% of patients undergoing carotid endarterectomy have significant coronary

artery disease, and cardiac complications are the most common cause of post-operative morbidity and mortality. Obviously, patients being considered for endarterectomy need a careful and thorough cardiac evaluation, including catheterization if the patient has angina. The issue of concomitant carotid endarterectomy and coronary bypass surgery arises when significant coronary and

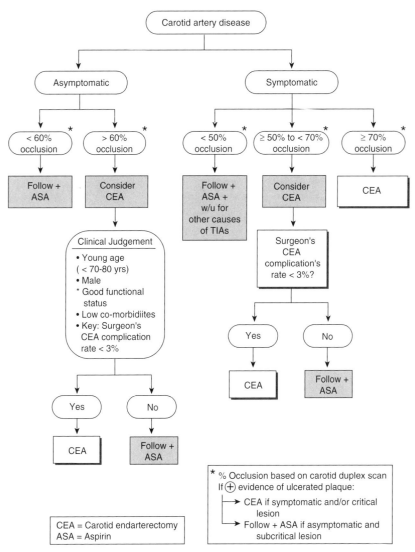

Algorithm 20.1.

carotid disease coexist. A rule of thumb is that the more symptomatic disease should be addressed first, reserving combined carotid and coronary surgery for patients with high-grade carotid stenosis or ulcerative plaque *and* severe unstable angina, significant left main coronary disease, or severe three-vessel coronary disease. Although combined procedures can be done safely, most studies have demonstrated higher stroke rates with combined procedures than with either procedure alone (19).

REFERENCES

1. Moore WS. Extracranial cerebrovascular disease. In: Moore WS, ed. Vascular Surgery: A Comprehensive Review. Philadelphia: Saunders, 1993:546.

2. Suave JS et al. Can bruits distinguish high-grade from moderate symptomatic carotid stenosis? The North American Symptomatic Carotid Endarterectomy Trial. Ann Intern Med 1994;120:8.

3. Ropper AH et al. Carotid bruit and the risk of stroke in elective surgery. N Engl J Med 1982;307:22.

4. Gerraty RP et al. Carotid stenosis and perioperative stroke risk in symptomatic and asymptomatic patients undergoing vascular or coronary surgery. Stroke 1993;24:8.

5. Liberopoulos K et al. Comparative study of magnetic resonance angiography, digital subtraction angiography, duplex ultrasound examination with surgical and histological findings of atherosclerotic carotid bifurcation disease. Int Angiol 1996;15:2.

6. North Medical Symptomatic Carotid Endarterectomy Trial Collaborators. Beneficial effect of carotid endarterectomy in symptomatic patients with high grade carotid stenosis. N Engl J Med 1991;325:445–453.

7. Executive Committee for the Asymptomatic Carotid Atherosclerosis Study. Endarterectomy for asymptomatic carotid artery stenosis. JAMA 1995;273:18.

8. Moneta GL, Masser PA. Randomized, multicenter trials of carotid endarterectomy. Ann Vasc Surg 1994;8:4.

9. Moore WS. Extracranial cerebrovascular disease. In: Moore WS, ed. Vascular Surgery: A Comprehensive Review. Philadelphia: Saunders, 1993:567.

10. McCarthy WJ et al. Carotid endarterectomy: lessons from intraoperative monitoring: a decade of experience. Ann Surg 1996;224:3.

11. Fiori L, Parenti G. Electrophysiological monitoring for selective shunting during carotid endarterectomy. J Neurol Anesth 1995;1:3.

12. Frawley JE et al. Carotid endarterectomy without a shunt for symptomatic lesions associated with contralateral sever stenosis or occlusion. J Vasc Surg 1996;23:3.

13. Katz D et al. Long term follow-up for recurrent stenosis: a prospective randomized study of expanded polytetrafluoroethylene patch angioplasty versus primary closure after carotid endarterectomy. J Vasc Surg 1994;19:2.

14. Myers SI et al. Saphenous vein patch versus primary closure for carotid endarterectomy: long-term assessment of a randomized prospective study. J Vasc Surg 1994;19:1.

15. Ricotta JJ, DeWesse JA. Is routine carotid surveillance after carotid endarterectomy worthwhile? Am J Surg 1996;172:2.

16. O'Donnell TF et al. Management of recurrent carotid stenosis: should asymptomatic lesions be treated surgically? J Vasc Surg 1996;24:2.

17. Coyle KA et al. Treatment of recurrent cerebrovascular disease: review of a 10-year experience. Ann Surg 1995;221:5.
18. Yadav JS et al. Angioplasty and stenting for restenosis after carotid endarterectomy. Stroke 1996;27:11.
19. Giangola G et al. Perioperative morbidity and mortality in combined vs. staged approaches to carotid and coronary revascularization. Ann Vasc Surg 1996;10:2.

Abdominal Aortic Aneurysm

Marc Norris

Mark Anderson is a 65-year-old retired army officer who was in good health until 2 years ago, when a routine physical examination revealed a pulsatile, nontender upper midline abdominal mass.

What is the differential diagnosis of a pulsatile abdominal mass?
Not every pulsatile mass is an aneurysm, although abnormal dilation of the aorta or one of its branch vessels (hepatic, splenic, superior mesenteric, renal, or iliac arteries) should be high on the list of possible diagnoses. A cystic or solid intraperitoneal or abdominal wall mass may also have referred aortic pulsations. A cystic mass in the small bowel mesentery, an inflammatory or neoplastic lesion in the colon, or a mass in the lesser sac related to previous pancreatitis may all have a presentation similar to Mr. Anderson's, especially if the patient is thin.

What is an aneurysm?
An aneurysm is a fixed, or permanent, enlargement of an artery to twice the normal diameter. The normal abdominal aorta averages 1.5 to 2.5 cm in diameter, depending on the age and sex of the person (1).

What causes abdominal aortic aneurysms?
Atherosclerosis is the cause of abdominal aortic aneurysms in approximately 95% of cases (2). The atherosclerotic process creates an intrinsic weakness in the arterial wall that leads to progressive dilation over time. Less common causes of abdominal aortic aneurysms include trauma, syphilis, mycotic infection, congenital defects, Marfan's syndrome, inflammation, and pregnancy. Aneurysms associated with reconstructive arterial surgery are being reported with increasing frequency (3).

How common are abdominal aortic aneurysms?
Abdominal aortic aneurysms are the most common of the atherosclerotic aneurysms, estimated to occur in as many as 2% of the elderly population in Western countries. Their incidence is increasing steadily, and they are the aneurysms most commonly diagnosed by physicians (4).

Mr. Anderson undergoes an abdominal ultrasound examination, which reveals a 3.5-cm abdominal aortic aneurysm. No further studies are performed, and he is monitored with serial ultrasound examinations.

Why is the size of an aneurysm important, and how does it guide surgical treatment?
Rupture of an aortic aneurysm ranks 10th as the cause of death in men more than 55 years old (5). Other complications of aneurysm include thrombosis, embolization, dissection, and obstruction of or erosion into an adjacent organ. Arterial wall tension, hence rupture risk, can be characterized by the law of La Place, in which tension is proportional to the product of the pressure and the radius (t = p × r). The risk of rupture increases considerably with aneurysm size. For an aneurysm less than 4 cm in diameter, the risk of rupture is generally thought to be negligible, although it can occur. Aneurysms 5 to 6 cm in diameter have a 5 to 15% annual risk, whereas those more than 8 cm in diameter have at least a 30 to 40% annual risk of rupture (6). Elective repair should be considered in most patients with an aneurysm 5 to 6 cm or larger and in young low-risk patients with 4- to 5-cm aneurysms (7).

How should a patient such as Mr. Anderson be managed?
A patient with a 3.5-cm aneurysm should be observed for symptoms and any evidence of growth. A 6-month follow-up ultrasound examination is routine. If the aneurysm is stable, yearly follow-up is recommended. Any indication of growth should prompt more frequent follow-up—for example every 3 months.

What is the best radiologic technique for monitoring an aneurysm?
There are essentially two options for surveillance: computed tomography (CT) and ultrasonography. Magnetic resonance imaging (MRI) is not cost effective. Plain radiography, such as cross-table lateral radiography (if sufficient calcification in the aortic wall is present), is occasionally useful in an emergency. On KUB radiography, the psoas shadow on the left may be obliterated. CT is also helpful for evaluating other intraabdominal lesions. Both CT and ultrasonography are noninvasive, but in most centers ultrasonography is accurate and cost effective. Regardless of the test chosen, the same test must be used for follow-up examinations. Aortography and MR angiography are not used for surveillance; they are discussed later.

Mr. Anderson is reevaluated 1 year later, at which time the abdominal ultrasound examination shows that the maximal transverse diameter of the abdominal aortic aneurysm is 3.7 cm and that it extends to the common iliac arteries bilaterally.

What is the average annual rate of growth of an abdominal aortic aneurysm?
Ultrasound studies show that expansion rates vary from 2 to 8 mm per year, with an average of 4 mm annually (3). Traditional belief was that almost all aneurysms

expand over time (8). However, it is now clear that some aneurysms show very little growth over a long period of follow-up, whereas others grow rapidly over a relatively short period (9). Certain risk factors, such as hypertension and chronic obstructive lung disease, are associated with rapidly growing aneurysms (10).

Mr. Anderson is scheduled for a repeat examination in 6 months, but he is lost to follow-up. He returns to the clinic 2 years later, at which time a follow-up abdominal ultrasound examination reveals enlargement of the aneurysm to 5 cm. Mr. Anderson is referred to surgery for further evaluation and elective surgical repair of his abdominal aortic aneurysm. Mr. Anderson does not have abdominal pain or tenderness, low back pain, extremity pain, hematuria, melena, or bloody stools. He has had no recent illness and has no history of angina, congestive heart failure, or cerebrovascular disease. He had a transurethral retrograde prostatectomy for benign prostatic hypertrophy 12 years ago. A physical examination shows Mr. Anderson appearing normal and in no apparent distress. His vital signs are blood pressure, 130/75 mm Hg; pulse, 78 beats per minute; respiratory rate, 18 breaths per minute; and temperature, 36.9°C. The only abnormal finding on physical examination is a large immobile pulsatile mass palpated in the midepigastrium just above the umbilicus. The mass is not tender, and there is no audible bruit. The stools are guaiac negative. The laboratory data are hematocrit, 41%; leukocyte count, 7200/mL; platelet count 284,000/mL; blood urea nitrogen, 33 mg/dL; creatinine 1.1 mg/dL; electrolytes, normal; and coagulation tests, normal. The electrocardiogram and chest radiograph are normal. Plain abdominal radiographs show a calcified aortic wall with infrarenal aneurysmal dilation to approximately 4.5 cm.

What is the most frequent presentation of an abdominal aortic aneurysm?
Abdominal aortic aneurysms are more common in men than in women by a ratio of 4:1, and they occur mainly in the sixth or seventh decade of life (3). In 75% of patients, the aneurysm presents as an asymptomatic pulsatile abdominal mass, and approximately 80% of these are found during a physical examination or are discovered by the patient. The remainder are detected during a radiologic examination performed for other reasons. With ultrasonography, an increasing number of smaller aneurysms are being detected (11). When symptoms are present, the most common complaint is vague abdominal pain, which may be caused by expansion or rupture of the aneurysm. The pain frequently begins in the epigastrium and penetrates to the back. Tenderness on direct palpation of the aneurysm and flank pain are other signs of rupture. On rare occasions, patients have flank pain from ureteral obstruction or gastrointestinal bleeding from a primary aortoenteric fistula. Ureteral obstruction should raise suspicion of an inflammatory aneurysm (12).

What are the important findings from a physical examination?
The physical examination is diagnostic in most cases. A large pulsatile immobile mass in the epigastrium is the most frequent finding. Because the bifurcation of the aorta is at the level of the umbilicus, the mass is usually at or above this level. Tenderness may be present on palpation, and a bruit may be found on auscultation of the abdomen. Distal pulses of the lower extremities may be diminished.

What is the natural history of abdominal aortic aneurysms?
The natural history of abdominal aortic aneurysms was described by Estes in 1950, before the advent of surgical repair (13). Of 102 patients with abdominal aortic aneurysms, only 67% were alive 1 year after diagnosis, 49% at 3 years, and 19% at 5 years. Rupture of the abdominal aneurysm caused the death of 63% of these patients. In a 1972 report on 156 patients who had been rejected for surgical repair, Szilagyi et al. (14) showed that among patients with aneurysms greater than 6 cm, 43% died of aneurysm rupture, and 37% died of myocardial infarction; among patients with aneurysms less than 6 cm, 36% died of myocardial infarction, and 31% died of rupture.

What are the guidelines for recommending repair of an aneurysm?
Treatment must be individualized, but the natural history of the condition provides general guidelines. Patients with an abdominal aortic aneurysm larger than 6 cm should be considered for elective repair unless they have severe uncorrectable coronary artery disease or severe chronic obstructive pulmonary disease. Most patients with an aneurysm that is 5 to 6 cm and no active coronary artery disease or chronic obstructive pulmonary disease should also be considered for elective repair. The treatment of aneurysms smaller than 5 cm is controversial and is being examined in three ongoing randomized prospective trials. At present, however, elective repair of aneurysms smaller than 5 cm is recommended only for patients less than 60 years old who are otherwise healthy.

What is the appropriate preoperative radiologic workup for an aneurysm?
The extent of disease and to some degree the experience of the surgeon determine the preoperative radiologic workup. Several authors have shown that contrast-enhanced CT is very accurate at defining both the extent of the aneurysm and its relation to important branch vessels, such as the renal arteries (15, 16). Spiral CT with multiplanar (three-dimensional) reconstruction is becoming the study of choice for accurate definition of abdominal aortic anatomy (17). Indications for aortography include the following:

• Unexplained impaired renal function or renovascular hypertension
• Suspected chronic visceral ischemia
• Abdominal or flank bruit

- Suspected suprarenal aneurysm
- Iliofemoral occlusive disease

Magnetic resonance angiography is also accurate at delineating abdominal aortic anatomy. It compares well with CT and aortography, especially with three-dimensional reconstruction (18). The definition and accuracy of spiral CT and magnetic resonance angiography depend on the ability to reconstruct images after they are acquired.

What is the appropriate cardiac workup before repair of an abdominal aortic aneurysm?
A good schema for cardiac workup is as follows (3):

Patient has no cardiac symptoms: repair aneurysm
Patient has mild but stable cardiac symptoms: perform noninvasive cardiac study
    Study positive: perform coronary angiography
    Study negative: repair aneurysm
Significant cardiac symptoms: perform coronary angiography
    Significant coronary artery disease: perform coronary artery bypass graft procedure and then repair aneurysm
    Insignificant coronary artery disease: repair aneurysm
Patient more than 80 years old, ejection fraction less than 30%, or coronary artery disease that cannot be reconstructed
    Aneurysm smaller than 6 cm: monitor patient
    Aneurysm larger than 6 cm: repair aneurysm with cardiac support

Before admission, digital subtraction aortography is performed on Mr. Anderson to confirm the infrarenal aneurysm with extension to the level of the common iliac arteries. This study also shows significant peripheral vascular disease involving the superficial femoral arteries bilaterally, with two-vessel runoff in the right lower extremity and single-vessel runoff in the left lower extremity. Extensive bilateral lower extremity collateral vessels are also noted.

What is the typical location of abdominal aortic aneurysms?
More than 95% of these aneurysms arise below the renal vessels (3). Approximately 66% extend inferiorly to involve the common iliac vessels (2). Rarely do they extend far enough to involve the internal iliac vessels.

Are prophylactic perioperative antibiotics indicated in patients undergoing repair of an aneurysm?
The infection rate without prophylactic antibiotic coverage approaches 7% and is reduced to about 1% with the use of antibiotics (19). Therefore, prophylactic antibiotics are indicated.

Mr. Anderson undergoes surgery the next day. Dissection is performed through a midline abdominal incision, down to and around the aorta. A fusiform aneurysm approximately 5.5 cm in diameter is noted. After aortic cross-clamping, an uncomplicated repair of the aneurysm is performed using a woven polyester (Dacron) bifurcating graft.

What precautions should be taken during repair of an abdominal aortic aneurysm?
Cardiovascular monitoring and management have utmost importance. A Swan-Ganz catheter should be inserted before the operation to help maintain fluid balance and monitor pressure. A radial arterial line should be placed for accurate blood pressure monitoring. Renal function must be monitored closely, and a Foley catheter is essential. Mannitol is occasionally administered to minimize the risk of renal failure during aortic cross-clamping.

What are the physiologic consequences of cross-clamping the aorta?
An acute interruption of the distal aortic flow increases afterload on the heart and decreases cardiac output. The systemic vascular resistance proximal to the cross-clamp also increases. A sudden decrease of blood flow to the lower extremity leads to lactate acidosis and a decreased venous return from the lower extremity. Heparin is administered prior to aortic cross-clamping to prevent arterial thrombosis.

What is the physiologic response after the aortic cross-clamp is released?
A sudden release of the cross-clamp sharply reduces the aortic blood pressure. In addition, there is a sudden increase of lactate-containing venous blood from the lower extremities. Particular attention must be given to acidosis, hypovolemia, and electrolyte abnormalities after the aorta is unclamped (3). Any fluid and bicarbonate should therefore be administered before the aortic cross-clamp is released.

What is the difference between woven and knitted polyester grafts?
Polyester grafts are textile fabrics developed by Debakey and others (20). The structural characteristics of these two types of grafts differ. Woven grafts have small interstitial holes and usually do not allow leakage through the fabric. They are stiffer and consequently more difficult to sew. Knitted grafts have larger interstitial holes in the fabric and require preclotting to reduce bleeding through the fabric. They are more supple and easier to sew than the woven grafts. Modern knitted grafts are coated with collagen, albumin, or gelatin, which obviates preclotting.

What is a meandering mesenteric artery, and why is it significant for abdominal aortic aneurysm surgery?
In patients with atherosclerosis of the abdominal aorta, either the superior mesenteric artery (SMA) or the inferior mesenteric artery (IMA) may be occluded at its

origin, requiring collateral vessels to supply the area of deficit. The meandering mesenteric artery is a large and tortuous collateral artery coursing from a branch of the SMA, the middle colic artery, to a branch of the IMA, the left colic artery, and is visible at the center of the abdomen on a preoperative angiogram in 25% of patients with abdominal aortic aneurysm (21). (The meandering mesenteric artery, also called the arc of Riolan, is a separate entity from the marginal artery of Drummond.) The IMA is the only major vessel usually involved in the aortic aneurysm. This vessel supplies blood to the left colon and rectosigmoid region of the bowel. It can be ligated without consequence during surgery on the abdominal aortic aneurysm in most patients, because of the rich collateral circulation from the superior mesenteric system. However, in patients with a meandering mesenteric artery visible on an angiogram arising as a result of previous SMA occlusion and a retrograde collateral flow from the IMA, inadvertent ligation of the IMA during surgery leads to severe mesenteric ischemia. In that case, preservation of the IMA during surgery is critical. If interruption of the IMA is unavoidable, reimplantation of the IMA onto the aortic graft may be necessary to avoid bowel ischemia. Measurement of mesenteric arterial stump pressure may be useful in identifying patients at risk for postoperative ischemic colitis (22).

Is the aneurysm removed during the operation?
The aneurysm is not removed. The anterior wall and thrombus are resected, with the posterior wall kept intact and undissected. The wall is then wrapped around the prosthetic graft and is reapproximated anteriorly by separating the graft from surrounding structures to prevent formation of aortoenteric or aortocaval fistulas.

Who performed the first successful repair of an abdominal aortic aneurysm?
Dubost performed the first successful repair of an abdominal aortic aneurysm in Paris in 1951. His repair included reconstruction of the aorta with an aortic homograft (23).

What are the alternatives to graft replacement of the aneurysm?
Nonresective treatment by ligation of the proximal and distal aneurysm and axillobifemoral reconstruction have been described in high-risk patients. These options are no longer recommended because of the high perioperative complication rate and mortality (combined rate, 10 to 18%) (24, 25). Transluminal placement of endovascular grafts is being evaluated for safety, efficacy, and longer-term results in phase II clinical trials. This procedure, which was developed by Parodi et al. (26, 27) in Argentina, may soon become the preferred treatment for this disorder. Problems with this technique include an endoleak rate of approximately 20%, with persistent flow in the native aorta. The procedure is used in only 30% of patients with an abdominal aortic aneurysm, but with ongoing follow-up and improvements in the device it will have wider applicability (28, 29).

Mr. Anderson remains hemodynamically stable through the rest of his surgery and is admitted to the surgical intensive care unit.

What is the prognosis after elective repair of an abdominal aortic aneurysm?
The operative and postoperative results of elective surgical repair of abdominal aortic aneurysms have improved in recent years. Most centers report an operative mortality of 1 to 5% after elective repair of these aneurysms (3). Furthermore, long-term survival reported by Debakey is 84% at 1 year, 72% at 3 years, and 58% at 5 years (30). Most of the deaths are associated with continued atherosclerosis of the coronary, renal, and cerebrovascular vessels. With successful repair of an aneurysm, the prognosis for a patient such as Mr. Anderson is very good.

What is the prognosis after emergency repair of an abdominal aortic aneurysm?
The operative morality for emergency repair of a ruptured abdominal aortic aneurysm is approximately 50% at most centers (31). Death is usually from massive intraoperative hemorrhage, cardiopulmonary complications, or acute postoperative renal failure.

Which potential postoperative complications should be discussed with the patient when obtaining consent for surgery?
Postoperative complications after repair of an abdominal aortic aneurysm are common in both elective and emergency cases. The following is a list of some of these complications and their relative frequencies (3, 4). When obtaining consent, the following problems should be discussed within appropriate limits.

Pulmonary atelectasis is seen in all patients to some degree and may lead to pneumonia in severe cases.

Acute renal failure occurs in approximately 2.5% of elective surgery and in more than 20% of cases of rupture. Mortality in these patients approaches 90%.

Abdominal distention arising from paralytic ileus occurs in most cases of intraperitoneal approach. This usually self-limited process requires nasogastric decompression until bowel function returns.

Embolization of thrombi to the lower extremities leads to acute ischemia in as many as 7% of patients. Treatment depends on the nature and extent of the obstruction and the ischemic tissues.

Bleeding may occur from the anastomosis site or through the interstices of the graft and mandates reexploration in some patients. Rupture of the suture line is rare but may occur with erosion into surrounding viscera. Emergency reoperation may be required in this situation.

Infection of the graft occurs in approximately 1% of patients in most studies. This requires removal of the graft material and ligation of the aorta below the renal vessels. Flow to the lower extremities is reestablished with an axillary-bifemoral graft. Treatment with appropriate antibiotics is essential.

False aneurysms may develop at the suture lines and may produce pain and a pulsatile mass. Diagnosis is by aortography. Reoperation with revision of the aortic repair may be indicated to reduce the risk of spontaneous rupture.

Cardiac arrhythmias are common and are usually due to underlying coronary artery disease with myocardial ischemia. Arrhythmias should be treated aggressively to maintain hemodynamic stability.

Bowel ischemia is rare but may result from ligation of the inferior mesenteric artery and inadequate collateral flow. Bowel movements within 48 hours of surgery should raise suspicion of colonic ischemia.

Sexual dysfunction in men is characterized by retrograde ejaculation in as many as 66% of patients and impotence in as many as 30% of patients. This results from disturbance or ligation of the sympathetic nerve plexus as it crosses the aortic bifurcation. Care in avoiding these nerves during surgical manipulation of the aorta reduces the risk of these complications.

Spinal cord ischemia is a rare complication characterized by an anterior spinal artery syndrome. In most cases, it is caused by hypotension or prolonged intraoperative ischemia. Some cases of spinal cord ischemia result from thrombosis or embolism.

What is the artery of Adamkiewicz, and what is its significance in surgery for abdominal aortic aneurysm?

Blood supply to the spinal cord is provided by the posterior spinal artery on the dorsal side and the anterior spinal artery on the ventral side. The posterior spinal artery is well collateralized through the entire length of the spinal cord, but the anterior spinal artery depends on a key collateral system from the aorta to supply the distal anterior spinal cord. This collateral artery, the artery of Adamkiewicz, arises from the aorta at the level of T8 to L2 in 85% of cases (it may occur as low as L4) (32) and is vulnerable to disruption during surgical dissection around the aorta or during aortic cross-clamping, which can lead to anterior spinal cord ischemia.

Mr. Anderson is transferred to the ward on postoperative day 2. His recovery is unremarkable except for transient ileus and mild pulmonary atelectasis. He is discharged home on postoperative day 10.

Should routine ultrasound screening be performed for abdominal aortic aneurysm?

Among persons who have a first-degree relative with an abdominal aortic aneurysm, men aged 55 and older have an approximately 20 to 25% risk of abdominal aortic aneurysm; in women, the risk is 6% (33). Screening on the basis of age alone is not cost effective (34); however, patients who have a first-degree relative with an abdominal aortic aneurysm should have a screening ultrasound examination at age 50 to 55.

Management Algorithm for Pulsatile Abdominal Mass

Algorithm 21.1.

REFERENCES

1. Ouriel K, Green RM, Donayre C, et al. An evaluation of new methods of expressing aortic aneurysm size: relationship to rupture. J Vasc Surg 1992;15:12.

2. Crisler C, Bahnson HT. Aneurysms of the aorta. In: Ravitch MM, ed. Current Problems in Surgery. St. Louis: Mosby–Year Book, 1989.

3. Rutherford RB. Infrarenal aortic aneurysms. In: Rutherford RB, ed. Vascular Surgery. 4th ed, vol 2. Philadelphia: WB Saunders, 1994:1032–1060.

4. Green RM, Ouriel K. Peripheral arterial disease. In: Schwartz SI, ed. Principles of Surgery. 6th ed. New York: McGraw Hill, 1994:925–987.

5. Vital Statistics of the United States, vol 2: Mortality, Part A. Department of Health and Human Service, Pub PHS 87–1101. Washington: US Government Printing Office, 1987.

6. Sampson LN, Cronenwett JL. Abdominal Aortic Aneurysms: Problems in General Surgery. Vol 2, Vascular Surgery. Philadelphia: Lippincott, 1995:385–417.

7. Cronenwett JL. When to Repair Abdominal Aortic Aneurysms: Advances in Vascular Surgery. Vol 4. St. Louis: Mosby–Year Book, 1996:7–21.

8. Darling RC, Messina CR, Brewster DC, et al. Autopsy study of unoperated abdominal aortic aneurysm. Circulation 1977;56(Suppl 2):II–161.

9. Cronenwett JL, Sargent SK, Wall MH, et al. Variables that affect the expansion rate and outcome of small abdominal aortic aneurysms. J Vasc Surg 1990;11:260.

10. Sterpetti AV, Cavallaro A, Cavallaro N, et al. Factors influencing the rupture of abdominal aortic aneurysms. Surg Obstet Gynecol 1991;173:175.

11. Bickerstaff LK, Hollier LH, Van Peenan HJ. Abdominal aortic aneurysms: the changing natural history. J Vasc Surg 1984;1:6.

12. Goldstone J, Malone JM, Moore WS. Inflammatory aneurysms of the aorta. Surgery 1978;83:425.

13. Estes JE Jr. Abdominal aortic aneurysm: a study of one hundred and two cases. Circulation 1950;2:258.

14. Szilagyi DE, Elliott JP, Smith RF. Clinical fate of the patient with asymptomatic aortic aneurysm and unfit for surgical treatment. Arch Surg 1972;104:600.

15. Pillari G, Chang JB, Zito J, et al. Computed tomography of abdominal aortic aneurysm. Arch Surg 1988;123:727.

16. Todd GJ, Nowygrod R, Benvensity A. The accuracy of CT scanning in the diagnosis of abdominal and thoracoabdominal aortic aneurysms. J Vasc Surg 1991;13:302.

17. Fillinger MF. Utility of Spiral CT in the Preoperative Evaluation of Patients with Abdominal Aortic Aneurysms: Advances in Vascular Surgery. Vol 5. St. Louis: Mosby–Year Book, 1997:115–131.

18. Pavone P, Di Cesare E, Di Renzi P. Abdominal aortic aneurysm evaluation: comparison of US, CT MRI, and aortography. Magn Reson Imag 1990;8:199.

19. Thompson JE, Hollier LH, Patman RD, Persson AV. Surgical management of abdominal aortic aneurysms: factors influencing mortality and morbidity: a 20 year experience. Ann Surg 1975;181:654.

20. Debakey ME, Jordan GL Jr, Abbot JP, et al. The fate of Dacron vascular grafts. Arch Surg 1964;89:757.

21. Ernst CB. Prevention of intestinal ischemia following abdominal aortic reconstruction. Surgery 1983;93:102–106.

22. Ernst CB, Hagihara PF, Daugherty ME, Griffen WO Jr. Inferior mesenteric artery stump pressure: a reliable index for safe IMA ligation during abdominal aorta aneurysmectomy. Ann Surg 1978;187:641.

23. Dubost C, Allary M, Oeconomos N. Resection of an abdominal aortic aneurysm: reestablishment of the continuity by a preserved human arterial graft, with results after five months. Arch Surg 1952;64:405.

24. Karmody AM, Leather RP, Goldman M. The current position on non-resective treatment for abdominal aortic aneurysm. Surgery 1983;94:591.

25. Inahara T, Geary GI, Mukherjee D. The contrary position to the nonresective treatment for abdominal aortic aneurysm. J Vasc Surg 1985;2:42.

26. Parodi JC, Palmaz JC, Garcia O, et al. Transfemoral intraluminal graft implantation for abdominal aortic aneurysms. Ann Vasc Surg 1991;5:491–499.

27. Parodi JC. Endovascular repair of abdominal aortic aneurysms. In: Advances in Vascular Surgery. Vol 1. St. Louis: Mosby–Year Book, 1993:85–106.

28. Matsumura JS, Pearce WH, McCarthy WJ, et al. Reduction in aortic aneurysm size after endovascular graft placement. J Vasc Surg 1997;25:113–123.

29. White GH, May J, McGahan T, et al. Historical control comparison of outcome for matched groups of patient undergoing endoluminal versus open repair of abdominal aortic aneurysms. J Vasc Surg 1996;23:201–212.

30. Debakey ME, Crawford ES, Cooley DA, et al. Aneurysm of abdominal aorta: analysis of results of graft replacement therapy one to eleven years after operation. Ann Surg 1964;160:622.

31. Lawrence MS, Crosby VG, Ehrenhart JL. Ruptured abdominal aortic aneurysm. Ann Thorac Surg 1966;2:159.

32. Ferguson LR, Bergan JJ, Conn J Jr, et al. Spinal ischemia following abdominal aortic surgery. Ann Surg 1975;181:267–272.

33. Webster MW, Ferell RE, St. Jean PI, et al. Ultrasound screening of first degree relatives of patients with abdominal aortic aneurysm. J Vasc Surg 1991;13:9.

34. Colin J, Araujo L, Lindsell D. Oxford screening programme for abdominal aortic aneurysm in men aged 65 to 74 years. Lancet 1988;2:613.

Peripheral Arterial Occlusive Disease

W. Charles Sternbergh III

David Brown is a 68-year-old retired carpenter who for the past 2 years has had cramps and aching in the right calf after walking. The discomfort has been gradually worsening and is now reproducible after he walks approximately two blocks; it subsides within 5 minutes of resting but reappears when he walks another two blocks. He denies having any pain in the left leg while walking or in the right calf or foot at rest, nor does he have any history of trauma to the extremities. He smokes two packs of cigarettes a day.

Mr. Brown's medical history is significant for coronary artery disease (CAD), for which he underwent coronary artery bypass grafting (CABG) 3 years ago. Since the CABG, he has had no angina, dyspnea on exertion, or orthopnea. He has no history of stroke, transient ischemic attacks, or hypercholesterolemia. He has mild chronic obstructive pulmonary disease because of smoking. His only medications are diltiazem and aspirin.

A physical examination indicates that Mr. Brown is normotensive and in sinus rhythm; findings of the neck, chest, abdominal, and neurologic examinations are normal. Evaluation of his peripheral pulse reveals a 2+ carotid pulse bilaterally without bruits, a 2+ radial pulse, and a 2+ femoral pulse without bruits. Mr. Brown is bilaterally pulseless in the popliteal, posterior tibial, and dorsalis pedis arteries, but these vessels produce a monophasic signal when evaluated with a Doppler study. The right leg has a well-healed longitudinal scar from the excision of the saphenous vein for the CABG. There is no muscle atrophy, ulceration, or any other sign of tissue loss in either leg; capillary refill in the toes is good.

What is claudication?
Claudication is exercise-induced intermittent discomfort in a particular muscle group that subsides within 1 to 5 minutes after the exercise is stopped. This dis-

comfort may be described by the patient as pain, cramping, burning, or weariness. In the lower extremities, the calves, thighs, and buttocks are most frequently affected. Because the pain is reproducible by the same degree of exertion, claudication is typically quantified by the distance a patient can walk before its onset (e.g., two-block claudication).

What causes claudication?
Claudication occurs when a particular muscle group becomes hypoxic because the increased metabolic demands for oxygen during exercise cannot be met. Normal arteries can increase flow 5- to 10-fold when regional metabolic demands rise; however, stenosed or occluded vessels have limited capacity to augment flow during exercise. The stenosis or occlusion is invariably caused by progressive atherosclerosis.

What is the differential diagnosis for lower extremity pain?
Claudication is a characteristic symptom in patients with significant arterial occlusive disease. Because of the reproducibility of hypoxic muscle pain after exercise, a history and physical examination should be sufficient to rule out most other causes, which may include the following:

Acute arterial embolism. The precipitous reduction of blood flow that results from acute arterial embolism causes an acute onset of diffuse lower extremity pain at rest in a patient with no history of arterial occlusive disease.
Diabetic neuropathy. Many patients with long-standing diabetes develop significant burning pain in the feet, which may be easily confused with ischemic rest pain.
Chronic venous disease. Venous valve incompetence and the resulting relative stasis cause chronic swelling, hyperpigmentation, and ulcers at or proximal to the malleoli.
Deep vein thrombosis. Characterized by swelling in the extremities or vague pain, deep vein thrombosis cannot be accurately diagnosed from the history and physical examination.
Musculoskeletal disorders. Patients with musculoskeletal disorders have a history of recent trauma or of pain associated with movement of a joint.
Neurologic disorders. Lumbar disc herniation or spinal stenosis may cause characteristic shooting pain or extremity weakness that is distinct from claudication.
Infection. Local erythema and tenderness that are not exacerbated by exercise are present.

What are some significant risk factors for arterial occlusive disease?
Hypercholesterolemia, tobacco use, hypertension, diabetes mellitus, male gender, age, and hereditary influences are all significant risk factors (1).

What are the signs of significant arterial occlusive disease?
These signs may be observed during a physical examination:

1. Lack of distal pulses
2. Pallor of the extremity on elevation and rubor on dependency
3. Trophic changes such as thinning of the skin, loss of hair, and thickening of the nails
4. Muscle atrophy
5. Tissue loss (e.g., ulcers distal to the malleolus or gangrene)

What is the natural course of lower extremity claudication?
Symptomatic arterial occlusive disease has a surprisingly benign course; 75 to 80% of patients have stable or diminished claudication with conservative management (2). Reported amputation rates for all patients with claudication who are managed without surgery range from 1.6 to 7% after a 6- to 8-year follow-up (3, 4). Approximately 20% of patients with claudication ultimately require invasive intervention for limb salvage.

What is an appropriate initial treatment for claudication?
Because of the benign natural course of this disease, a conservative approach is warranted initially. This includes the following measures:

Cessation of smoking. Tobacco use is clearly associated with a significant exacerbation of vascular occlusive disease. Smoking doubles an elderly patient's risk of claudication (5). Most smokers with claudication show a significant improvement in exercise tolerance after quitting (6).

Exercise. A graded exercise program stimulates formation of collateral vessels. The resulting increase in blood flow can increase the walking distances by 80 to 120%.

Analysis and control of blood lipids. Patients with claudication should maintain their ideal body weight. A lipid profile should be obtained, and lipid levels should be controlled with an appropriate diet and, if needed, drug therapy.

Rheologic agents. By increasing erythrocyte flexibility or decreasing platelet aggregation, medications such as pentoxifylline (Trental) offer moderate benefit in increasing walking distance. Cilostizol, a new agent in clinical trials, may offer greater clinical benefit.

Mr. Brown's physician instructs him to stop smoking and begin a graded exercise program, but his interest and participation in exercise are limited, and he does not stop smoking. He does not go to scheduled follow-up visits. Over the next 2 years, his walking distance before onset of the characteristic right calf pain gradually shortens.

He also begins to have pain in his right foot at rest, especially at night; the discomfort is relieved by dangling the foot off the bed. The intensity and duration of the pain gradually increase, and after 3 weeks, he seeks help.

What is rest pain, and what causes it?
Rest pain is caused by inadequate delivery of oxygen to the tissues during rest. This hypoperfusion inevitably manifests as ischemic pain in the foot at rest. The lower extremity muscles that are prone to claudication (the calf, thigh, and buttock muscles) rarely exhibit rest pain because they are not at the end of the arterial tree. Conversely, the foot does not claudicate because it has relatively little muscle mass that is susceptible to exercise-induced hypoxia. By definition, the pain caused by claudication is intermittent, whereas rest pain can be continuous. Rest pain is characteristically worst at night, when the patient is supine, because the arterial flow to the foot is not aided by gravity. The pain is relieved by dangling the foot off the bed, walking a few paces, or sleeping in a chair.

What is the natural history of rest pain?
In contrast to claudication, true ischemic rest pain ultimately progresses to limb loss in most untreated patients. An aggressive treatment regimen is therefore warranted in the absence of prohibitive comorbid medical conditions.

What are the indications for treatment of arterial occlusive disease?
The classic indications include the following:

Rest pain.
Tissue loss. This may be a nonhealing inframalleolar ulcer, nonhealing distal amputation, or pregangrenous changes in toes.
Disabling claudication. The availability of minimally invasive endovascular treatments has resulted in a more liberal policy for treatment of claudication in many centers, although it is still controversial.

How is arterial occlusive disease evaluated?
A thorough history and physical examination are essential, and any comorbid medical conditions must be addressed. Segmental arterial Doppler studies and angiography of the lower extremities are performed if surgery or other invasive interventions are indicated.

What does an arterial Doppler study measure? What is the ankle-brachial index (ABI)?
Segmental arterial Doppler studies measure the systolic pressure at several locations on the extremity. A pressure difference greater than 20 mm Hg between levels suggests significant occlusive disease. The ABI (obtained by dividing the ankle pressure by the highest brachial pressure) provides a value indicating distal

perfusion. A normal ABI is 0.9 to 1.1; an ABI of 0.5 to 0.7 is typical of claudication; and an ABI of less than 0.5 may accompany rest pain or tissue loss. The ABI is only a relative number, and many patients with an ABI of 0.5 have no symptoms. Because diabetic patients sometimes have heavily calcified arteries that are poorly compressible, their ABI may be misleadingly high.

At what point does arterial stenosis become hemodynamically significant?
The cutoff point is a 75% reduction of the cross-sectional area, which is equivalent to a 50% reduction of the diameter. At this level of stenosis, poststenotic pressure and blood flow are maintained at 90 to 95% of normal values; however, any further stenosis causes a precipitous fall in distal perfusion.

Mr. Brown's physician orders a lower extremity segmental arterial Doppler study. It reveals a reference right brachial pressure of 130 mm Hg, high thigh pressure of 140 mm Hg, above-knee pressure of 73 mm Hg, below-knee pressure of 60 mm Hg, ankle pressure of 51 mm Hg, and toe pressure of 45 mm Hg. The ABI is calculated to be 0.39. The contralateral leg has fairly similar pressures and an ABI of 0.5.

What is the anatomy of the vascular tree in the lower extremities?
The vascular anatomy of the lower extremity is shown in Figure 22.1.

How does the location of the pain suggest the probable area of stenosis or occlusion?
In 60 to 70% of patients, the arterial lesion is one level above the claudicating muscle group. Calf claudication, as in Mr. Brown's case, therefore suggests superficial femoral artery (SFA) or popliteal artery disease, whereas thigh or buttock claudication indicates more proximal occlusive disease. However, up to 40% of patients with aortoiliac disease have calf claudication.

What is Leriche's syndrome?
In 1940, Leriche described a group of patients with distal aortic occlusion resulting from progressive atherosclerotic disease. These patients exhibited characteristic signs and symptoms: impotence, symmetric lower extremity muscle wasting, pallor of the legs and feet, and easy fatigability. Impotence is caused by the greatly decreased flow to the hypogastric arteries. Because of the extensive formation of collateral vessels, these patients can remain asymptomatic for as long as 5 to 10 years, but many ultimately need surgery.

What is the most likely location of Mr. Brown's lesion?
Both the Doppler studies, which reveal a large decrease in pressure between the high and the low thigh, and the patient's initial symptom (right calf claudication) suggest an occlusion of the SFA. The most common site of occlusion in the lower extremities is the distal SFA as is passes through the adductor canal.

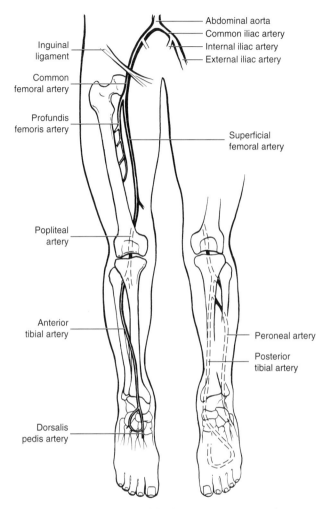

Figure 22.1.   Anatomy of the lower extremity arterial tree.

The patient is referred to a vascular surgeon for further evaluation and definitive treatment. An aortogram with bilateral runoff is obtained.

What are the indications for arteriography?
Arteriography is performed only if the patient is to undergo invasive intervention. It should not be used as a screening tool. Arterial Doppler studies are a good noninvasive tool for this purpose.

What are the risks of arteriography, and how can they be minimized?
The risk of a life-threatening reaction to the contrast medium is 1 in 14,000. The reported incidence of renal dysfunction from contrast toxicity ranges from

0 to 10% in low-risk patients. The most important measure for minimizing contrast medium–induced renal dysfunction is judicious use of intravenous hydration, both before and after the study.

Mr. Brown's arteriogram reveals mild to moderate atherosclerotic changes in the distal aorta and common iliac arteries in the absence of hemodynamically significant stenoses. The right extremity has a patent profunda femoris, but the SFA has a 15-cm occlusion, with distal reconstitution at the popliteal artery below the knee. There is one vessel runoff (anterior tibial artery). The left extremity has diffuse mild to moderate occlusive changes; there is a 3-cm occlusion at the distal SFA, with popliteal reconstitution.

If an arteriogram reveals significant occlusive disease in both extremities but the patient has symptoms on only one side, should both extremities undergo invasive treatment?
Only symptomatic lesions should be treated.

What type of cardiac evaluation before surgery is appropriate for a patient who has had a myocardial infarction?
Perioperative myocardial infarction is the most common cause of postoperative death in patients operated on for peripheral arterial occlusive disease. The prevalence of severe CAD in this patient population is high; 34% of patients with clinically suspected coronary disease have severe correctable CAD, as do 14% of patients with no history of CAD (7). It is therefore important to identify patients at risk for a perioperative cardiac event. Any history of CAD, angina, or congestive heart failure necessitates further study. An abnormal electrocardiogram in the absence of clinical symptoms should also prompt further investigation. Frequently used cardiac stress tests include the dobutamine-stressed echocardiogram and the Persantine-stressed thallium (radionuclide) scan. If a significant portion of myocardium is found to be at risk for ischemia, cardiac catheterization is indicated.

When in the perioperative period is a myocardial infarction most likely?
A myocardial infarction is most likely to occur 3 to 5 days postoperatively. Although reasons for this temporal relation are not completely understood, a major contributing factor may be the mobilization of third-space fluid that accumulates intraoperatively. This internal fluid challenge may overwhelm a marginally vascularized heart and cause ischemia and infarction.

What is the mortality from an acute myocardial infarction in the perioperative period in a patient undergoing noncardiac surgery?
Mortality associated with a myocardial infarction in the perioperative period is 20 to 50%, in contrast to 8 to 14% mortality after acute myocardial infarction

in nonsurgical patients. These statistics underscore the importance of aggressive preoperative cardiac risk assessment.

Mr. Brown has a standard electrocardiogram that reveals a normal sinus rhythm of 80, Q waves in leads II, III, and AVF, but no other Q waves or ST segment abnormalities. Because of his history of CAD, he undergoes a Persantine-thallium cardiac stress test that reveals no redistribution and thus indicates that the risk of perioperative myocardial infarction is low.

What is the treatment for severe symptomatic occlusive peripheral vascular disease?
Revascularization of the limb at risk for ischemia is essential. This may be accomplished by the surgical placement of a conduit that bypasses the area of disease or, in selected cases, by percutaneous endovascular techniques, specifically balloon angioplasty. Percutaneous endovascular treatment reduces the morbidity, mortality, and cost associated with conventional surgery. However, the lack of durability after treatment with some endovascular techniques limits their application.

What is the role of balloon angioplasty in the treatment of peripheral occlusive arterial disease?
Angioplasty is a useful technique for treating vascular disease. The ideal lesion for successful primary angioplasty is a proximal lesion less than 5 cm long with no significant distal occlusive disease. After successful angioplasty of an isolated common iliac stenosis, the 5-year patency rate is 80 to 85%. Angioplasty may also be useful as a secondary procedure, such as dilating a discrete stenosis in a failing graft. A vessel with an occluded segment longer than 10 cm, more distal location, and multilevel disease all impede the initial and long-term success of angioplasty.

Do stents improve the patency rate after angioplasty?
Stents, or metal scaffolds placed within the lumen of the vessel, are most useful when the initial angioplasty leads to less than optimal technical results. In this situation, stenting may improve patency rates, particularly in iliac vessels. However, stents in the femoral, popliteal, or tibial vessel have not met with much success.

How does balloon angioplasty affect an atheromatous plaque?
An increase in the cross-sectional diameter of the vessel occurs primarily through disruption or cracking of the plaque. Extrusion of the plaque contents contributes 6 to 12% to this increase, whereas compression of the plaque, which earlier was considered to be the primary mechanism, is now believed to contribute only about 1%.

What factors determine successful revascularization?
Three elements are essential for a durable revascularization: inflow of blood, a conduit for the blood, and an outflow tract. A bypass of an SFA occlusion from the common femoral to the popliteal artery is destined for early thrombosis if there is a significant iliac stenosis (inflow problem). The same bypass will also fail early if there is extensive occlusive disease in the tibioperoneal trunk (outflow problem). Clearly, the vasculature of the entire limb must be studied to plan an effective and long-lasting revascularization.

What are the types of conduits used for peripheral revascularization procedures, and how durable are they?
The choice of conduit is based on the long-term patency of the grafts. Grafts for revascularization in decreasing order of preference:

Autogenous vein. The greater saphenous vein is preferred to the basilic, cephalic, and lesser saphenous veins because of its superior patency.
Synthetic material (polytetrafluoroethylene [PTFE] or polyester [Dacron]). PTFE conduits also have good patency rates in bypasses from the common femoral to the popliteal artery above the knee. After 2 years, reversed saphenous vein and PTFE bypasses have a similar patency rate, approximately 80%; however, after 4 years the patency of PTFE decreases to 54%, whereas the patency of the reversed vein graft is still 76% (8). Arterial reconstruction to the tibial vessels with PFTE leads to very low patency rates—12% with PTFE versus 49 to 75% with vein—at 4 years (8) and should be avoided. A composite graft consisting of a proximal PTFE graft sewn to a distal vein may be used for a bypass to the tibial vessels when available vein is insufficient.
Cryopreserved or glutaraldehyde-preserved umbilical vein. Cryopreserved veins are a poor choice for a conduit because of their uniformly low patency rate.

What is the difference between a reversed saphenous vein bypass graft and an in situ graft?
For a reversed saphenous vein bypass, the vein is removed from the leg, the branches are ligated, and the vessel is reversed so that the distal end of the vein is used as the proximal origin of the bypass conduit. The vein is reversed so that arterial flow is not impeded by its numerous valves. For in situ saphenous vein grafts, the greater portion of the vein is left in position; only the most proximal and distal aspects are dissected free for the arterial anastomoses. The valves are excised with special instruments. These valve cutters, or valvulotomes, are inserted through a side branch or through the distal end of the vein. Finally, all of the branches of the vein are ligated, with minimum dissection in surrounding areas.

What are the advantages of the in situ technique?
Most of the advantages of the in situ technique are predicated on the concept of endothelial cell preservation. The endothelium has remarkable antithrom-

botic properties that are easily compromised by ischemia and reperfusion. Therefore, avoiding the ischemic damage caused by surgical excision of the vein segment has great theoretic appeal. The vasa vasorum, which supply the media and adventitia with blood, are minimally injured. Manipulation-induced spasm and the resulting need for hydrostatic dilation, which may lead to additional damage, are avoided. Also, a smaller-caliber vein may be used.

Do in situ techniques give better long-term patencies than standard reversed bypasses? Although some proponents of in situ techniques claim better patency rates (9), the emerging consensus is that with precise attention to detail, the two techniques produce equivalent results. Controlled trials have shown no differences in long-term patency between them (10).

What are the types of vascular procedures for lower extremity occlusive disease? What is the usual choice of conduit? What are their approximate 5-year patency rates? The various procedures, together with the conduits and duration, are listed in Table 22.1. The indicated patency rates are only average rates. Thus, bypasses performed for claudication have a higher patency rate than those done for rest pain or tissue loss. Finally, limb salvage rates are higher than the 5-year patency rates.

Mr. Brown undergoes surgery, during which the left greater saphenous vein is harvested, reversed, and anastomosed to the common femoral artery proximally and to the popliteal artery below the knee distally. An arteriogram obtained after completion of surgery reveals no technical defects and excellent runoff. The right dorsalis pedis artery has a palpable pulse.

Table 22.1.   RELATION OF LOCATION OF ARTERIAL BYPASS TO LONG-TERM PATENCY

Arterial Bypass Type	Conduit Type	5-year Patency (%)
Aortobifemoral or aortoiliac	Polyester or PTFE	85–95
Axillary-femoral	PTFE or polyester	35–35
Femoral-bifemoral	PTFE or polyester	50–70
Femoral-femoral	PTFE or polyester	50–80
Femoral-popliteal	Vein or PTFE	60–80
		35–60
Femoral-tibial or femoral-peroneal	Vein or PTFE	50–70
		<20

PTFE, polytetrafluoroethylene.

What is the role of intraoperative arteriography or duplex ultrasound?
Both modalities can be used to assess the technical adequacy of a bypass. Duplex ultrasound may be more sensitive than arteriography to technical problems with the graft, particularly with the in situ technique (11, 12). Sometimes the preoperative angiogram does not provide sufficient detail of the distal vasculature. In these cases, an intraoperative arteriogram, directed specifically to the area of interest, may guide the arterial reconstruction.

What are some important considerations in the postoperative management of a patient who has had vascular surgery?
Aspects of postoperative management that require particular attention are the following:

Careful management of coexisting medical problems. As a group, patients who have undergone vascular surgery have a higher prevalence of coexisting diseases than does any other subset of surgical patients. Accordingly, meticulous attention must be paid, especially to cardiac, pulmonary, and renal disease.

Frequent assessment of graft patency. The functioning bypass should produce a palpable pulse or a strong Doppler signal in the distal vessels. This pulse should be checked hourly for the first 12 hours and then several times a day for the next few days. A baseline ABI should also be recorded at the bedside. Any sign of graft thrombosis demands an imaging study (duplex study or angiography) and immediate surgical reexploration.

Use of anticoagulation. Routine perioperative anticoagulation with dextran or heparin is usually not indicated. Exceptions are patients with high-risk grafts from technical difficulties, marginal conduit, or poor runoff; patients with grafts that are prone to thrombosis; and patients with hypercoagulable conditions. These patients may be treated with heparin postoperatively, and they can be maintained on warfarin indefinitely.

Administration of antibiotics. Patients undergoing vascular surgery are typically treated with a single preoperative and one to three postoperative intravenous doses of a first-generation cephalosporin (e.g., cefazolin). If a prosthetic graft is used, many surgeons prolong the postoperative coverage to 5 days. If the patient has an infected foot or ulcer, the antibiotic therapy is prolonged and the coverage is widened.

Walking. Most patients should be encouraged to begin walking a day or two after surgery.

Mr. Brown's right ABI increases from 0.39 preoperatively to 0.8, and he maintains a good right dorsalis pedis pulse. His rest pain is gone. He begins limited walking the day after the operation and is discharged on the fifth day with continued good distal pulse.

What is the 5-year survival for patients such as Mr. Brown, who have had surgery for peripheral arterial disease?
The 5-year survival rate for patients after peripheral arterial reconstruction ranges from 22 to 85% (Table 22.2). Survival of individual patients depends on the severity of any CAD, status of the CABG, gender, and any diabetes mellitus. Stratification of the patients according to gender and diabetes reveals that nondiabetic men gain the greatest benefit from CABG. This subgroup has 81% 5-year survival after CABG, compared with 58% in women and diabetic patients (13). Thus, Mr. Brown, who is not diabetic and who has undergone CABG, has approximately a 70 to 80% chance of surviving 5 years.

Why is it important to maintain long-term surveillance for a failing graft?
The patency rates for grafts that are threatened and revised before thrombosis sets in are 15 to 25% higher than patency rates for grafts that are revised after thrombosis (14, 15). A discrete area of stenosis may be treated with balloon angioplasty, open patch angioplasty, or a short jump graft. After total occlusion and thrombosis, the revision is more difficult and the outcome less favorable.

What causes bypass graft failure?
These factors can induce graft failure:

Technical problems with the graft. Most graft thromboses within the first 30 days of surgery are due to technical problems such as a kinked graft, an inadequate venous conduit, or an unrecognized intimal flap. Prompt surgical revision is indicated.
Intimal hyperplasia at the anastomosis. For reasons that are not well understood, significant stenosis caused by intimal hyperplasia may occur at the distal anastomosis. The pathogenesis may be related to shear stress, operative

Table 22.2. EFFECT OF CORONARY ARTERY DISEASE ON SURVIVAL AFTER PERIPHERAL ARTERIAL RECONSTRUCTION

Status of CAD	5-year Survival (%)
No significant CAD	85
Severe CAD with CABG	72
Advanced compensated CAD (no CABG)	64
Severe CAD without CABG	43
Severe inoperable CAD	22

CABG, coronary artery bypass grafting; CAD, coronary artery disease.
From Hertzer NR. The natural history of peripheral vascular disease: implications for its management. Circulation 1991;83(Suppl):12–19.

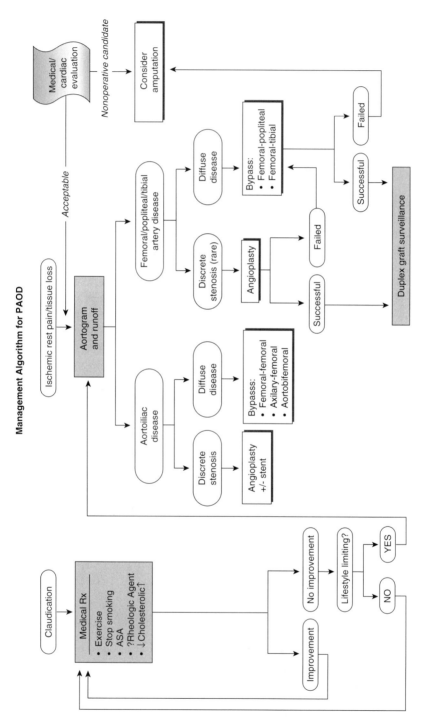

Management Algorithm for PAOD

Algorithm 22.1.

handling of the anastomosis, and the degree of compliance mismatch between the conduit and recipient artery. Intimal hyperplasia is the most frequent cause of graft failure 2 to 24 months after a bypass operation.

Progression of arterial disease. Atherosclerotic disease may progress proximal or distal to the bypass, compromising its inflow, outflow, or both. Progression of atherosclerotic disease is the most common cause of graft occlusion after 3 to 4 years.

Degenerative changes in the graft. The body of the graft can also be affected by intimal thickening, atherosclerotic changes, and fibrosis, especially at the old valve sites. These degenerative changes may appear within months or many years after surgery.

How is a failing graft detected?
Patients with significant graft stenoses may have recurring rest pain, claudication, or tissue loss; however, many patients have no symptoms. Although examination of the strength and character of the pulses is important for monitoring a patient after peripheral vascular reconstruction, variation between examinations and the difficulty in comparing pulses over time may make the physical examination unreliable. Duplex ultrasound is therefore important in surveillance of these patients. Changes in pulse volume or Doppler velocity usually precede a drop in the ABI. Any suspicion of impending graft failure should be cause for prompt arteriography and any necessary correction for the best long-term results.

REFERENCES

1. Dawber TR. The Framingham Study: The Epidemiology of Atherosclerotic Disease. Cambridge: Harvard University Press, 1980:105–110.
2. Imparato AM, Kim GE, Davidson T, Crowley JG. Intermittent claudication: its natural course. Surgery 1975;78:795–799.
3. Kannel WB, Skinner JJ, Schwartz MJ, et al. Intermittent claudication: incidence in the Framingham study. Circulation 1970;41:875–883.
4. Mcallister FF. The fate of patients with intermittent claudication managed nonoperatively. Am J Surg 1976;132:593–595.
5. Kannel WB, Shurtleff D. Cigarettes and the development of intermittent claudication. Geriatrics 1973;28:61–65.
6. Quick CRG, Cotton LT. The measured effect of stopping smoking on intermittent claudication. Br J Surg 1982;69:S24–S26.
7. Hertzer NR, Bever EG, Young JR, et al. Coronary artery disease in peripheral vascular patients: a classification of 1000 coronary angiograms and results of surgical management. Ann Surg 1984;199:223–233.
8. Keith FJ, Gupta SK, Ascer E, et al. Six-year prospective multicenter randomized comparison of autologous saphenous vein and expanded polytetrafluoroethylene grafts in infrainguinal arterial reconstruction. J Vasc Surg 1986;3:104–114.
9. Leather RP, Veith FJ. In situ vein bypass. In: Haimovici H, ed. Vascular Surgery. Norwark, CT: Appleton & Lange, 1989:524–526.

10. Wengerter KR, Veith FJ, Gupta SK, et al. Prospective randomized multicenter comparison of in situ and reversed vein infrapopliteal bypasses. J Vasc Surg 1991;13: 189–199.
11. Papanicolaou G, Aziz I, Yellin AE, Weaver FA. Intraoperative color duplex scanning for infrainguinal vein grafts. Ann Vasc Surg 1996;10:347–355.
12. Bandyk DF, Johnson BL, Gupta AK, Esses GE. Nature and management of duplex abnormalities encountered during infrainguinal vein bypass grafting. J Vasc Surg 1996; 24:430–438.
13. Hertzer NR. The natural history of peripheral vascular disease: implications for its management. Circulation 1991;83(Suppl 1):I-12–I-19.
14. Berkowitz HD, Greenstein SM. Improved patency in reversed femoral infrapopliteal autogenous vein grafts by early detection and treatment of the failing graft. J Vasc Surg 1987;5:755–761.
15. Caps MT, Cantwell-Gab K, Bergelin RO, Strandness DE. Vein graft lesions: time of onset and rate of progression. J Vasc Surg 1995;22:466–75.

CHAPTER

23

Adrenal Tumors

K. Francis Lee

Tony Perez is a 41-year-old factory foreman who has been referred to the surgical service by a neurosurgeon. He has been undergoing evaluation for chronic back pain, which has become worse in the past few weeks and because of which he has been on medical leave for the past 2 weeks. Computed tomography (CT) of the lumbar spine obtained the previous week showed a lumbar disc herniation. The CT also showed a 3-cm solid mass in the right adrenal gland. He is referred for evaluation of this adrenal mass.

What is the clinical significance of an adrenal mass in a patient with no signs or symptoms of adrenal disease?
Adrenal gland disease in the absence of abnormal symptoms or signs is being observed increasingly as CT has come into widespread use. Adrenal masses of varying sizes are incidental findings in up to 0.6% of CT obtained for unrelated reasons (1), and their clinical significance should be ascertained.

What is the differential diagnosis for an incidentally discovered adrenal mass?
The possibilities include tumor of the adrenal cortex, such as adenoma, carcinoma, or aldosteronoma; tumor of the adrenal medulla, such as benign or malignant pheochromocytoma; and tumor of neuroectodermal origin, such as neuroblastoma and neuroganglioma (2). Metastatic tumors are also found in the adrenal gland.

How is an adrenal mass in an otherwise asymptomatic patient treated?
The clinical algorithm at the end of chapter outlines the recommended approach. Management of an incidental adrenal mass depends on two factors: its secretory status and its size. If the history, physical examination, and laboratory tests indicate that the tumor is secreting a physiologically active biochemical factor, the mass should be resected regardless of the size. If the mass is large, it should be resected. Some surgeons consider it appropriate to resect a nonsecretory mass larger than 3 cm, whereas others believe resection should be reserved for tumors larger than 6 cm. A nonsecretory mass smaller than 3 cm should be

monitored. Masses between 3 and 6 cm should be carefully followed with bio-chemical tests and CT. A mass larger than 6 cm has a significant risk of being a carcinoma, and it should be resected regardless of secretory function (1).

What are some important anatomic features of the adrenal gland?
Each adrenal gland is two organs: (*a*) The *adrenal cortex,* the outer structure, is derived from mesothelial cells. (*b*) The *adrenal medulla,* the inner structure, is de-rived from ectodermal neural crest cells that have differentiated specifically from a group of sympathetic ganglionic cells. The adrenal cortex consists of three zones: (*a*) The zona glomerulosa (outer cortex) produces aldosterone in response to angiotensin II. (*b*) The zona fasciculata (middle cortex) produces cortisol in response to adrenocorticotrophic hormone (ACTH). (*c*) The zona reticularis (inner cortex) produces the androgen dehydroepiandrosterone (DHEA) in re-sponse to ACTH. The adrenal medulla secretes catecholamines, such as epi-nephrine (80%), norepinephrine (20%), and dopamine (small amounts). Diseases of the adrenal cortex include Cushing's syndrome, hyperaldosteronism, adreno-cortical insufficiency, and adrenogenital syndrome; diseases of the adrenal medulla include pheochromocytoma and neuroblastoma (1).

Which blood vessels supply the adrenal glands?
Three arterial branches supply both right and left adrenal glands: the superior suprarenal artery from the inferior phrenic artery, the middle suprarenal artery from the aorta, and the inferior suprarenal artery from the renal artery. The ve-nous drainage consists of the right adrenal vein, which empties directly into the inferior vena cava, and the left adrenal vein, which empties into the left renal vein.

Mr. Perez reports that his blood pressure has been high recently—160/90 mm Hg. His primary care physician attributes the hyperten-sion to work stress and is treating him with diuretics and angiotensin-converting enzyme inhibitors.

What is the differential diagnosis for Mr. Perez's hypertension?
A simple way to determine the cause of hypertension is to differentiate between medically treatable and surgically correctable hypertension. Essential hyperten-sion comprises the majority of cases of medically treatable hypertension. How-ever, surgically correctable causes must be considered if (*a*) the onset of hyper-tension, especially severe hypertension, is sudden; (*b*) relatively well-controlled hypertension becomes malignant and uncontrollable; or (*c*) other symptoms and signs of associated hormonal excess become apparent.

What is the differential diagnosis for surgically correctable hypertension?
Pheochromocytoma, renovascular stenosis, coarctation of the aorta, hyper-adrenocorticism, and primary hyperaldosteronism must all be considered in the differential diagnosis (3).

On further questioning, Mr. Perez reveals that for 6 months he has had occasional anxiety attacks at night that awaken him with sweat and palpitation. The attacks have become worse, and they seem to appear more frequently during the day, especially when he is walking around the factory floor at work.

What is the interpretation of a clinical situation such as Mr. Perez's?
The history of paroxysmal attacks of palpitation, diaphoresis, and hypertension in the presence of an adrenal mass makes pheochromocytoma a likely diagnosis.

Are there other symptoms of pheochromocytoma?
The symptoms and signs of pheochromocytoma are the physiologic manifestations of sudden releases of catecholamines from the tumor into the bloodstream. In addition to hypertension, diaphoresis, and palpitations, features include headache, anxiety, tremor, chest pain, epigastric pain, dyspnea, skin pallor, and chronic symptoms such as weight loss, fatigue, and nausea (1). The growing tumor may press on local structures and cause abdominal or flank pain.

Is pheochromocytoma a component of any familial syndrome?
Approximately 10% of pheochromocytomas are part of the multiple endocrine neoplasia syndrome (MENS) (Table 23.1). This condition is transmitted as an autosomal dominant trait (1), affecting 50% of the offspring of carriers.

Table 23.1. CONDITIONS ASSOCIATED WITH THE THREE TYPES OF MULTIPLE ENDOCRINE NEOPLASIA

	MEN I (Wermer's Syndrome)	MEN IIa (Sipple's Syndrome)	MEN IIB
Adrenal gland		Pheochromocytoma (50%)	Pheochromocytoma (31%)
Thyroid gland		Medullary carcinoma (95%)	Medullary carcinoma (95%)
Parathyroid gland	Hyperplasia (95%)	Hyperplasia (60%)	
Pancreas	Islet cell tumor (80%)		
Pituitary gland	Adenoma (70%)		
Neuroectodermal tissue			Cutaneous and mucosal neuromas
Other			Marfanoid habitus

What are the priorities for management of a patient with three diseases—pheochromocytoma, medullary thyroid carcinoma, and primary hyperparathyroidism?
Pheochromocytoma should be surgically treated first, followed by the other two diseases.

Mr. Perez has no knowledge of a relative having any cancer or endocrine problems.

What physical signs should be sought during physical examination of a patient suspected of having pheochromocytoma?
When pheochromocytoma is a consideration, one should look for signs of chronic high levels of catecholamines, such as weight loss, skin discoloration, livedo reticularis, tachycardia, hypertension, and cardiac failure. Other causes of surgically correctable hypertension should be ruled out by checking for Cushing's physical features, renovascular bruit, and right-to-left arm blood pressure differential, although they are unlikely in the presence of an adrenal mass. Other possible related causes of hypertension, such as features of hyperthyroidism, Cushing's disease, and carcinoid syndrome, should also be sought (1).

Mr. Perez's physical examination is unremarkable, except for a blood pressure of 170/95 mm Hg and a pulse of 105 beats per minute. Blood tests are ordered.

Which blood tests should be ordered for evaluation of pheochromocytoma?
Routine blood tests may show a slightly increased hematocrit and blood glucose level. The urinary levels of catecholamines and their metabolites—epinephrine, norepinephrine, metanephrine, normetanephrine, and vanillylmandelic acid (VMA)—should be measured.

Which urinary test offers the most useful diagnosis?
It is easiest to screen the urine for the metabolite metanephrine, and its measurement offers the most reliable diagnosis. VMA is the least specific measurable metabolite (1).

Can any other laboratory tests reveal pheochromocytoma?
No other laboratory tests are available. In a small subset of patients in whom the likelihood of pheochromocytoma is high but who have equivocal or normal urinary catecholamine levels, a pharmacologic stimulation test may induce catecholamine release. The stimulants can be histamine or glucagon, both of which activate a sudden sympathetic response. By contrast, in a Regitine test, α-adrenergic blockade may be induced to cause sudden severe hypotension.

Neither test is specific or sensitive; both pose a significant risk of complications, and they are no longer an important part of diagnostic workup in most patients.

Mr. Perez's urinary tests show elevated levels of metanephrine, norepinephrine, and epinephrine.

What is the next step in management?
The elevated catecholamine levels in urine confirm the diagnosis of pheochromocytoma. The patient should be considered for surgery.

In preparation for surgery, Mr. Perez's CT is reviewed again with the radiologist. It appears that the CT for lumbar disc evaluation is inadequate for intraabdominal and retroperitoneal examination. The radiologist recommends repeating the CT and suggests magnetic resonance imaging (MRI) or other radiologic tests.

What are the roles of CT, MRI, and metaiodobenzylguanidine (MIBG) scans in evaluating patients with pheochromocytoma?
CT finds 90 to 95% of all pheochromocytomas larger than 1 cm (1) and is sufficient in most cases. MRI has a similar resolution. ^{131}I-MIBG scanning, a nuclear test in which radioactive MIBG accumulates more rapidly in pheochromocytoma than in other chromaffin tissues, has 80% accuracy. Because the nuclear scan examines the entire body, it can be a useful initial diagnostic tool or a follow-up test to assess recurrent tumor growth (1).

A repeat CT of the abdomen shows no abnormal mass in the abdomen except for the right adrenal mass.

What is the incidence of pheochromocytoma outside the adrenal gland?
In 10% of patients, pheochromocytomas are found outside the adrenal gland, along the paravertebral ganglia.

What is the rule of 10 for pheochromocytoma?
The rule of 10 refers to the observation that the following features occur in 10% of patients:

• Tumor outside the adrenal gland
• Bilateral adrenal tumors
• Familial trait (MEN II)
• Malignancy
• Young age (in children, the incidence of bilaterality is 30%)

Mr. Perez is scheduled to undergo surgery in 2 weeks. He is prescribed an oral regimen of phenoxybenzamine and encouraged to drink plenty of liquids.

Why is preoperative preparation important in patients with pheochromocytoma?
The patient must be treated with antiadrenergic drugs to block the effects of a severe catecholamine crisis. α_1-receptors cause postsynaptic adrenergic vaso-constriction, whereas α_2-receptors effect presynaptic negative feedback on nor-epinephrine release. α_1-antagonists block catecholamine-induced hypertension, whereas α_2-antagonists have the opposite effect. Selective α_1-antagonists are therefore preferred. Drugs used for a blockade include the following:

1. Phenoxybenzamine has a greater effect on α_1-receptors than on α_2-receptors, and it has been widely used for preoperative adrenergic blockade in patients with pheochromocytoma.
2. Prazosin is another selective α_1-antagonist.
3. Phentolamine is nonselective but is also used.
4. α-methyl tyrosine blocks the enzyme tyrosine hydrolase and inhibits catecholamine synthesis. It is used in combination with the α-adrenergic antagonists (1).

β-adrenergic antagonists such as propranolol are used to control catecholamine-induced tachycardia, reflex tachycardia induced by the α-blockade, and any cardiac arrhythmia. The patient is usually treated with α-blockers for 2 weeks, and β-blockers such as propranolol are added to the regimen a few days before surgery.

Mr. Perez's preoperative preparation is uneventful. On the evening before surgery, he is admitted to the surgical floor. A large infusion of intravenous fluids is administered, and an additional dose of propranolol is given. Surgery is performed the next morning.

What are some important intraoperative strategies?
Attention should be directed to the following points during the operation:

1. The patient should be closely monitored, especially arterial and central venous pressures and, if appropriate, pulmonary artery pressure. The anesthesiology team should be ready to manage sharp decreases as well as sudden increases in blood pressure by maintaining intravenous drips of norepinephrine and nitroprusside, adjusting doses as necessary, and administering a number of adrenergic antagonists and antiarrhythmic drugs in the event of sudden catecholamine release during operation. Adequate hydration should be maintained to optimize the cardiac preload.

2. All anesthetic agents that cause sympathetic stimulation, such as cyclopropane, ether, and curare, should be avoided. Agents that do not cause sympathetic stimulation, such as pentothal, nitrous oxide, succinylcholine, halothane, and penthrane, should be used preferentially.
3. Close communication between the anesthesiology team and the surgeon is necessary because surgical procedures can profoundly affect the hemodynamic stability of the patient. For example, blood pressure may fall when the adrenal vein is clamped. When the tumor is being manipulated, blood pressure may increase because of catecholamine release. It is important that the anesthesiologists anticipate these physiologic changes so that no untoward events occur.
4. Tissues should be handled carefully to avoid stimulating the release of catecholamines from the tumor mass.

What is the recommended incisional approach for resection of pheochromocytoma?
An anterior approach should be used, so that a full exploratory laparotomy can be performed if needed. This is because of the 10% likelihood that the tumor is bilateral, malignant, or extraadrenal. Tumors outside the adrenal gland are found along the paravertebral ganglia. Adrenal tumors secrete both norepinephrine and epinephrine, but paraganglion tumors secrete norepinephrine almost exclusively.

How is a pheochromocytoma determined to be malignant or benign?
Pheochromocytoma is one of the few neoplasms in which differentiation between a malignant and a benign tumor under the microscope is difficult. The diagnosis of malignancy is made by intraoperative evaluation of local invasion and distant spread. Malignant tumors should be resected with a cure in mind, because aggressive extirpation may result in either significant palliation of symptoms or in a cure.

What is the long-term prognosis for malignant and benign pheochromocytomas?
The 5-year survival rates are 44 and 96% for patients with malignant and benign tumors, respectively (1).

Mr. Perez has a single right adrenal pheochromocytoma that is resected uneventfully. There are no other tumors in the abdomen, and surgery is finished without any hemodynamic problems. He recovers without complication and is discharged five days after the operation.

How should patients be monitored postoperatively?
Careful follow-up is very important because of the risk of recurrent disease or incomplete resection of multifocal disease. Urinary catecholamine levels should be measured 3 months after surgery and every 6 months thereafter for 2 to 3 years. If the tumor was malignant and resection was incomplete because of metastasis, the patient must be maintained on α- and β-blockade for life. There

is no effective chemotherapy for malignant pheochromocytoma. In patients with familial pheochromocytoma, follow-up is even more important, especially for concomitant manifestations of abnormal thyroid or parathyroid functions. Families should be instructed to be vigilant for onset of hypertension also.

During his first clinic visit 2 weeks after surgery, Mr. Perez reports that his abdominal incision has healed well and that he is tolerating diet well and taking daily walks. He is satisfied with his care. *See Algorithm 23.1 at the end of this chapter.*

Jenny Curran is a 54-year-old woman who has had hypertension for several years. She complains of fatigue, muscle weakness, and weight gain. She reports that her primary care physician has just diagnosed her as having Cushing's syndrome, and she needs advice on management. The physical examination shows that she has a round face, hirsutism, truncal obesity, and leg and ankle edema.

What is Cushing's syndrome?
Named after a famous neurosurgeon who reported the condition in 1912, Cushing's syndrome is a systemic manifestation of high serum cortisol levels. Fat deposits are mobilized to the face, neck, shoulders, and trunk, leading to a moon face, buffalo hump, and truncal obesity with relatively thin extremities. Cushing's syndrome causes thinning of hair, hirsutism, acne, and abdominal striae. It also causes other hormonal effects, such as menstrual or sexual dysfunction, osteoporosis and bony fractures, glucose intolerance, and diabetes. Arteriosclerosis and hypertension are common.

What causes Cushing's syndrome?
Cushing's syndrome can arise from three sources:

1. The most common cause of Cushing's syndrome today is iatrogenic, from the administration of exogenous corticosteroids for other medical conditions.
2. Excessive production of corticosteroids as the result of an abnormality in the hypothalamus-pituitary-adrenal axis leads to endogenous Cushing's syndrome.
3. Production of ACTH by ectopic tumors, such as medullary carcinoma of the thyroid, lung cancer, and carcinoids, may also cause Cushing's syndrome.

Regardless of the cause, the syndrome is the same.

What is the difference between Cushing's syndrome and Cushing's disease?
Cushing's syndrome is the collective symptoms and signs of cortisol excess. Cushing's disease refers to a specific cause of that syndrome, namely a ba-

sophilic tumor of the pituitary gland leading to increased pituitary ACTH production, which in turn stimulates the adrenal production of cortisol.

Other than antihypertensive drugs, Ms. Curran does not take any medication that might cause Cushing's syndrome. Measurement of her urinary cortisol level confirms overproduction of endogenous cortisol. Two further tests are ordered: a dexamethasone suppression test and serum ACTH measurement.

What physiologic principle guides the approach to determining the cause of Cushing's syndrome?
The hypothalamus-pituitary-adrenal axis normally maintains a balance in the production of cortisol. The hypothalamus secretes corticotrophic hormone-releasing hormone (CRH), which stimulates the pituitary gland to secrete corticotrophic hormone, or ACTH. ACTH then stimulates the end organ of the axis, the adrenal cortex, to produce cortisol. As cortisol is produced, it down-regulates ACTH production by the pituitary gland through a negative feedback mechanism, maintaining cortisol homeostasis in the blood.

What is a dexamethasone suppression test?
Dexamethasone is a potent synthetic corticosteroid that suppresses ACTH secretion from the pituitary gland. Low-dose (1 mg orally) dexamethasone suppresses ACTH production in normal subjects only. High-dose (2 mg orally every 6 hours for 48 hours) dexamethasone suppresses ACTH production in normal subjects and in most patients with a pituitary tumor (Cushing's disease). Patients with an adrenal tumor or an ectopic ACTH-producing tumor do not show suppression by dexamethasone at any dose.

How is the serum ACTH test interpreted?
Because ACTH stimulates cortisol production and cortisol in turn down-regulates ACTH production, adrenal tumors are associated with high serum cortisol levels but almost undetectable serum ACTH levels. By contrast, with pituitary tumors and ectopic tumors that secrete ACTH, the serum ACTH level remains very high despite the high cortisol level.

How is the cause of Cushing's syndrome determined from the results of these two tests?
If the iatrogenic cause is excluded, the three causes of Cushing's syndrome can be differentiated as follows:

• Cushing's disease (pituitary tumor) is associated with excessive levels of ACTH that are not easily suppressed by the end hormone cortisol and is therefore marked by increased ACTH and cortisol levels. ACTH production is not suppressed by low-dose dexamethasone, but high-dose dexamethasone suppresses ACTH production by most pituitary tumors, and thus the cortisol level is suppressed.

- Adrenal tumors (adenomas or carcinomas) produce excessive cortisol, which suppresses ACTH production via the negative feedback mechanism. Adrenal tumors are therefore characterized by an undetectable ACTH level in the presence of a high cortisol level. Exogenous dexamethasone does not suppress cortisol production by the tumor.
- Ectopic tumors produce ACTH, which increases the adrenal production of cortisol. Ectopic tumors are typified by increased levels of both ACTH and cortisol. Exogenous dexamethasone does not suppress cortisol or ACTH production.

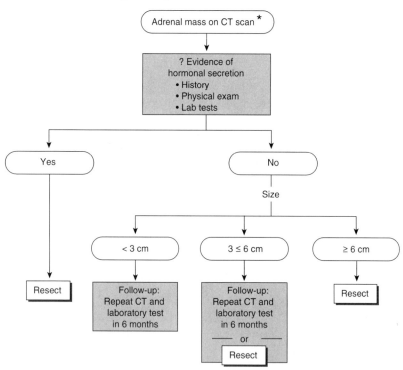

Management Algorithm for Incidental Adrenal Mass

* If cystic, aspiration should be performed.
If aspiration is clear, follow.
If aspiration is bloody, do further work-up.

Algorithm 23.1.

Management Algorithm for Cushing's Syndrome

Algorithm 23.2.

Ms. Curran's laboratory results show a low ACTH level, high cortisol level, and failure of both low- and high-dose dexamethasone suppression tests. A cortisol-producing adrenal tumor is suspected, and this is confirmed by the finding of a 4-cm right adrenal mass on CT. She undergoes surgical resection and is found to have an adrenal adenoma. Her symptoms gradually resolve under the care of an endocrinologist.

REFERENCES

1. Gann D, DeMaria E. Pituitary and adrenal glands. In: Schwartz SI, Shires GT, Spencer FC, eds. Principles of Surgery. 6th ed. New York: McGraw Hill, 1994:1561–1609.

2. Kamel N, Corapcioglu D, Uysal AR, et al. The characteristics of nine patients with adrenal incidentalomas. Endocr J 1995;42:497–503.

3. Fry WJ, Fry RE. Surgically correctable hypertension. In: Schwartz SI, Shires GT, Spencer FC, eds. Principles of Surgery. 5th ed. New York: McGraw Hill, 1989: 1041–1052.

Coronary Artery Disease

Michael McGrath and Cornelius M. Dyke

Harry Stein is a 55-year-old accountant who complains to his family physician of chest pains that have been troubling him for several months. He describes the feeling as heaviness that begins in the middle of his chest and spreads to his neck and throat. He has no back pain, arm pain, or nausea. Although he has a sedentary lifestyle, the pain usually occurs when he walks uphill to his office and occasionally after meals. He also has noticed that stress from work brings on the symptoms. Mr. Stein smokes cigarettes at work and when he feels stressed. He has no diabetes and only mild hypertension.

What is this patient's diagnosis?
Mr. Stein has angina pectoris. Usually substernal or centered in the left chest, the feeling has been described as crushing, pressure, or heaviness, occasionally radiating to the neck, left shoulder, or left arm. Typical symptoms come on slowly, reach maximal intensity within minutes, and reside with rest and nitrates within minutes. Noncardiac causes of chest pain should be considered in patients with a sharp or stabbing pain, pain that lasts only seconds, or pain associated with specific movements of the arms or shoulders. Changes in position or posture usually do not affect anginal chest pain. However, breathlessness, fatigue, belching, and epigastric discomfort may also indicate anginal "equivalents." Some patients (e.g., diabetics) are asymptomatic. The New York Heart Association's functional classification of angina pectoris is useful to quantitate and compare anginal symptoms (Table 24.1).

What other causes of chest pain mimic angina?
The differential diagnosis of chest pain includes esophageal disorders, biliary disease, costochondritis, musculoskeletal pain, cervical radiculopathy, pericarditis, pulmonary hypertension, pulmonary embolism, and acute aortic dissection. Acute myocardial infarction must be excluded in any patient with a long episode of chest pain.

Table 24.1. NEW YORK HEART ASSOCIATION FUNCTIONAL CLASSIFICATION OF ANGINA PECTORIS

Class	Activity Level
I	No limitations in physical activity; ordinary activity does not precipitate symptoms.
II	Slight limitation in physical activity; comfortable at rest; ordinary activity may precipitate anginal symptoms.
III	Marked limitation in physical activity; comfortable at rest; less than ordinary activity precipitates anginal symptoms.
IV	Severe limitation in physical activity; symptoms occur even at rest; any activity exacerbates anginal symptoms.

What does angina indicate?
Angina is caused by myocardial ischemia, or a mismatch between myocardial oxygen supply and demand. It usually accompanies an increase in myocardial oxygen demand brought about by physical activity. Most patients with angina have fixed obstructive lesions in their coronary arteries as well as defects in the ability of the coronary arteries to dilate and compensate for increased activity. When the demands on the myocardium exceed the threshold at which the coronary arteries can supply oxygenated blood, myocardial ischemia occurs and symptoms may develop.

What are the determinants of myocardial oxygen consumption?
Myocardial oxygen consumption is determined by the workload placed on the heart. The determinants are complex; they include the tension within the wall of the heart, the contractile state of the heart, the heart rate, and the energy costs of maintaining the integrity of the myocardial cells. The heart rate is particularly important because conditions that increase heart rate (e.g., exercise, stress, hyperthyroidism, sepsis) significantly increase myocardial oxygen consumption. When myocardial oxygen delivery is limited (e.g., with fixed coronary atherosclerotic obstruction), myocardial ischemia occurs.

What is unstable angina?
Unstable angina and acute myocardial infarction are two manifestations of acute ischemic syndromes distinct from stable angina. An anginal pattern that is increasing in intensity or frequency is considered unstable, and it puts the patient at risk for acute myocardial infarction. Unstable angina, which may be considered a different pathophysiologic process from stable angina, occurs when existing atherosclerotic plaques rupture or develop fissures, leading to acute thrombosis of the coronary artery. If the thrombus is not lysed, acute

myocardial infarction results. This process is the basis of thrombolytic therapy for the treatment of acute myocardial infarction. The critical role of platelets in the development of acute ischemic syndromes has recently been recognized. That discovery led to the development of potent platelet inhibitors for the treatment of acute myocardial infarction and unstable angina.

Mr. Stein is managed medically with β-blockers, nitrates, and aspirin with good success. He is strongly advised to quit smoking. About 2 years later, he awakens at night with typical angina pain. Despite taking three sublingual nitroglycerin tablets, the pain persists. After 30 minutes, he calls 911 and is taken to the emergency department. There, an electrocardiogram (ECG) demonstrates significant ST elevation in the inferior leads consistent with an acute inferior myocardial infarction; he is started on nitroglycerin and heparin intravenously and given an aspirin by mouth. Thrombolytic therapy is initiated and he is admitted to the coronary care unit with a diagnosis of acute myocardial infarction. Cardiac enzymes are measured and diagnostic cardiac catheterization is performed.

Describe the anatomy of the coronary arteries.
The right and left coronary arteries are the first branches off the aorta. The left coronary artery, or left main artery, soon branches into the left anterior descending (LAD) artery and the circumflex artery. The LAD artery supplies the anterolateral left ventricular wall and the interventricular septum. The obtuse marginal branches of the circumflex artery supply the posterolateral wall of the left ventricle. The right coronary artery and its branches supply the right ventricular free wall and in 85 to 90% of patients provide blood to the posterior left ventricular wall and posterior septum through the posterior descending artery. The origin of the posterior descending artery determines the *dominance* of the coronary circulation: 10 to 15% of the population have a left dominant coronary circulation in which the posterior descending artery arises from the circumflex system. It is important to understand the blood supply of several vital cardiac structures. The artery to the sinus node usually arises from the right coronary artery, but in up to 40% of patients it arises from the left system. The atrioventricular node is usually supplied by a branch of the right coronary artery. The anterolateral papillary muscle of the left ventricle is usually supplied by branches of the left anterior descending artery, whereas the posteromedial papillary muscle may arise from either the right or left systems, depending on which is dominant.

Mr. Stein's catheterization reveals a 90% stenotic lesion of the proximal right coronary artery and a 50% lesion in the proximal LAD artery. The first obtuse marginal of the circumflex artery has a 20 to 30% stenosis. Left ventricular function is normal.

Which of these lesions are hemodynamically significant?
A 75% reduction in area of the is required to restrict flow. Because coronary arteriograms are displayed in cross-section, this translates into a 50% reduction in cross-sectional area; therefore, more than 50% stenosis is generally considered significant. Furthermore, determining the severity of stenosis is relatively subjective, and in general coronary angiography tends to underestimate severity of the lesions.

What are the treatment options for this patient?
A complete discussion of the management of coronary artery disease is beyond the scope of this chapter, which provides only a review; reference texts provide more detailed coverage. Patients with atherosclerotic coronary disease may be successfully treated with medications, percutaneous angioplasty, or coronary artery bypass surgery, depending on the severity of the disease and the patient's overall health. Patients with significant symptoms and one- or two-vessel coronary disease with suitable coronary angiographic morphology are usually considered for percutaneous revascularization. Patients with multivessel coronary disease, left main coronary disease, or significant left ventricular dysfunction have better long-term survival with surgical revascularization than with angioplasty. Also, patients with diabetes have a greater long-term survival benefit with surgical revascularization [1]. Elective coronary revascularization may also be necessary in patients who develop restenosis of the coronary artery after angioplasty. Emergency coronary bypass surgery is occasionally needed after acute angioplasty failures (1 to 4% of percutaneous transluminal coronary angioplasty [PTCA]).

Are there any randomized trials comparing PTCA with coronary artery bypass grafting (CABG)?
Revascularization for ischemic heart disease is probably the most intensely studied disease treatment. During the 1970s, several large, randomized trials, including the Veterans Administration Cooperative Study [2], the CASS Study [3], and the European Cooperative Study, compared PTCA with CABG [4]. Although these trials highlighted several important lessons (e.g., the importance of surgery for multivessel and left main disease), dramatic changes in practices and advancement in surgical and catheter-based techniques have since occurred; other advances include the ubiquitous use of the internal mammary artery (IMA) as a conduit and the use of intracoronary stenting and pharmacologic support for percutaneous interventions. These caveats must be considered even in the interpretation of recent trials.

Recently, a number of trials comparing CABG with PTCA have been reported. In a 15-year follow up from the CASS trial, a significant number of patients originally receiving PTCA crossed over, such that at 15 years 70% of patients had undergone CABG. High-risk patients had significantly better survival after

CABG than after PTCA. In 1996, the BARI trials found an equivalent 5-year survival in patients following CABG and PTCA; however, PTCA patients required more frequent revascularizations (1). Furthermore, patients with diabetes had significantly better survival with CABG than with PTCA. In the CABRI trial, patients had fewer anginal symptoms and took less medication after CABG surgery than after PTCA. In the EAST trial, patients had equivalent survival at 3 years (5).

In summary, long-term survival for patients with multivessel coronary artery disease is probably equivalent after PTCA and CABG; however, in certain subgroups (e.g., diabetics, high-risk patients) survival after surgical revascularization is superior. Additionally, most of the data demonstrate an increased need for multiple procedures after PTCA and an increased incidence of symptoms of angina and need for antianginal medications. Cost implications are difficult to quantify. These and other issues remain the focus of intense study.

Mr. Stein undergoes successful percutaneous revascularization with angioplasty and intracoronary stenting of the right coronary artery. He recovers and remains pain free for 12 months. Then he returns to his cardiologist with new complaints of angina. He has tried to quit smoking several times but has been unsuccessful. Evaluation and recatheterization demonstrate that the right coronary artery has restenosed with a 90% lesion, and the LAD artery is 80% stenosed. The first obtuse marginal branch (OM1) of the left circumflex artery has a 50 to 60% stenosis. His left ventricular function is still normal.

What is restenosis?
Restenosis occurs in approximately 30% of patients after balloon angioplasty (intracoronary stenting is a major advance and reduces the incidence of restenosis to less than 10%). Restenosis is a pathophysiologic response to an iatrogenic injury. By definition, angioplasty creates a local vascular injury at the site of the coronary stenosis. The disruption of the endothelial layer and injury to the subendothelial tissues that occurs with angioplasty promotes a strong wound healing response. Intimal hyperplasia occurs and fibroblasts proliferate and when unchecked may lead to restenosis of the vessel 3 to 12 months after initially successful angioplasty. The pathogenesis of restenosis and methods of prevention are subjects of intense investigation.

What are Mr. Stein's treatment options at this point?
Again, the choice for revascularization is between a percutaneous and surgical method. Repeat angioplasty of one or more vessels is frequently successful, with a similar incidence of restenosis. CABG should be considered more strongly now than previously, because Mr. Stein has two severely stenotic le-

sions (the right coronary artery and the LAD artery) with an additional lesser but hemodynamically significant lesion (OM1). The choice of therapy should be thoroughly discussed with the patient.

Mr. Stein elects to try angioplasty again. He undergoes successful PTCA of the right coronary artery and LAD artery lesions and is discharged home. However, he returns 3 months later with recurrent angina. Catheterization reveals significant restenosis, and Mr. Stein requests consultation with a surgeon.

What are the risks of CABG?
Kirklin (6) has demonstrated that the risk of death after CABG surgery is time related; the hazard function for death has an early perioperative phase, a middle and constant phase from 2 to 3 months to about 6 years, and a late rising phase beyond 6 years. The early risk of death relates to problems that occur during and immediately after surgery, such as stroke, perioperative myocardial infarction, wound complications, bleeding, and technical problems during surgery. After recovery from surgery, the risk of death is rather low and does not begin to increase again for 5 to 6 years. Thereafter, the progressive nature of atherosclerotic coronary disease must be accounted for; angina or acute myocardial infarction may recur as native coronary disease progresses and vein grafts become stenotic.

What are risk factors for morbidity and mortality following CABG?
Preoperative low ejection fraction, acute myocardial infarction, cardiogenic shock, advanced age, female gender, and significant comorbid conditions (e.g., transient ischemic attacks, stroke, renal dysfunction, severe obstructive pulmonary disease) increase the risk of surgery. However, these risk factors may not be prohibitive, as these sicker patients may derive the greatest relative benefit from surgical revascularization compared with medical therapy.

Mr. Stein is scheduled for elective CABG. Hemodynamic monitoring consists of an arterial pressure line, central line, and pulmonary artery catheter. The IMA is anastomosed to the LAD artery and reversed saphenous vein grafts are placed in the posterior descending branch of the right coronary artery and the obtuse marginal branch of the circumflex artery.

Why is the IMA the preferred conduit for revascularization?
In a landmark article in 1986, Loop (7) demonstrated the superiority of the IMA for coronary bypass. Use of the IMA for bypass was associated with improved long-term survival, reduced incidence of myocardial infarction, and reduced need for subsequent revascularization in all groups of patients. Patency

of the IMA-LAD artery graft is at least 95% at 15 years, compared with a 50% patency rate for saphenous vein grafts at 10 years. These data led to the widespread use of the left internal artery to bypass stenotic disease of the LAD artery in virtually all cases. There are few contraindications for its use.

What features of the IMA make it such a good conduit?

1. The IMA is a branch of the subclavian artery. It has a well-formed internal elastic membrane, a very thin tunica media with few smooth muscle cells, and a highly metabolic and active endothelium.
2. Atherosclerosis of the internal mammary artery is virtually nonexistent.
3. The IMA is quite reactive, with the ability to vasodilate to accommodate the metabolic needs of the heart.

Occasionally a patient has a proximal subclavian stenosis that precludes use of the IMA as a pedicled graft.

There are two IMAs, right and left. Should they both be used for bypass?
Perhaps. Although it has not been demonstrated that bilateral IMA grafting improves survival over unilateral IMA grafting, there is intuitive appeal to the use of both arteries as conduits. Use of bilateral IMAs has its drawbacks: the sternum is significantly devascularized after harvest of the right and left IMAs. This devascularization may predispose certain patient groups (e.g., diabetics, obese patients) to serious infectious complications. Other vessels that may be considered for grafting include the right gastroepiploic artery, the radial arteries, and the inferior epigastric arteries. It is unclear whether these other conduits match the quality of the IMAs.

What is cardioplegia?
Cardioplegic solutions arrest the heart in diastole, allowing the surgeon to operate within a still, bloodless field. Stopping mechanical activity reduces myocardial oxygen consumption to basal levels. There is tremendous variety in the particular solutions, mode of delivery, temperature, and timing of delivery of cardioplegia. Use of a high concentration of potassium (15 to 30 mEq/L) to induce depolarized arrest is a unifying concept. Cardioplegic solutions may be crystalloid or blood based and may contain additives such as Krebs cycle substrates or buffers. They may be delivered antegrade through the aortic root of the cross-clamped aorta, down completed vein grafts, or retrograde through a catheter within the coronary sinus. Most centers use cold solutions to cool the heart, although tepid or warm cardioplegia may also be used. Some surgeons use fibrillatory arrest without cardioplegia with good results. Using standard techniques of myocardial protection, cross-clamp times of up to 2 hours, sometimes more, can be well tolerated.

Immediately postoperatively, Mr. Stein is putting out 300 mL of blood from his mediastinal chest tubes in his first hour in the intensive care unit (ICU). He remains hemodynamically stable, although he appears mildly hypovolemic.

What conditions contribute to excessive bleeding after cardiopulmonary bypass?
Bleeding requiring reoperation occurs in approximately 1% of patients undergoing cardiopulmonary bypass, although this incidence is higher in patients with reoperations, endocarditis, and those requiring hypothermic circulatory arrest. Any of several factors may be causative. The potential for surgical bleeding is significant and requires strict attention to technical detail. Hypothermia, excessive heparin, and platelet dysfunction after bypass all contribute to varying degrees of coagulopathy. Coagulation factor deficits are not usually problematic because of the innate redundancy of the coagulation cascade.

Do any pharmacologic agents reduce bleeding after cardiopulmonary bypass?
Aprotinin (Trasylol), a serine protease inhibitor first studied as an antiinflammatory agent, reduces mediastinal bleeding after cardiopulmonary bypass. Aprotinin reduces platelet dysfunction typical with cardiopulmonary bypass and inhibits kallikrein activation, hence fibrinolysis, perhaps through its action on protein C, a naturally circulating fibrinolytic. Most surgeons reserve aprotinin for patients at risk for excessive bleeding (e.g., reoperation patients, those with endocarditis, Jehovah's Witnesses). Other agents, such as tranexamic acid, ε-aminocaproic acid (Amicar), and desmopressin, have also been used as adjuncts to hemostasis, although their efficacy after cardiac surgery is less clear.

What are the indications for reexploration?
Chest tube output of 400 mL for the first hour or persistent bleeding of 200 to 300 mL/hour for several hours should prompt the surgeon to consider reexploration. Cardiac tamponade and hemodynamic instability are the inevitable result of significant mediastinal bleeding and are best avoided by early rather than late reexploration.

Mr. Stein's bleeding gradually subsides during the next few hours with warming and platelet transfusion. He remains hemodynamically stable, is extubated uneventfully, and is transferred from the ICU to a monitored bed the day after surgery. On postoperative day 3, his heart rate suddenly increases to 130 beats per minute and he is slightly short of breath.

What is the likely cardiac rhythm?
Atrial fibrillation with a rapid ventricular response is the likely rhythm; it occurs in up to 30% of patients following cardiac surgery. The cause is unclear

but may involve the significant fluid shifts that occur after bypass and their effect on atrial stretch receptors. Atrial flutter is less common; 2:1 atrial flutter may be differentiated from a sinus rhythm by the heart rate or by an atrial electrocardiographic tracing with the temporary atrial wires. Atrial flutter may be terminated by rapid atrial pacing. Atrial fibrillation is treated in a variety of ways; the ventricular response is usually slowed pharmacologically (e.g., with diltiazem, β-blocker, or digoxin) before conversion with a class IA antiarrhythmic (e.g., procainamide or quinidine). Anticoagulation and cardioversion are required in refractory cases. Antiarrhythmics are usually continued for 4 to 6 weeks postoperatively, at which point they may be discontinued if the patient has remained in normal sinus rhythm.

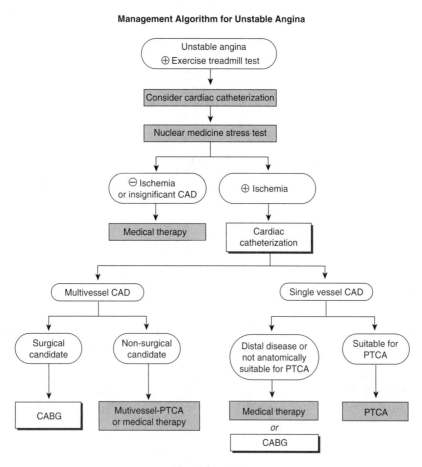

Management Algorithm for Unstable Angina

Algorithm 24.1.

Mr. Stein is treated with diltiazem and procainamide and converts to a normal sinus rhythm. The rest of his recovery is uneventful. By postoperative day 5, he is walking without difficulty, no longer on oxygen, eating a regular diet, and ready for discharge.

What is his risk of developing recurrent angina or myocardial infarction?
Several recent trials have demonstrated an 85 to 90% event-free survival 5 years after CABG (5, 8). Atherosclerosis is a relentless disease, however; progression of native coronary artery disease distal to the bypass grafts or the development of atherosclerotic plaques within saphenous bypass grafts may bring back the symptoms. As mentioned, use of the IMA-LAD artery bypass graft improves late survival in all patient groups.

Atherosclerosis being a chronic systemic disease, what can Mr. Stein do to prevent recurrence of angina?
Cessation of smoking is the primary step patients can take to improve their long-term survival and avoid recurrence of symptoms. Management of their serum cholesterol and triglycerides, antiplatelet therapy, and positive lifestyle changes, such as weight loss and exercise, are also important.

REFERENCES

1. Bypass Angioplasty Revascularization Investigation (BARI) Investigators. Comparison of coronary bypass surgery with angioplasty in patients with multivessel disease. N Engl J Med 1996;335:217–225.
2. The Veterans Administration Coronary Artery Bypass Surgery Cooperative Study Group. Eleven year survival in a Veterans Administration randomized trial of coronary bypass surgery for stable angina. N Engl J Med 1984;311:333–339.
3. Davis KB, Chaitman B, Ryan T, et al. Comparison of 15 year survival for men and women after initial medical or surgical treatment for coronary artery disease: a CASS registry study. J Am Coll Cardiol 1995;25:1000–1009.
4. European Surgery Study Group. Long term results of a prospective, randomized study of coronary artery bypass surgery in stable angina pectoris. Lancet 1982;2:1173.
5. First year results of CABRI (coronary angioplasty versus bypass revascularization investigation). Lancet 1995;346:1179–1184.
6. Kirklin JW, Barratt-Boyes BG, eds. Stenotic arteriosclerotic coronary artery disease. In: Cardiac Surgery. 2nd ed. New York: Churchill Livingstone, 1992:285–381.
7. Loop FD, Lytle BW, Cosgrove DM, et al. Influence of the internal mammary artery on 10-year survival and other cardiac events. N Engl J Med 1986;314:1–6.
8. Pocock SJ, Henderson RA, Seed P, et al. Quality of life, employment status, and anginal symptoms after coronary angioplasty or bypass surgery: three year follow up in the Randomized Intervention Treatment of Angina (RITA). Circulation 1996;94:135–142.

Valvular Heart Disease

James S. Gammie and Cornelius M. Dyke

AORTIC STENOSIS

Stanley Osis is a 75-year-old man with no significant medical history. While mowing his lawn, he suffers a brief syncopal event. He is taken to the local emergency department and evaluated. He has no symptoms, and a careful review of systems is unrevealing. On physical examination, his heart rate is 80 beats per minute and regular. Auscultation reveals a harsh crescendo-decrescendo systolic murmur that is best heard in the right second intercostal space and along the left sternal border. The murmur radiates to both carotid arteries. His peripheral pulse has a delayed upstroke and low volume (pulsus parvus et tardus). The lungs are clear, and the examination is otherwise normal. The electrocardiogram shows normal sinus rhythm and left ventricular hypertrophy. The chest radiograph shows mild left ventricular enlargement.

What is the most likely diagnosis?
On the basis of the characteristic murmur on physical examination, the most likely diagnosis is a syncopal event caused by severe aortic stenosis.

Mr. Osis is admitted to the hospital for 24 hours. Continuous electrocardiographic monitoring shows no evidence of arrhythmia. Serial creatine phosphokinase levels are normal. Carotid Doppler studies show only mild stenosis of the left internal carotid artery. A two-dimensional transthoracic echocardiogram reveals concentric left ventricular hypertrophy with severe aortic stenosis. The calculated aortic valve area is 0.7 cm². Mitral valve function is normal, and the ejection fraction is estimated to be 60%.

What are the three most common causes of aortic stenosis, and what is the most likely cause in this patient?
The following are the three most common causes of aortic stenosis:

Degenerative (senile) calcific aortic stenosis is the most common cause of aortic stenosis in patients undergoing aortic valve replacement. It is characterized by immobilization of the aortic valve cusps by dense deposits of calcium. The calcium prevents normal opening of the valve during systole. Degenerative aortic stenosis is seen most commonly in patients over age 65.

Congenital bicuspid aortic valve affects as many as 2% of infants at birth. Although a bicuspid valve usually does not cause symptoms early in life, it does generate turbulent flow that ultimately leads to fibrosis of the leaflets and to valvular stenosis. Patients with congenital bicuspid aortic valves usually develop symptoms in their 50s and 60s. Congenital bicuspid aortic valve is the most common cause of aortic stenosis in patients under 65 years of age.

Rheumatic aortic stenosis usually occurs in a previously normal valve. It is characterized by commissural fusion (attachment of the valve cusps to each other in the clefts between the cusps). Some aortic regurgitation is common in patients with rheumatic aortic stenosis, and the mitral valve is almost always diseased.

What are the three cardinal symptoms of aortic stenosis, and what is the pathophysiology of each?
Angina, syncope, and congestive heart failure are the three cardinal symptoms of *aortic stenosis*. Progressive obstruction to left ventricular outflow by the stenotic valve causes compensatory concentric left ventricular hypertrophy. This permits maintenance of cardiac output despite a significant obstruction. The hypertrophied left ventricle can maintain a large pressure gradient across the valve without a decrease in cardiac output, left ventricular dilation, or symptoms.

Angina occurs in two-thirds of patients with critical aortic stenosis and in 50% of cases is associated with coronary occlusive disease. Angina is typically associated with exertion. In patients without coronary artery disease, angina results from an imbalance in myocardial oxygen supply and demand. Oxygen demand increases as a result of the increased left ventricular mass and wall tension, whereas myocardial blood flow is compromised by compression of intramyocardial coronary arteries. Epicardial coronary artery obstruction secondary to atherosclerotic plaque further contributes to ischemia in patients with aortic stenosis.

Syncope is a result of inadequate cerebral perfusion. Syncope normally occurs during exertion, when arterial blood pressure decreases as a result of systemic vasodilation in the presence of a fixed cardiac output.

Left ventricular failure is caused by increased left ventricular filling pressures. As the ventricle progressively hypertrophies to compensate for the aortic valvular obstruction, it becomes less compliant (stiffer), and left ventricular filling pressures increase. In turn, elevated left ventricular filling pressure is transmitted to the left atrium and the pulmonary capillary bed, which results

in clinical symptoms of left ventricular failure, including dyspnea with exertion, paroxysmal nocturnal dyspnea, and orthopnea. Synchronized left
atrial contraction is especially important for filling of the thickened, non-
compliant ventricle in aortic stenosis. The onset of atrial fibrillation and loss
of this atrial kick can lead to significant hemodynamic and clinical deterioration in patients with advanced aortic stenosis.

*What is the natural history of aortic stenosis, and what is the characteristic time interval
between onset of each of the cardinal symptoms and death?*
Patients with severe aortic stenosis can remain hemodynamically compensated
for years. However, the onset of symptoms is an ominous event that portends
a poor prognosis. Once patients develop angina or syncope, the average survival is 2 to 3 years. Average survival with congestive heart failure is 1.5 years.
The characteristic natural history of this disease (prolonged compensated survival in the absence of symptoms, with rapid deterioration and dismal survival
after the onset of symptoms) was defined by Ross and Braunwald (1) in a classic article in 1968 (Fig. 25.1). Death is rare among patients who have aortic
stenosis but do not display symptoms. Thus, the indication for operation in a
patient with severe aortic stenosis is the development of symptoms.

What is the next step in the workup for patients with aortic stenosis?
Cardiac catheterization is mandatory to assess the coronary anatomy. Significant coronary artery disease is common among patients with aortic stenosis, and

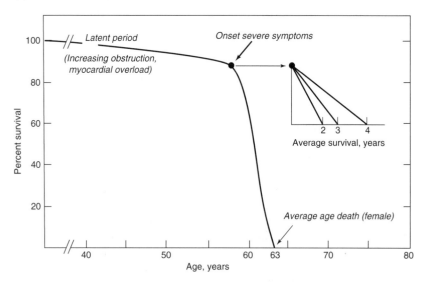

Figure 25.1.   Natural history of patients with aortic stenosis. (Reprinted with permission
from Ross J, Braunwald E. Aortic stenosis. Circulation 1968;38[Suppl 5]:V61–67.)

these patients require coronary artery bypass grafting at the time of aortic valve replacement. Cardiac catheterization allows simultaneous measurement of pressure within the left ventricle and in the proximal aorta. Measurement of the pressure gradient across the aortic valve allows precise determination of aortic valve area. Catheterization also allows estimation of left ventricular function and rules out coexisting valvular heart lesions.

What is the Gorlin formula?
Developed by Richard Gorlin and his father at Peter Bent Brigham Hospital in Boston, this formula allows accurate calculation of the aortic valve area on the basis of hemodynamic data obtained during cardiac catheterization (2):

$$AVA = \frac{CO \div (SEP)(HR)}{44.3 \sqrt{(P)}}$$

where AVA is the aortic valve area (cm^2), CO is the cardiac output in liters per minute, SEP is the systolic ejection period in seconds per beat, HR is the heart rate, C is a constant, and (P) is the pressure gradient across the aortic valve. The normal aortic valve area is 3 to 4 cm^2. Symptoms generally do not develop until aortic valve area is less than 1 cm^2.

Are there any medical alternatives to aortic valve replacement?
There are no medical alternatives to aortic valve replacement. In percutaneous balloon aortic valvuloplasty, the stenotic aortic valve is dilated with a balloon. Patients generally have a reduction of peak transvalvular gradient of about 50% and an increase in valve area of 0.5 to 1 cm^2. However, 50 to 75% of patients develop restenosis within 9 months, and the 1-year mortality is 30% (3). Thus, aortic valvuloplasty should be considered only a palliative procedure applicable to patients who are not candidates for aortic valve replacement.

Mr. Osis is scheduled for elective aortic valve replacement. After a detailed discussion of the risks and benefits of surgery, he agrees to proceed.

Do patients undergoing valve surgery need any special preoperative preparation?
All patients planning to have elective heart valve surgery should undergo a careful dental examination. Severely diseased teeth (abscess, periodontal disease) should be extracted before operation to remove a source of sepsis. Other possible sources of sepsis, such as urinary tract infections, respiratory infections, or septic processes within the gastrointestinal tract should be identified and treated prior to operation.

What are the ideal characteristics of a valve substitute?
An ideal replacement valve would have hemodynamic characteristics similar to those of native human cardiac valves, which are characterized by minimal

transvalvular gradients during forward flow and freedom from regurgitation during closure. The perfect valve would be nonthrombogenic and durable, completely free of structural degeneration, resistant to infection, nondestructive to blood elements, readily available, and low in cost. Such a valve substitute has yet to be created.

What are the different types of replacement aortic valves? What factors guide the choice of a valve?
The two main categories of replacement valves are mechanical prostheses and bioprostheses. In special cases, homograft aortic valves may be used.

Bioprostheses. The most commonly used bioprostheses are the stented porcine type, constructed from glutaraldehyde-fixed porcine aortic valves. Bioprostheses have the advantage of not requiring chronic anticoagulation. This benefit is offset by a limited valve lifespan, 10 to 12 years, in the aortic position. Bioprostheses last longest in older patients, and they are therefore commonly implanted in patients older than 70 years of age and in patients with a life expectancy less than 10 to 12 years.
Mechanical prostheses. The most commonly implanted mechanical prosthesis is a bileaflet tilting disc valve made of pyrolytic carbon. Mechanical prostheses have excellent long-term durability, but this advantage is offset by the requirement for long-term anticoagulation with warfarin (Coumadin). This results in a 2 to 3% rate of anticoagulant-related hemorrhage per patient-year and 0.2% annual mortality. Women of childbearing age should not receive a mechanical valve because warfarin is teratogenic. In general, mechanical valves should be implanted in patients without contraindications to anticoagulation who have a life expectancy longer than 10 years and in whom childbearing is not a concern. Both bioprosthetic and mechanical valves carry a risk of thromboembolism of 1% to 2% per year. Older patients, whose risk of anticoagulation is greater and who have a life expectancy of less than 10 years, generally benefit from a bioprosthetic valve. Most surgeons would probably choose a bioprosthetic valve for Mr. Osis.
Homograft aortic valves. These are aortic valves obtained from a cadaver and preserved, usually by deep-freezing (cryopreservation). The homograft has a durability of about 90% at 10 years, does not require anticoagulation, and has an extremely low rate of thromboembolism. The chief disadvantages of homografts are limited availability and technical complexity of insertion. Homografts are commonly inserted in young patients with contraindications to anticoagulation, and because of the resistance of these grafts to infection, they are often used in patients with bacterial endocarditis.

What is the Ross procedure?
In 1967, Donald Ross first replaced a diseased aortic valve with a pulmonary autograft. The aortic valve was excised and replaced with the patient's own pul-

monic valve, which was transposed into the aortic position. The pulmonic valve was replaced with a homograft (cadaveric) valve. His first patient remains well 30 years later. The Ross procedure is unique because the diseased aortic valve is replaced with native tissue. Advantages of this procedure include excellent durability (in one study, only 15% of patients required reoperation 18 years after valve replacement), freedom from anticoagulation (particularly important for women of childbearing age), normal growth characteristics in children, resistance to infection, and a low incidence of thromboembolism (4). The Ross procedure is generally applied to young patients with isolated aortic valve disease and a life expectancy greater than 20 years. It is technically demanding, and an experienced surgeon is necessary.

Mr. Osis undergoes uncomplicated aortic valve replacement. A 25-mm bioprosthesis is inserted in the aortic position. He is extubated 4 hours after surgery and is discharged home on the fourth day postoperatively.

What are the key technical considerations in aortic valve replacement?
After cardiopulmonary bypass is in place and the heart has been arrested, the aorta is opened and the diseased valve is exposed. The valve leaflets are excised, and calcium deposits are removed. Great care must be taken to remove all loose debris to avoid a stroke. A valve of appropriate size is chosen and sutured in place.

What postoperative complications are unique to aortic valve replacement surgery?
The conduction system passes inferiorly and close to the aortic annulus near the junction of the right coronary and noncoronary valve leaflets (Fig. 25.2). Sutures placed too deep at this location can produce temporary or permanent postoperative heart block. Heart block that requires a permanent pacemaker occurs in about 1% of cases.

What is the average mortality for an aortic valve replacement?
Mortality averages 3 to 5%.

What is the long-term prognosis after aortic valve replacement?
The 5-year survival after aortic valve replacement is 75%, and the 10-year survival is 60%.

How should anticoagulation be managed in the early postoperative period? What is the target international normalized ratio (INR) for patients with artificial heart valves?
Most patients are given intravenous heparin starting 24 to 48 hours after operation. Warfarin is also administered, and heparin is stopped when the INR is therapeutic, which is 2.5 to 3.5 for prosthetic heart valves (5). Anticoagulation in patients who have received bioprosthetic valves usually consists of warfarin

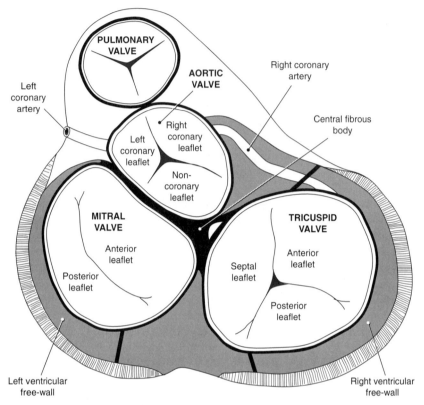

Figure 25.2. Anatomy of the aortic valve. (Reprinted with permission from Siavosh Khonsari. Cardiac Surgery: Safeguards and Pitfalls in Operative Technique. 2nd ed. Philadelphia: Lippincott-Raven, 1997.)

for 3 months after the operation and aspirin only thereafter. Mechanical valves require lifelong anticoagulation.

When can a patient resume normal activities after aortic valve replacement surgery? Light work can generally be resumed 4 to 6 weeks after operation; heavy work, such as lawn mowing, can be resumed 3 to 4 months after operation.

AORTIC REGURGITATION

Fred Smith is a 54-year-old peanut farmer who is referred by his family physician because of an abnormal chest radiograph, which was obtained because of a recent fever and cough. Although there is no evidence of pneumonia or pulmonary disease on radiograph, the physician thought the ascending aortic silhouette looked abnormal.

Mr. Smith says he has no symptoms, and his cough has resolved. He works up to 10 hours daily on his farm and has not noted any decrease in his exercise tolerance or activity level. On physical examination, he appears in general good health. His blood pressure is 160/60 mm Hg with a heart rate of 84 beats per minute. His pulses are prominent and brisk. On auscultation, a diastolic murmur is audible, apparently at the beginning of diastole. No systolic or carotid murmurs are appreciated, and no third or fourth heart sounds are heard. The rest of his examination is unremarkable.

What is the significance of Mr. Smith's blood pressure?
The pulse pressure is abnormally wide, suggesting an incompetent aortic valve. This suggestion is supported by the diastolic murmur and the bounding, or water hammer, pulses. Systolic hypertension is also common.

What other pertinent findings (or lack of findings) should be elucidated from the patient's history and physical examination?
The patient should be carefully evaluated for symptoms of congestive heart failure. Patients with aortic regurgitation are asymptomatic for long periods; however, when symptoms do occur, dyspnea on exertion, orthopnea, and paroxysmal nocturnal dyspnea are common. Anginalike symptoms may occur even with normal coronary arteries. Onset of symptoms is a significant turning point for patients with aortic regurgitation, and it should prompt physicians and patients to seek consultation with a cardiac surgeon.

Why are the pulses bounding?
The pulse characteristics of aortic regurgitation reflect the abrupt filling of the arterial tree with the increased volume at end-diastole and the abrupt decrease in the pulse pressure due to the incompetent aortic valve. In end-stage aortic regurgitation, water hammer pulses may not be present because ventricular systolic function decreases and end-diastolic pressure increases (less regurgitant flow into the left ventricle as the pressure differential across the valve decreases).

What is an Austin-Flint murmur?
Using a stethoscope, skilled practitioners can distinguish subtle differences in the diastolic murmurs associated with aortic regurgitation. The murmur of aortic insufficiency is early in diastole and trails off in late diastole except in severe aortic insufficiency, in which the diastolic murmur may be holodiastolic. The diastolic murmur is best heard along the left and right sternal borders. The Austin-Flint murmur, a middiastolic murmur best heard at the apex, is a result of turbulence caused by the regurgitant stream of blood hitting the anterior leaflet of the mitral valve. It may be distinguished from a mitral stenosis murmur by the absence of an opening snap and loud S_1 (heard with mitral stenosis).

What are the common causes of aortic regurgitation?
Rheumatic valve disease with leaflet retraction used to be the most common cause of aortic regurgitation, but as rheumatic disease becomes less common in the United States, annuloaortic ectasia has become the most common cause of aortic valve incompetence. The cause of the aortic root dilation is idiopathic in the vast majority of patients, although Marfan's syndrome is an important cause in a subset of these patients. Acute causes of aortic valve incompetence include Stanford type A aortic dissection and acute endocarditis.

How does an incompetent aortic valve affect loading conditions within the heart?
Severe acute aortic regurgitation causes a volume overload on the left ventricle that is poorly tolerated and requires urgent surgical intervention. Chronic aortic regurgitation, however, produces both volume and pressure overload upon the heart. End-diastolic volume is increased, raising systolic pressure as well. Over time, the heart dilates to maintain normal systolic function and to compensate for the increased regurgitant volume. Left ventricular hypertrophy occurs to normalize left ventricular wall stress. These compensatory mechanisms work well, providing a normal cardiac output and keeping the patient asymptomatic for years. However, continued aortic valve incompetence tests the limits of these compensatory changes; eventually, left ventricular end-diastolic pressure increases, left ventricular systolic wall stress increases, and systolic and diastolic impairment ensues. At this point, symptoms occur. If treated (e.g., restoring valvular competence), these changes do not progress and, if corrected early enough, may regress. Untreated aortic regurgitation results in continued and worsening symptoms, irreversible myocardial damage, and death.

What is the natural history of mild to moderate aortic regurgitation?
Patients with mild to moderate aortic regurgitation have a 90% 10-year survival rate. Once symptoms develop, however, mean survival is only 2 years.

Is medical therapy effective treatment for aortic regurgitation?
Although medical therapy can provide temporary relief of congestive symptoms, medications do not address the underlying problem of the leaky valve. Aortic valve replacement is required to stop the volume overload and break the vicious cycle of ventricular dilation, hypertrophy, and failure.

When is aortic valve replacement indicated for aortic regurgitation?
Timing of valve replacement is critical. It depends on the balance of two competing risks: the risks of valve replacement itself with the consequences of living with a prosthetic valve versus the risk of further left ventricular damage due to continued valvular incompetence. It is generally agreed that truly asymptomatic patients with normal ventricular function should be observed. Additionally, symptomatic patients with moderate to severe aortic regurgitation should un-

dergo surgery to avoid irreversible left ventricular damage and to alter the natural history of rapidly progressive congestive heart failure. Treatment of asymptomatic patients who are beginning to show evidence of left ventricular impairment is controversial. Most surgeons and cardiologists agree that objective evidence of progressive left ventricular dysfunction is an indication for aortic valve replacement and signifies the end of the effective compensatory period.

What objective tests are useful in assessing the need for aortic valve replacement with aortic regurgitation?
Echocardiography is the most useful tool. Two critical echocardiographic criteria are the left ventricular end-systolic dimension and the ejection fraction. A left ventricular end-systolic dimension larger than 55 mm and an ejection fraction below 55% signify the beginning of left ventricular failure and the near-onset of symptoms. Surgery should be considered at this point. Radionuclide scanning and cardiac catheterization also provide useful information.

How is the ascending aorta managed in patients with annuloaortic ectasia?
If the aorta is smaller than 5 cm, it does not need repair, and valve replacement only may be performed. In patients *without* Marfan's syndrome, an ascending aorta larger than 5 cm is an indication for repair at the time of valve replacement to prevent progressive dilation and rupture. Repair can be performed via:

• A supracoronary aortic graft
• Use of a valved conduit and reimplantation of the coronary arteries as buttons onto the sidewall of the aortic conduit, increasing the complexity and risk of the operation

Mr. Smith undergoes an echocardiogram and chest computed tomography to assess his heart and ascending aorta. His ventricular function is normal, with a 65% ejection fraction and a left ventricular end-systolic diameter of 4.1 cm. His aortic valve leaflets appear normal, but the annulus is enlarged and the degree of regurgitation is estimated as moderate. The ascending aorta has a widest diameter of 3.8 cm. Mr. Smith is advised to return to his cardiologist every 6 months for examination.

MITRAL STENOSIS

Lydia Neal is a 55-year-old woman who complains to her family physician of increasing shortness of breath, which she has noticed for several months. She works at home, and she has become increasingly fatigued and out of breath while doing her housework as well as when

she is on her feet for long periods while shopping. This is a relatively new problem, because she does not recall feeling breathless the previous summer. She has never been hospitalized, and her only medication is an oral hypoglycemic agent for non–insulin-dependent diabetes. She has no chest pain, hemoptysis, fevers, stroke, weight fluctuations, or pulmonary disease. She does not smoke.

On physical examination, Mrs. Neal appears healthy, is in no distress, and has normal vital signs. Her heart rate is regular. Her head and neck examination reveals no carotid bruits, and there is a prominent jugular venous pulsation. Her lungs are clear. On cardiac auscultation, the first heart sound is loud, and the second is split normally. A soft diastolic murmur is heard. The examiner carefully listens for an opening snap but is unsure whether one is present or not. Her pulse is normal, as is the rest of her physical examination.

What are the symptoms of mitral stenosis?
Dyspnea, the classic symptom of mitral stenosis, is caused by pulmonary venous engorgement and reduced pulmonary compliance. Hemoptysis and chest pain that can mimic angina pectoris may also be troublesome. Hemoptysis is usually a symptom of longer-standing and more severe mitral stenosis that has resulted in a variable degree of pulmonary hypertension. Thromboembolic events, especially stroke, may be the presenting symptom. Before the advent of anticoagulant therapy and surgical treatment, thromboembolic events were a major cause of death in patients with mitral stenosis, nearly always occurring in patients who had developed atrial fibrillation. With current therapy, this complication is much less common.

What are the classic signs of mitral stenosis?
A prominent *a* wave in the jugular venous pulse reflects the increased transmitted force of atrial contraction in patients with mitral stenosis who are in normal sinus rhythm. Patients in atrial fibrillation do not have a detectable *a* wave. The first heart sound is usually prominent and the second heart sound is normally split, at least until the development of severe pulmonary hypertension, when only a single S_2 is audible. An opening snap due to the sudden tensing of the subvalvular chordae may be heard if the leaflets are pliable. The classic murmur of mitral stenosis is low and rumbling and is a reflection of the pressure gradient across the mitral valve orifice. As the mitral valve becomes more stenotic, the murmur lengthens and consumes more of diastole. The murmur is relatively low pitched because the pressure gradients across the mitral valve are relatively low (e.g., compared with the high-pitched and high-pressure gradients of aortic stenosis). Maneuvers that reduce flow across the valve (e.g., Valsalva) reduce the intensity of the murmur.

What is the most common cause of mitral stenosis?
Rheumatic fever is the only known cause of mitral stenosis, although only 50% of patients have a history of rheumatic fever. Patients with a history of rheumatic fever develop symptoms after a latency period that may last 20 to 25 years. Once symptoms develop, the disease progresses quickly; patients may develop severe disability in a few years. It should be noted that left atrial myxoma may cause many of the signs and symptoms of mitral stenosis because of obstruction of the mitral valve orifice.

According to the New York Heart Association (NYHA) classification (see Table 24.1), what functional class is Mrs. Neal in?
Although unavoidably subjective and not strict, the NYHA classification is a convenient, universal, and quick way to categorize symptoms. Mrs. Neal is fatigued with exercise and therefore falls into NYHA class II.

As an outpatient, Mrs. Neal has a normal chest radiograph and an electrocardiogram (ECG) that demonstrates normal sinus rhythm without ischemia. A transthoracic echocardiogram shows moderate left atrial enlargement and normal left ventricular size and function. No thrombus is visible within the left atrium. Pulmonary artery pressure is estimated to be 35/20 mm Hg. The mitral valve leaflets are noted to be thickened, with limited excursion. Calcification is minimal. The mitral valve area (MVA) is calculated to be 1.4 cm^2, with a transvalvular gradient of 8 mm Hg.

What is the normal MVA?
The normal MVA is 4 to 6 cm^2 with no pressure gradient across the valve during diastole. Stenosis of the valve must be significant for any hemodynamic consequence; the MVA must decrease to less than 2 cm^2 (mild mitral stenosis) before left atrial pressure begins to increase. As the MVA decreases, the pressure gradient across the valve increases, so that with critical mitral stenosis (MVA <1 cm^2), the gradient approaches 20 mm Hg.

What are the hemodynamics of significant mitral stenosis?
As the MVA decreases into the severe and critical range, left atrial pressure rises, creating a pressure gradient across the valve. The elevated left atrial pressure is transmitted retrograde into the pulmonary veins and capillaries, increasing the hydrostatic pressure within the pulmonary circulation. Pulmonary edema and hemoptysis may result. Pulmonary vascular resistance increases and pulmonary hypertension develops, with severe mitral stenosis due to the increased passive transmission of the increased left atrial pressure and arteriolar vasoconstriction triggered by increased left atrial pressure. Pathologic changes within the pulmonary arteriolar tree may be seen with long-standing severe mitral stenosis.

Right-sided abnormalities, such as right ventricular dysfunction and tricuspid valvular disease, may result.

Why is the development of atrial fibrillation in patients with mitral stenosis a significant event?
In patients with mitral stenosis in normal sinus rhythm, left atrial contraction augments the transvalvular pressure gradient by approximately 30%, helping to maintain cardiac output in the normal range. The development of atrial fibrillation may be manifested by symptoms of congestive heart failure, because this atrial boost to left ventricular filling is lost.

Why does exercise or exertion make patients worse (e.g., shorter of breath)?
Exercise demands an increase in flow across the valve (cardiac output) to keep up with the metabolic demands of the body. Laws of fluid dynamics dictate that at any orifice size, the gradient across the orifice is a function of the square of the transvalvular flow rate (6). Doubling the flow rate (increasing the cardiac output) quadruples the pressure gradient across the valve; this dramatic increase in left atrial pressure is transmitted to the lungs, resulting in dyspnea on exertion.

Mrs. Neal is in NYHA functional class II and has echocardiographic evidence of mild to moderate mitral stenosis. How should she be treated?
Although Mrs. Neal has recently developed symptoms and her mitral valve is stenotic, the natural history of patients with mild to moderate mitral stenosis is quite good. Patients may survive for years before the inevitable deterioration in symptoms begins; that is, the 10-year survival rate for patients with mitral stenosis and NYHA class I or II symptoms is approximately 85%. Patients with more severe symptoms (NYHA classes III and IV) have 5-year survival rates that are much worse (40% and 15%, respectively). Therefore, Mrs. Neal should be treated medically and closely followed.

Mrs. Neal is started on furosemide and digoxin and, on follow-up several weeks later, she says she feels better. She does well for the next 2 years, but at that time returns to her physician complaining that she can't do as much as she used to. She gets short of breath in the grocery store and has to take a break while doing her laundry. A repeat echocardiogram at this time demonstrates that her MVA is 0.9 cm^2, with a transvalvular gradient at rest of 12 mm Hg.

What are the indications for mitral valve replacement or repair?
In general, surgery is recommended for patients who are significantly symptomatic (NYHA class III or IV) with severe mitral stenosis (MVA less than 1 cm^2). Patients who have had a thromboembolic event should also be considered for

surgery, because the risk of recurrent thromboembolism from the left atrium is high.

Are there any alternatives to surgical repair or replacement of the mitral valve?
Percutaneous balloon mitral valvotomy is a catheter-based technique for performing mitral commissurotomy. In selected patients, balloon valvotomy can double the effective mitral orifice and halve the gradient. The major benefit of balloon valvotomy is the avoidance of median sternotomy and cardiopulmonary bypass; this can be especially useful in patients for whom surgery poses a high risk. Echocardiographic scores help identify patients in whom balloon valvotomy is most effective: younger patients with minimal valvular calcification, good leaflet morphology (not much leaflet chordal thickening), and minimal mitral regurgitation may benefit from balloon valvotomy. Significant mitral regurgitation, unacceptable echocardiographic score, and known left atrial thrombus discourage balloon valvotomy.

What are the surgical options for the treatment of mitral stenosis?

Closed mitral commissurotomy was initially performed in 1923 and successfully applied by Harken and Bailey in 1948. Closed mitral commissurotomy is accomplished without cardiopulmonary bypass. It consists of inserting a finger through a hole in the left atrial appendage to separate the fused commissures. In some cases, a mechanical dilator is introduced via the apex of the left ventricle to assist with commissurotomy. Closed mitral commissurotomy is particularly effective for patients with minimal valvular calcification, absent mitral regurgitation, and no left atrial thrombus. The requirement for reoperation averages 50% at 10 years. The development of safe and effective techniques for cardiopulmonary bypass lets open mitral commissurotomy largely replace closed techniques. Closed mitral commissurotomy is still commonly used in developing nations, where access to cardiopulmonary bypass is limited.

Open mitral commissurotomy is performed via a median sternotomy: the left atrium is opened and examined for the thrombus. The left atrial appendage is oversewn to prevent formation of further thrombi. The fused commissures are divided with a scalpel to within 2 mm of the annulus, and the underlying subvalvular apparatus (the chordae tendinea and the papillary muscles) are inspected. Areas of fusion of the chordae or papillary muscles are incised. The operative risk of open mitral commissurotomy is less than 1%, and the incidence of reoperation for recurrent mitral stenosis is 10 to 20% at 10 years.

Mitral valve replacement is required when the degree of disease of the mitral valve or subvalvular apparatus makes mitral valve repair impossible. The choice between a bioprosthetic and a mechanical replacement valve is dictated by similar considerations for aortic valve replacement (discussed earlier). If possible, the posterior leaflet and chordae of the mitral valve are preserved during mitral valve replacement; the posterior leaflet is folded between the sewing ring of the valve and the annulus. Preservation of this structure improves postoperative ventricular function and long-term survival.

Describe the surgical anatomy of the mitral valve. What key structures surrounding the mitral valve are at risk for injury during operation, and where are they?
The mitral valve is the doorway to the left ventricle. It consists of two leaflets, the anterior and posterior, which are anchored by the circumferential mitral annulus. The anterior leaflet is attached to the anterior third of the annulus, whereas the posterior leaflet is anchored to the remaining two-thirds of the annulus. Prolapse of the mitral valve into the left atrium during systole is prevented by the subvalvular apparatus, which consists of the chordae tendineae, the papillary muscles, and the left ventricle. The chordae are anchored to the papillary muscles, which in turn arise from the left ventricle. Key structures surrounding the mitral valve include the left circumflex coronary artery, the coronary sinus, the atrioventricular node, and the noncoronary leaflet of the aortic valve.

Mrs. Neal successfully undergoes open mitral commissurotomy. Findings at operation include fused commissures that are easily incised and several fused chordae that are similarly incised. She is discharged from the hospital on postoperative day 4. At follow-up examination, she is symptom free (NYHA class I) and has resumed normal activities. A follow-up echocardiogram demonstrates a mitral valve of 3 cm² and no evidence of mitral regurgitation. Ventricular function is normal.

Should Mrs. Neal take an anticoagulant?
No. After valve repair, only patients with atrial fibrillation or with a preoperative history of a thromboembolic event require anticoagulation.

MITRAL REGURGITATION

James Hovis is a 54-year-old National Park ranger with a 4-month history of progressive shortness of breath. He notes that he is becoming increasingly fatigued at work, especially walking up hills. He has no chest, back, or arm pain and says that 6 months ago he was completely asymptomatic. He does not smoke and takes no medications. He has a family history of heart disease. Pertinent findings on physical examination include a holosystolic murmur best heard at the apex of the heart and radiating to the axilla. It is high pitched, with little respiratory variation. His lungs are clear to auscultation. The re-

mainder of his examination is unremarkable. An ECG demonstrates atrial fibrillation and no evidence of ischemic injury. The chest radiograph demonstrates clear lungs and a slightly enlarged cardiac silhouette. No significant annular calcification is present.

What is the working diagnosis?
Mr. Hovis's symptoms and cardiac examination suggest mitral valve disease. It is likely that Mr. Hovis has had some degree of mitral regurgitation for many years and has only recently had symptoms. The character of the cardiac murmur helps differentiate it from aortic stenosis, which is harsher, radiates to the neck rather than the axilla, and is associated with a diminished upstroke of the central pulses.

Is this a chronic or acute process?
It is likely that Mr. Hovis's mitral regurgitation is chronic. The left atrial fibrillation suggests that the mitral regurgitation is long-standing and has led to atrial distention, enlargement, and fibrillation. Acute mitral regurgitation is usually associated with a normal left atrial chamber, increased pulmonary artery pressures, and sometimes flash pulmonary edema. Important causes of acute mitral regurgitation that may be elicited from the history and physical examination include bacterial endocarditis (with ruptured chordae tendineae) and ischemic heart disease resulting in papillary muscle dysfunction or rupture.

What should be the next diagnostic test?
Echocardiography is a powerful tool for examining valvular heart disease and is useful in determining the causation and hemodynamic consequences of mitral regurgitation. It is also useful in evaluating the other heart valves and left ventricular function.

What important anatomic features of the mitral valve should be assessed?
The mitral annulus, leaflets, and subvalvular apparatus (chordae tendineae and papillary muscles) may all contribute to mitral regurgitation. The normal mitral annulus is approximately 4 cm^2, but any disease process causing left ventricular dilation may cause annular dilation. Annular dilation reduces the coapting surface area of the anterior and posterior leaflets and may result in a central jet of regurgitation. It is also critical to assess the degree of annular calcification, particularly in the elderly. Severe mitral annular calcification may preclude valve repair or replacement. Causes of chordal rupture include endocarditis, rheumatic disease, and ischemic heart disease; it may also be idiopathic. Posterior chordae rupture more frequently and may result in a flail leaflet segment, causing an eccentric regurgitant jet; this anatomic detail is detectable with echocardiography. A ruptured papillary muscle head produces a similar regurgitant picture. Leaflet abnormalities causing valve retraction or thickening may

occur with rheumatic heart disease (although stenosis is more common), systemic lupus erythematosus, and healed endocarditis.

**Mr. Hovis has an echocardiogram, which shows a dilated mitral an-
nulus, a flail segment of the posterior leaflet with an eccentric regurgitant jet tracking posteriorly along the left atrial wall. The left atrium
is dilated, and there is no significant calcification of the valve or subvalvular apparatus. The degree of regurgitation is severe. His left ventricular function is normal.**

Why is Mr. Hovis short of breath and easily fatigable?
Left atrial compliance and effective forward cardiac output are two principal
factors that determine symptoms in patients with mitral regurgitation. When

Management Algorithm for Mitral Stenosis

History & physical exam

Severe symptoms:
• CHF
• Emboli
• Severe arrythmias

Mild to moderate
symptoms

• ECG
• Echo

• ECG
• Echo
• Cath if > 40 years old

MVA
$1.0\text{-}2.0\ cm^2$

MVA
$< 1.0\ cm^2$

Serial exam and
echo in 6 months

Assess
valvuloplasty score

Suitable
valvuloplasty score

Unsuitable
valvuloplasty score

Suitable

Unsuitable

Percutaneous
balloon valvuloplasty

Mitral valve repair
or replacement

Percutaneous
balloon valvuloplasty

Mitral valve repair
or replacement

Algorithm 25.1A.

mitral regurgitation has sudden onset, the normally small atrium is loaded with a large regurgitant volume, and the left atrial pressure may increase dramatically. Pulmonary congestion and hypertension may result, with sudden shortness of breath or flash pulmonary edema. With chronic mitral regurgitation, the left atrium enlarges with time, sometimes to quite massive dimensions, allowing large volumes of regurgitant flow to enter the left atrium with little change in pressure (increased compliance). This is one reason patients may tolerate mitral regurgitation for years without symptoms.

Mitral regurgitation places an increased volume load on the heart. In addition to the forward cardiac output across the aortic valve, a significant portion of the stroke volume is regurgitant and enters the left atrium. To maintain cardiac output, end-diastolic volume increases, and the heart dilates progressively, which over time exacerbates the regurgitation (hence the saying "mitral regurgitation begets more mitral regurgitation"). However, because the left ventri-

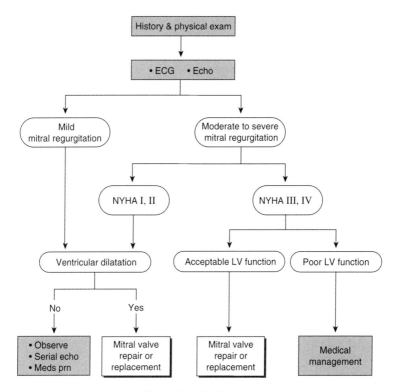

Management Algorithm for Mitral Regurgitation

Algorithm 25.1B.

cle is unloaded, left ventricular wall tension does not increase or increases very slowly, which is why patients tolerate significant degrees of mitral regurgitation for years without symptoms. Eventually, however, these compensatory mechanisms are exhausted; exercise intolerance and easy fatigability occur because the left ventricle cannot maintain an adequate cardiac output to meet the systemic demands of exercise. Hence, exertional dyspnea occurs.

Management Algorithm for Aortic Stenosis

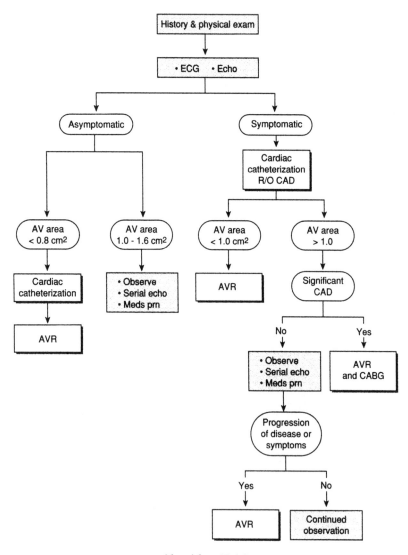

Algorithm 25.1C.

What medical management of patients with mitral regurgitation is available?
Diuretics are important because they reduce pulmonary artery pressure and reduce stroke volume, hence left ventricular dimension. This allows improved
leaflet coaptation and can significantly reduce the degree of mitral regurgitation.

Should Mr. Hovis have his valve surgically repaired or replaced?
Definitive treatment requires surgical replacement or repair of the flail segment.
Patients with class III or IV heart failure or patients whose ventricle is progres-
sively dilating on serial echocardiographic exams are candidates for surgery.

What is the difference between mitral valve repair and mitral valve replacement?
Replacement of the mitral valve with a prosthesis effectively cures mitral regurgitation. The choice of prosthesis is critical; mechanical valves last a lifetime
but require systemic anticoagulation. A bioprosthesis in a young patient like Mr.

Management Algorithm for Aortic Regurgitation

History & physical exam

→ Asymptomatic
→ Symptomatic

Asymptomatic → Echo

- LV end systolic diameter > 55 mm
- EF < 55%
→ Consider surgery
  - Ascending aorta > 5 cm → AVR & replacement of ascending aorta
  - Ascending aorta < 5 cm → AVR only

- LV ESS < 55 mm
- LV ES normal
→ • Observe • Serial echo

Symptomatic:
Acceptable surgical candidate → Aortic valve replacement
  - Ascending aorta > 5 cm → AVR & replacement of ascending aorta
  - Ascending aorta < 5 cm → AVR only

Unacceptable surgical candidate *or* end-stage cardiomyopathy → Medical therapy
Consider transplant if < 65 years old

Algorithm 25.1D.

Hovis is not likely to last for the remainder of his life, exposing him to the risk of re-replacement in 10 to 15 years. Carpentier initiated the concept of aggressive mitral valve repair as a superior alternative to replacement. Successful valve repair obviates the dilemma of valve choice by leaving the patient with a normal mitral valve with lifelong usefulness and no need for anticoagulation.

How should Mr. Hovis's valve be repaired?
Using cardiopulmonary bypass and cardioplegia, the left atrium is entered and the valve carefully inspected. If the surgeon determines intraoperatively that the valve is reparable, repair proceeds. The flail segment of the posterior leaflet is excised and the edges reapproximated. An annuloplasty ring is sewn to the annulus (taking care not to reduce the annular size excessively), and the valve is tested. Transesophageal echocardiography is critical to assess valve function in the operating room after weaning from cardiopulmonary bypass. Trace to mild mitral insufficiency is an acceptable result. Other types of valve repair are frequently used.

Mr. Hovis undergoes successful mitral valve repair and recovers uneventfully. After a 6-week recuperative period, he returns to work.

REFERENCES

1. Ross J Jr, Braunwald E. Aortic stenosis. Circulation 1968;38(Suppl 5):V61–67.
2. Gorlin R, Gorlin G. Hydraulic formula for calculation of area of stenotic mitral valve, other cardiac values and central circulatory shunts. Am Heart J 1951;41:1.
3. Desnoyers MR, Isner JM, Pandian NG, et al. Clinical and noninvasive hemodynamic results after balloon angioplasty for aortic stenosis. Am J Cardiol 1988;62:1078–1084.
4. Ross D, Jackson M, Davies J. Pulmonary autograft aortic valve replacement: long-term results. J Cardiac Surg 1991;6:529–533.
5. Stein PD, Alpert JS, Copeland J, et al. Antithrombotic therapy in patients with mechanical and biological prosthetic heart valves. Chest 1995:108:371s–379s.
6. Olsean KH. The natural history of 271 patients with mitral stenosis under medical treatment. Br Heart J 1962;24:349–357.

CHAPTER
26

Lung Cancer

Pasquale Ferraro and André Duranceau

**Derek Ferguson is a 59-year-old auto mechanic who is admitted
to the hospital with a fever, persistent cough, and blood-streaked sputum. He was treated by his family doctor with oral antibiotics for
an episode of acute bronchitis 2 weeks ago. He has a 40 pack-year
smoking history and his medical history is significant for non–
insulin-dependent diabetes mellitus and peptic ulcer disease. Over
the years, he has had several episodes of what he calls bronchitis. He
is mildly short of breath on exertion but denies any chest pain or
wheezing. His weight is stable and he maintains an active 40-hour
work week.**

What are the possible diagnoses on the basis of this history?
The differential diagnosis at this point includes community-acquired pneumonia, acute bronchitis, exacerbated chronic bronchitis, and lung cancer.

Is fever a common finding with lung cancer?
Fever, which affects only 10% of patients with lung cancer, is usually associated with postobstructive atelectasis or pneumonia. An abscess can develop in
a tumor cavity, but this is rare.

What are the clinical manifestations of lung cancer?
More than 90% of patients with lung cancer have symptoms (pulmonary,
metastatic, systemic, or paraneoplastic) at the time of diagnosis. Bronchopul-
monary symptoms, including coughing, dyspnea, chest pain, and hemoptysis,
are found in up to 80% of patients. Some 30% of patients have metastatic disease at presentation, and the usual symptoms are those associated with central
nervous system (CNS), bone, or liver metastases. Although common, adrenal
gland metastases are rarely symptomatic. Systemic symptoms such as malaise,
weight loss, and anorexia are found in 34% of patients. Paraneoplastic syndromes (found in 2% of patients) secondary to lung cancer are among the
most varied in clinical presentation. The different types of syndromes include

endocrine (hypercalcemia, Cushing's syndrome, syndrome of inappropriate antidiuretic hormone secretion, gynecomastia), neurologic (encephalopathy, peripheral neuropathy, polymyositis, Eaton-Lambert syndrome), skeletal (clubbing, pulmonary hypertrophic osteoarthropathy), cutaneous (acanthosis nigricans), and hematologic disorders. Only 5% of patients with lung cancer are asymptomatic at the time of diagnosis (1, 2).

On physical examination, Mr. Ferguson appears healthy. He is mildly overweight and shows no signs of respiratory distress. His heart rate, blood pressure, and respiratory rate are normal, and his temperature is 38°C. There is no clubbing, and the head and neck examination shows no suspicious lymph nodes. Chest auscultation reveals some crackles over the left lung; the right lung is clear; heart sounds are normal; and the liver is not tender.

Which tests should be ordered initially?
Blood tests should include a complete blood count and electrolyte, blood urea nitrogen, and creatinine levels. A chest radiograph and electrocardiogram (ECG) should be ordered as well.

The results of the initial blood tests and electrocardiography are normal. The chest radiograph shows a 4-cm mass in the left upper lung and a clear right lung field.

What is the differential diagnosis on the basis of these findings?
Included in the differential diagnosis are the following:

1. Inflammatory or infectious conditions such as abscess, granuloma, tuberculosis, fungal infection, or pneumonia
2. Neoplastic disorders, including benign lung tumors and malignant tumors (primary lung cancers and secondary or metastatic lesions)
3. Congenital lesions
4. Traumatic lesions

What are other pertinent findings on a simple chest radiograph in a patient suspected of having lung cancer?
Important radiologic findings include a mass with irregular borders, no calcifications, a pleural effusion, an elevated diaphragm, a widened mediastinum, and contralateral nodules. Areas of pneumonitis often surround central tumors with an endobronchial component. When possible, comparison with older radiographs is essential to establish the evolving nature of a nodule or mass.

Which radiologic features characterize a benign lesion in a patient with a solitary pulmonary nodule?
Features of a benign nodule include a smooth border, homogenous appearance, fat within lesion, calcifications in a benign pattern (central, laminated, or diffuse), and stable size over 2 years (3).

What is the likelihood that a radiologically detected mass in a patient such as Mr. Ferguson is cancer?
In a 59-year-old man with a history of heavy smoking and a newly discovered 4-cm mass, the likelihood is greater than 90% that the lesion is a bronchogenic carcinoma. Generally, in the adult population any new pulmonary nodule carries a 50% risk of being a malignancy if the patient has a significant smoking history (1).

What is the incidence of lung cancer in the United States?
The estimated total number of new cases in 1996 was 177,000, and the estimated number of lung cancer deaths was 158,700. The probability of developing lung cancer is 1 in 12 for men and 1 in 19 for women (4).

What factors have been linked to the development of lung cancer?
Tobacco smoking is undoubtedly the most important causative factor in lung cancer. The lung cancer mortality is 20- to 70-fold higher in smokers than in nonsmokers. Although generally believed to be an important factor, air pollution independent of tobacco use increases the risk of lung cancer only slightly. Exposure to uranium, asbestos, arsenic, nickel, chromium, or beryllium carries proven occupational risk. Certain organic compounds (aromatic hydrocarbons, chlormethyl ether, and isopropyl oils) have also been implicated. The association of dietary factors with lung cancer is less convincing. The consumption of vegetables or fruits containing β-carotene is considered to be protective, whereas dietary animal fat is believed to promote the development of lung cancer (5).

What additional workup does a patient with probable lung cancer require?
Additional workup is needed to (a) confirm the diagnosis, (b) establish the extent and resectability of the lesion, and (c) assess operability.

How is the diagnosis of lung cancer confirmed?
The diagnosis may be confirmed with sputum cytology, bronchoscopy, or transthoracic needle biopsy. Histologic confirmation may be obtained with a more invasive procedure, such as cervical mediastinoscopy, scalene node biopsy, thoracoscopy, or an exploratory thoracotomy.

What is the yield from and the importance of these different diagnostic tests?
Sputum cytology is the most useful test for central hilar lesions, endobronchial tumors, and squamous cell carcinoma, with an overall diagnostic yield of 82%

when three early morning specimens are analyzed; with peripheral tumors, the yield is 40 to 50%. The overall rate of false-positive results with sputum cytology is 1 to 3% (6). Bronchoscopy is diagnostic in 25 to 50% of patients with small cell or squamous cell carcinoma. Additional analysis of brushings and washings increases the yield to 90% (2). Bronchoscopy also provides information on tumor location and extent that helps in staging the tumor, and it helps identify a synchronous cancer in another lobe or in the contralateral lung in 1 to 2% of patients. A transthoracic needle biopsy should not be performed as part of the routine workup for lung cancer because the results seldom affect management, it has no value in the staging process, and the procedure is associated with a 30% risk of pneumothorax. Furthermore, the rate of false-negative findings can be as high as 15 to 25% (7). Transthoracic needle biopsy should be limited to patients with a clinically unresectable lesion, to high-risk patients who are inoperable for medical reasons, and to patients who refuse surgery.

How are patients assessed for operability?
Determination of operability necessitates a cardiac workup in patients with symptoms of heart disease, a significant medical history, or risk factors for coronary artery disease. Pulmonary function tests, exercise tolerance, and overall performance status must be assessed in all patients. Renal function and presence of other major systemic diseases also should be evaluated in selected patients.

How is lung cancer classified and staged?
The tumor, node, metastasis (TNM) staging classification is based on a number of specific criteria with respect to the tumor (T) (size, site, local invasion, associated atelectasis), the lymph nodes (N) (hilar, mediastinal, or extrathoracic nodes; ipsilateral or contralateral nodes), and the presence of distant metastases (M). The TNM classification is shown in Table 26.1. The staging of lung tumors according to the TNM classification is shown in Table 26.2.

Why is the TNM classification important?
The TNM system serves several purposes, such as selecting the most appropriate therapy, establishing the prognosis, and permitting the comparison of data and results.

How are the extent of the lesion and its resectability evaluated?
Bronchoscopy and computed tomography (CT) of the chest are the best techniques for evaluating the local and regional extent of lung cancer. A bronchoscopic finding that suggests unresectability is invasion of the trachea or main carina. On CT of the chest, indications of unresectability include bulky N_2 disease (metastatic ipsilateral mediastinal adenopathy), N_3 disease (contralateral mediastinal or extrathoracic metastatic adenopathy), or any T_4 lesion (invasion of the heart, great vessels, esophagus, trachea, or vertebral body).

Table 26.1. TUMOR, NODE, METASTASIS CLASSIFICATION FOR LUNG CANCER

Primary Tumor (T)

T_0	No evidence of primary tumor
TIS	Carcinoma in situ
T_1	Tumor 3 cm or smaller, not involving the visceral pleura and not invading proximal to the lobar bronchus
T_2	Tumor larger than 3 cm; tumor with invasion of visceral pleura or extending into mainstem bronchus but more than 2 cm from carina; or tumor with lobar atelectasis
T_3	Tumor of any size with invasion of parietal pleura, chest wall, pericardium, mediastinal pleura, or diaphragm; tumor in mainstem bronchus within 2 cm of carina but not involving carina; tumor with atelectasis of entire lung; or superior sulcus (Pancoast) tumor
T_4	Tumor of any size with invasion of mediastinum, heart, great vessels, esophagus, vertebral body, trachea, or carina; or tumor with malignant pleural effusion

Nodal Involvement (N)

N_0	No metastases to regional lymph nodes
N_1	Metastases to peribronchial or ipsilateral hilar lymph nodes
N_2	Metastases to ipsilateral mediastinal lymph nodes
N_3	Metastases to contralateral hilar or mediastinal lymph nodes or to extrathoracic lymph nodes (scalene or supraclavicular)

Distant Metastases (M)

M_0	No known distant metastases
M_1	Distant metastases present

Table 26.2. STAGING OF LUNG CANCER WITH TUMOR, NODE, METASTASIS CLASSIFICATION

Stage	Classification
I	T_1, N_0, M_0; T_2, N_0, M_0
II	T_1, N_1, M_0; T_2, N_1, M_0
IIIA	T_3, N_0, M_0; T_3, N_1, M_0; T_1, N_2, M_0; T_2, N_2, M_0; T_3, N_2, M_0
IIIB	T_4, N_0, M_0; T_4, N_1, M_0; T_4, N_2, M_0; T_1, N_3, M_0; T_2, N_3, M_0; T_3, N_3, M_0
IV	Any T; any N; M_1

Which tests should be included in the workup for metastatic disease?
Blood tests should consist of liver function tests and determination of the serum calcium level. CT of the chest should also include imaging of the liver and adrenal glands, both frequent sites of lung metastases. Unsuspected metastases

have been found in the liver or adrenal glands in 3 to 7% of patients (8, 9). A bone scan and head CT should be obtained in selected cases and in all symptomatic patients.

What are the most frequent sites of metastases from a lung cancer?
In descending order of occurrence, the most frequent sites are the mediastinal lymph nodes, the contralateral lung, the adrenal glands, the liver, the brain or CNS, and the bones.

Mr. Ferguson's blood tests, including liver enzymes, are normal. CT shows a 4-cm mass in the anterior segment of the left upper lobe. The hilar or mediastinal nodes are not enlarged, there is no pleural effusion, and the left lower lobe and the right lung appear normal. Both the liver and the adrenal glands are free of metastases. Bronchoscopy shows a large, friable, irregular mass in the left upper lobe bronchus 2 cm from its origin on the left main stem bronchus. Biopsy of the lesion reveals a squamous cell carcinoma.

What is the clinical stage of Mr. Ferguson's disease?
According to the TNM classification, the tumor is T_2, N_0, M_0. It is stage I.

How are malignant tumors of the lung classified histologically?
The histologic classification of lung tumors is presented in Table 26.3.

Table 26.3.   HISTOLOGIC CLASSIFICATION OF LUNG TUMORS

Primary malignant tumors
  Bronchogenic carcinoma
    Squamous cell carcinoma (spindle cell, exophytic endobronchial)
    Adenocarcinoma (acinar, papillary, bronchoalveolar)
    Large cell carcinoma (giant cell, clear cell, neuroendocrine)
    Small cell carcinoma (oat cell, intermediate, mixed)
    Adenosquamous carcinoma
    Bronchial gland carcinoma (carcinoid tumors, adenoid cystic, mucoepidermoid)
  Nonbronchogenic carcinoma
    Sarcoma
    Lymphoma
    Melanoma
    Pulmonary blastoma
Secondary malignant tumors
  Metastatic lesions from primary tumors outside the lung

Which are the most common metastatic tumors to the lung?
The most common tumors responsible for lung metastases are breast, prostate, kidney, and colon tumors; soft tissue sarcoma; and thyroid carcinoma.

What is the incidence of the different types of bronchogenic carcinomas?
The frequencies of the different types of bronchogenic carcinomas are as follows: adenocarcinoma (the most common type), 40 to 45%; squamous cell carcinoma, 30 to 35%; large cell carcinoma, 5 to 15%; and small cell carcinoma, 20 to 25% (10).

What are some important characteristics of each of the four types of bronchogenic carcinoma?

Squamous cell carcinoma was once the most frequent type of bronchogenic carcinoma but now accounts for approximately a third of cases. Typically located in major bronchi (lobar or first segmental bronchus), it is often perihilar, slow growing, and large when diagnosed. Central necrosis with cavitation is possible, and distant metastases occur late in the evolution.

Adenocarcinoma is the most common type of lung cancer. Most lesions arise from peripheral bronchial branches rather than from major bronchi and present initially as solitary nodules less than 3 cm in diameter. Endobronchial central adenocarcinomas are much less common. Spread to hilar and mediastinal nodes occurs readily, and 20% of patients with this tumor have distant metastases at the time of diagnosis. A subtype known as bronchoalveolar carcinoma presents as multicentered nodules or as a diffuse infiltrate with air bronchograms. Although local recurrences after surgery are common with bronchoalveolar carcinomas, these tumors have a more favorable prognosis.

Large cell carcinoma is a peripheral lesion in 60% of patients, and two thirds of these tumors are larger than 4 cm. Some 10% of patients have metastatic mediastinal adenopathy at the time of diagnosis. These poorly differentiated carcinomas are believed by some experts to be anaplastic adenocarcinomas.

Small cell carcinoma accounts for 20 to 25% of bronchogenic cancers. These tumors arise in major bronchi and are generally central. Half of patients have metastatic hilar and mediastinal adenopathy. Subtypes include oat cell, intermediate cell, and combined oat cell carcinomas. Features of squamous cell carcinoma or glandular differentiation are common (1, 2, 10).

After the clinical stage and histology of the tumor have been determined, how is preoperative pulmonary functional status assessed?
All patients undergoing a thoracotomy must have pulmonary function tests (PFTs) (spirometry and diffusing capacity for carbon monoxide [DL_{CO}]) to establish the extent of resection (wedge, lobectomy, or pneumonectomy) that will be tolerated. Selected patients may require more advanced testing, including

arterial blood gas analysis, quantitative ventilation and perfusion (V/Q) scanning, and exercise testing to determine maximal oxygen consumption (VO_{2max}). The V/Q scan allows calculation of the amount of functional residual lung tissue after a resection by establishing the percentage blood flow to each segment before the surgery. Echocardiogram and right heart catheterization with pulmonary artery measurements may be indicated in the rare patient with clinical signs of pulmonary hypertension or right ventricular failure.

What PFT values constitute an acceptable operative risk for pneumonectomy?
Risk associated with pneumonectomy is considered acceptable if preoperative forced expiratory volume in 1 second (FEV_1) is greater than 60% (2 L), the maximal voluntary ventilation is greater than 50%, and DL_{CO} is more than 60%; or if predicted postoperative values are FEV_1 higher than 40% and DL_{CO} higher than 40%. Most patients with a preoperative FEV_1 of more than 40% tolerate lobectomy well (11, 12).

How does the VO_{2max} help in assessing operability?
Patients whose predicted postoperative FEV_1 is less than 30 to 40% should undergo formal exercise testing and a desaturation study. The VO_{2max} alone has been used as an independent predictor of postoperative morbidity. A VO_{2max} greater than 15 to 20 mL/kg per minute is generally associated with low mortality and acceptable operative risk, whereas a VO_{2max} less than 10 mL/kg per minute contraindicates any resection other than a biopsy or wedge (12, 13).

Mr. Ferguson's PFTs show an FEV_1 of 1.5 L (50%), MVV of 45%, and DL_{CO} of 40%. The PFT results prompt ABG analysis and quantitative V/Q scanning. The ABG determinations on room air are normal, and the V/Q scan shows 57% of the perfusion to the right lung and 43 to the left lung with an equal distribution to the left upper and left lower lobe. VO_{2max} measurement reveals oxygen consumption of 12 mL/kg per minute.

What is the appropriate resection for a patient with these pulmonary test results?
The patient can tolerate a wedge resection, segmentectomy, or lobectomy. A pneumonectomy would probably be associated with poor postoperative pulmonary function and should not be carried out.

Should a cervical mediastinoscopy be performed in a case such as Mr. Ferguson's?
Before the advent of CT, mediastinoscopy was performed as a staging procedure in all patients with lung cancer. However, the routine use of mediastinoscopy is associated with a positive yield of 30 to 35% for central lesions and only 5% for peripheral tumors. Metastases are rarely detected with nodes that are smaller than 1 cm on the chest CT (in only 2 to 7% of patients). How-

ever, with nodes larger than 1 cm, mediastinoscopy reveals metastases in 60 to 80% of patients (14–16). Mr. Ferguson's CT shows no nodes larger than 1 cm, so he should probably not undergo a mediastinoscopy before thoracotomy.

In what circumstances is a mediastinoscopy recommended?
Mediastinoscopy is recommended in patients with (*a*) nodes larger than 1 cm in the paratracheal region, (*b*) nodes larger than 1.5 cm in the subcarinal area, (*c*) large hilar masses, (*d*) chest wall involvement, (*e*) recurrent lung cancer prior to surgery, or (*f*) bilateral lesions. Mediastinoscopy may also be used to exclude small cell lung cancer.

Mr. Ferguson is taken to the operating room and a left posterolateral thoracotomy is performed. Exploration shows no signs of metastatic disease. A standard lobectomy with a mediastinal nodal dissection is carried out. The left lower lobe is free of nodules and masses.

Why is it important to do frozen section analysis during the procedure?
The resection margins must be verified by pathologic analysis to be free of tumor, and any suspicious nodules in the remaining lobe must be sampled for biopsy. Also, the status of the hilar and interlobar nodes should be established, and whether there is N_2 disease must be determined during the procedure because this may influence the type and extent of resection.

What should be done if a pleural effusion is discovered at the time of thoracotomy?
If pleural effusion is present, metastatic seeding of the parietal pleura must be ruled out. A malignant effusion is classified as a T_4 tumor (stage IIIB) and contraindicates resection. If the pleura appears normal, a sample should be sent for immediate cytologic examination. Lung cancer patients may have an inflammatory effusion (transudate), which does not preclude a pulmonary resection. Despite an extensive preoperative workup, 2 to 5% of patients are found at the time of thoracotomy to have unresectable lesions (1, 2).

The final pathologic examination shows that Mr. Ferguson's tumor is a moderately differentiated squamous cell carcinoma with metastases to two peribronchial lymph nodes (T_2, N_1, M_0, stage II). Resection margins on the bronchus are free of tumor.

Is a lobectomy optimal therapy for Mr. Ferguson's lung cancer?
For a stage II non–small cell lung cancer, a complete surgical resection with negative margins is sufficient treatment. Although the incidence of local or regional recurrences is reduced with postoperative radiation therapy, survival is not improved. Trials with neoadjuvant chemotherapy and radiation therapy are under way. Adjuvant therapy after a complete resection is not recommended (17–19).

What are the survival rates for stage I and stage II disease, and what are some prognostic factors?
Stage I (T_1, N_0 and T_2, N_0) tumors are associated with a 5-year survival rate of 60 to 80%. Lesions less than 3 cm in diameter have a significantly better prognosis than do larger T_2 lesions. Adjuvant therapy is not recommended for patients after a complete resection. Recurrences, mainly distant metastases, are found in 20% of patients. Stage II (T_1, N_1 and T_2, N_1) lung cancers are associated with a 40% 5-year survival rate. Prognostic factors include size of the tumor, histology (squamous cell carcinoma has a more favorable prognosis than does adenocarcinoma), and the number of N_1 nodes. The location of the tumor and invasion of the visceral pleura do not affect survival. The sites of recurrence appear to depend on tumor histology. Squamous cell carcinomas recur locally, whereas adenocarcinomas have a tendency to recur at distant sites (20–22).

What is recommended therapy for stage IIIA cancers, especially for N_2 disease?
For locally advanced stage IIIA lesions (T_3, N_0 and T_3, N_1), the mainstay of therapy is complete surgical resection with a mediastinal node dissection. Peripheral tumors with chest wall involvement should be resected en bloc. Prognostic factors with T_3 tumors include complete resectability, extent of chest wall invasion, and any regional lymph node metastases. The 5-year survival rate varies from 20 to 40% (23–25). The management of N_2 disease remains controversial. Symptomatic N_2 disease with rare exceptions is considered unresectable. Median survival in these patients varies from 6 to 12 months. Asymptomatic patients with bulky N_2 disease as determined by CT or bronchoscopy also have a poor prognosis, with a 10% 5-year survival rate (26). A number of trials to evaluate the role of neoadjuvant chemotherapy and radiation therapy are under way (27–31). Surgery alone is not recommended in this situation. Patients in whom N_2 disease is discovered at mediastinoscopy are an interesting subset of patients with stage IIIA disease. Generally, 80% of such patients have unresectable tumors. However, a number of prognostic factors (number of nodes, number of nodal stations, location of nodes, and extracapsular extension) have been identified, and surgery may therefore be indicated in selected patients. In patients with micrometastases, aortopulmonary window involvement, or metastasis limited to one node in whom the tumor is completely resected, 5-year survival rates of 15 to 20% have been reported. Overall, the prognosis remains poor, and neoadjuvant therapy in combination with surgery should be recommended for most patients (32, 33). Patients with unsuspected but completely resectable N_2 disease discovered at thoracotomy have a more favorable outcome. Prognostic factors include the number of nodes, number of nodal stations, location of nodes, and any extracapsular invasion. The tumor status also influences survival. A 5-year survival rate of 20 to 30% has been reported in selected patients after a complete resection (34–36). T_1, N_2 lesions are associated with survival as high as 45%, and a rate of 10% has been reported

with larger T_3, N_2 lesions. Postoperative radiation therapy for N_2 disease discovered at thoracotomy seems beneficial in patients at high risk for local recurrence and in patients with an incomplete resection (37).

How should stage IIIB tumors be managed?
With stage IIIB disease (T_4 or N_3 lesions), therapy is limited, prognosis is poor, and patients should be considered inoperable (20, 21). Neoadjuvant therapy is being studied and may be favorable (30). Within this subgroup, a T_4 lesion invading the superior vena cava with negative mediastinal nodes may be considered resectable in selected patients. Unfortunately, local recurrences ultimately develop in most patients even after a complete resection (22).

Mr. Ferguson's immediate postoperative course is uneventful. Chest tubes are removed on the fourth postoperative day. He is comfortable, walking, and mildly short of breath on exertion. A chest radiograph shows a well-reexpanded left lower lobe with a small residual pleural effusion. However, on the day before his discharge, he suddenly becomes markedly short of breath as he is getting out of bed. His vital signs are heart rate, 110 beats per minute; blood pressure, 160/85 mm Hg; respiratory rate, 24 breaths per minute; and O_2 saturation, 88% on room air. Both lung fields are relatively clear on auscultation.

What is the most likely diagnosis, and what measures should be taken?
The most likely diagnosis is a pulmonary embolus or pneumothorax. Included in the differential diagnosis are atelectasis, aspiration pneumonia, and acute myocardial infarction. Supplemental oxygen should be administered to maintain saturation at more than 92%, a peripheral intravenous line should be inserted, and blood tests, arterial blood gas measurements, chest radiographs, and ECG should be ordered.

With a 50% oxygen face mask, the patient's respiratory rate decreases to 18 breaths per minute and oxygen saturation increases to 94%. The ECG and chest radiographic findings are normal. ABG testing shows a pH of 7.31, partial pressure of carbon dioxide of 34 mm Hg, partial pressure of oxygen of 68 mm Hg, and bicarbonate level of 24.

How should the patient be managed?
The most probable diagnosis is a pulmonary embolus. If the patient has no contraindications, heparin should be started and a V/Q scan should be ordered to confirm the diagnosis. Monitoring in an intensive care unit may be necessary if the patient becomes hemodynamically unstable or develops progressive hypoxemia. Although pulmonary emboli are relatively uncommon after thoracic surgery (fewer than 2% of patients), they are associated with a mortality that may be as high as 50% (38).

Mr. Ferguson's V/Q scan shows perfusion defects in both left and right lower lobes, suggesting a high probability of pulmonary emboli. He remains clinically stable, with only mild hypoxemia and no signs of right ventricular failure. A Doppler ultrasound study of his lower extremities does not reveal any signs of deep venous thrombosis. He is eventually discharged home 10 days after the incident and is treated with oral anticoagulation for 6 months.

What are the morbidity and mortality after pulmonary resection for lung cancer?
Major complications occur in 10% of patients with stage I and II disease. A complication rate of 20% is reported in patients who require an extended resection for locally advanced tumors (stage III). Mortality after lobectomy and

Management Algorithm for Lung Cancer

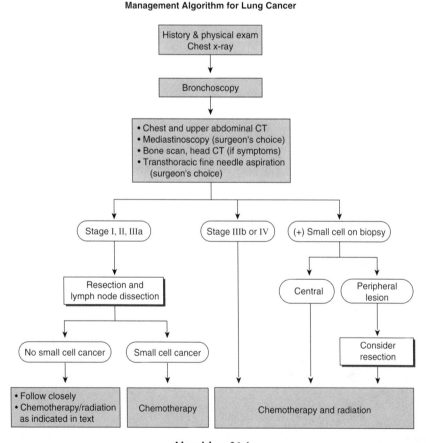

Algorithm 26.1.

pneumonectomy is 1 to 2% and 4 to 7%, respectively. Risk factors for postoperative complications include age over 70 years, restricted pulmonary reserve, and the need for pneumonectomy (39, 40).

REFERENCES

1. Shields TW. Presentation, diagnosis, and staging of bronchial carcinoma and the asymptomatic solitary pulmonary nodule. In: Shields TW, ed. General Thoracic Surgery. 4th ed. Philadelphia: Williams & Wilkins, 1994:1122–1154.

2. Maddaus M, Ginsberg RJ. Lung cancer: diagnosis and staging. In: Pearson FG, ed. Thoracic Surgery. New York: Churchill Livingstone, 1995:671–90.

3. Khouri NF, Meziane MA, Zerhouni EA, et al. The solitary pulmonary nodule: assessment, diagnosis and management. Chest 1987;91:128–133.

4. American Cancer Society. Cancer statistics 1996. CA Cancer J Clin 1996:46:5–27.

5. Miller AB. Lung cancer: epidemiology. In: Pearson FG, ed. Thoracic Surgery. New York: Churchill Livingstone, 1995:648–661.

6. Ng A, Horak GC. Factors significant to the diagnostic accuracy of lung cytology in bronchial washings and sputum samples. Acta Cytol 1983;27:397.

7. Wescott JL. Direct percutaneous needle aspiration of localized pulmonary lesions: results in 422 patients. Radiology 1980;137:31.

8. Lewis JW et al. Can computed tomography of the chest stage lung cancer: yes or no? Ann Thorac Surg 1990;49:591.

9. Pagani JJ. Non–small cell lung carcinoma adrenal metastases: computed tomography and percutaneous needle biopsy in their diagnosis. Cancer 1984;53:1058.

10. Zaman MB. Lung cancer: pathology. In: Pearson FG, ed. Thoracic Surgery. New York: Churchill Livingstone, 1995:661–670.

11. Arroglia AC, Buzaid AC, Mattay RA. Which patients can safely undergo lung resection? J Respir Dis 1991;12:1080.

12. Epstein SK, Faling JL, Daly B, Celli BR. Predicting complications after pulmonary resection: preoperative exercise testing vs a multi-factorial cardiopulmonary risk index. Chest 1993;104:694.

13. Bechard D, Wetstein L. Assessment of exercise oxygen consumption as preoperative criterion for lung resection. Ann Thorac Surg 1987;44:344.

14. Luke WP, Pearson FG, Todd TRJ, et al. Prospective evaluation of mediastinoscopy for assessment of carcinoma of the lung. J Thorac Cardiovasc Surg 1986;91:53–56.

15. Gross BH, Glazer GM, Orringer MB, et al. Bronchogenic carcinoma metastatic to normal sized lymph nodes: frequency and significance. Radiology 1988;166:71–74.

16. Backer CL, Shields TW, Lockhart CG, et al. Selective preoperative evaluation for possible N$_2$ disease in carcinoma of the lung. J Thorac Cardiovasc Surg 1987;93:337–343.

17. Martini N, Burt ME, Bains MS, et al. Survival after resection in stage II non–small cell lung cancer. Ann Thorac Surg 1992;54:460.

18. Holmes EC, Gail M. Surgical adjuvant therapy for stage II and stage III adenocarcinoma and large cell undifferentiated carcinoma. J Clin Oncol 1986;4:710–715.

19. Lung Cancer Study Group. Effects of postoperative mediastinal radiation on completely resected stage II and stage III epidermoid cancer of the lung. N Engl J Med 1986; 315:1377–1381.

20. Mountain CF. Value of the new TNM staging system for lung cancer. Chest 1989;96:47S.

21. Naruke T et al. Prognosis and survival in resected lung carcinoma based on the new international staging system. J Thorac Cardiovasc Surg 1988;96:440.

22. Martini N, Ginsberg RJ. Lung cancer: surgical management. In: Pearson FG, ed. Thoracic Surgery. New York: Churchill Livingstone, 1995:690–705.

23. McCaughan BC, Martini N, Bains MS, McCormack P. Chest wall invasion of carcinoma of the lung: therapeutic and prognostic implications. J Thorac Cardiovasc Surg 1985;89:836.

24. Piehler JM, Pairolero PC, Weeland LH, et al. Bronchogenic carcinoma with chest wall invasion: factors affecting survival following en-bloc resection. Ann Thorac Surg 1982; 34:684.

25. Allen MS, Mathisen DJ, Grillo HC, et al. Bronchogenic carcinoma with chest wall invasion. Ann Thorac Surg 1991;51:948–51.

26. Shields TW. The significance of ipsilateral mediastinal lymph node metastasis (N_2 disease) in non–small cell carcinoma of the lung. J Thorac Cardiovasc Surg 1990;99: 48–53.

27. Faber LP, Kittle CF, Warren WH, et al. Preoperative chemotherapy and irradiation for stage III non–small cell lung cancer. Ann Thorac Surg 1989;47:669–77.

28. Weiden PL, Piantadosi S, The Lung Cancer Study Group. Preoperative chemotherapy and radiation therapy in stage III non–small cell lung cancer: a phase II study of the Lung Cancer Study Group. J Natl Cancer Inst 1991;83:266–72.

29. Burkes RL, Ginsberg RJ, Shepherd F, et al. Induction chemotherapy with mitomycin, vindesine and cisplatin for stage III unresectable non–small cell lung cancer: results of the Toronto phase II trial. J Clin Oncol 1992;10:580–86.

30. Rusch VW, Albain KS, Crowley JJ, et al. Surgical resection of stage IIIA and stage IIIB non–small cell lung cancer after concurrent induction chemoradiotherapy: a Southwest Oncology Group trial. J Thorac Cardiovasc Surg 1993;105:97–106.

31. Martini N, Kris MG, Flehinger BJ, et al. Preoperative chemotherapy for stage IIIA (N_2) lung cancer: the Sloan Kettering experience with 136 patients. Ann Thorac Surg 1993; 55:1365–1374.

32. Roth JA, Fossella F, Komaki R, et al. A randomized trial comparing perioperative chemotherapy and surgery with surgery alone in resectable stage IIIA non–small cell lung cancer. J Natl Cancer Inst 1994;86:673–680.

33. Rosell R, Gomez-Codina J, Camps C, et al. A randomized trial comparing preoperative chemotherapy plus surgery with surgery alone in patients with non–small cell lung cancer. N Engl J Med 1994;330:153–158.

34. Martini N, Flehinger BJ. The role of surgery in N_2 lung cancer. Surg Clin North Am 1987;67:1037.

35. Naruke T, Goya T, Tsuchuya R, et al. The importance of surgery to non–small cell carcinoma of the lung with mediastinal lymph node metastasis. Ann Thorac Surg 1988; 46:603.

36. Patterson GA, Piazza D, Pearson FG, et al. Significance of metastatic disease to subaortic lymph nodes. Ann Thorac Surg 1987;43:155.

37. Swayer TE, Bonner JA, Gould PM, et al. Effectiveness of postoperative irradiation in stage IIIA non–small cell lung cancer according to regression tree analyses of recurrence risks. Ann Thorac Surg 1997;64:1402–1408.

38. Tedder M, Anstadt MP, Tedder SD, Lowe JE. Current morbidity, mortality and sur-
    vival after bronchoplastic procedures for malignancy. Ann Thorac Surg 1992;54:387.
39. Ginsberg RJ, Hill LD, Eagan RT, et al. Modern thirty-day operative mortality for sur-
    gical resections in lung cancer. J Thorac Cardiovasc Surg 1983;86:498.
40. Deslauriers J, Ginsberg RJ, Dubois P, et al. Current operative morbidity associated with
    elective surgical resection for lung cancer. Can J Surg 1989;32:335.

Surgery for Chronic Obstructive Pulmonary Disorder

Pasquale Ferraro and André Duranceau

Jerry Robinson, a retired 52-year-old postal worker, goes to his local hospital's emergency department for shortness of breath. Mr. Robinson states that while lifting boxes in his garage, he suddenly felt an intense pain over his right chest and began breathing heavily. He says he has never had this type of pain before in his life, and he describes it as worsening with deep breathing. His medical history is significant only for hypertension and a cholecystectomy. He admits to having smoked two packs of cigarettes a day since age 20 years, but he has not smoked a single cigarette during the past 18 months. He denies any chest pain, coughing, or hemoptysis before this episode. He has been short of breath on mild exertion (dyspnea scale, 2.75) for a number of years, and he has used bronchodilators occasionally for what he calls a wheezing problem. The patient has no drug allergies, and his medication includes a calcium channel blocker for high blood pressure.

What is the most likely diagnosis in Mr. Robinson's case?
The most likely diagnosis with this history is spontaneous pneumothorax. The differential diagnosis at this point includes pulmonary embolus, acute bronchospasm, myocardial infarction, and less probably, dissecting aortic aneurysm.

On physical examination, Mr. Robinson is agitated, diaphoretic, and tachypneic. He is conscious, well oriented, and not cyanotic. His vital signs are as follows: heart rate, 112 beats per minute, regular sinus; blood pressure, 168/94 mm Hg; respiratory rate, 24 breaths per minute; temperature, 37.3°C; and oxygen saturation, 90% on room air. His jugulars are not distended, his heart sounds are normal, and chest auscultation reveals decreased breath sounds diffusely, no wheezing, and increased resonance on percussion over his right chest. Examination of his abdomen and lower extremities is unremarkable.

What should be included in Mr. Robinson's initial workup?
The workup on admission should consist of a complete blood count, electrolytes, blood urea nitrogen and creatinine levels, cardiac enzymes, a chest radiograph, and an electrocardiogram (ECG).

Mr. Robinson's blood work, cardiac enzymes, and ECG are within normal limits. The chest radiograph shows a 3-cm pneumothorax starting at the apex of his chest cavity and extending down to his diaphragm. There is no cardiomegaly, and the left lung appears to be normal.

How should the patient be managed at this point?
The chest radiograph confirms the diagnosis suggested by the history and physical examination. A 3-cm pneumothorax in a symptomatic patient necessitates drainage. Supplemental oxygen should be administered to maintain an oxygen saturation above 92%, and a peripheral intravenous line should be started. Information about Mr. Robinson's arterial blood gases is not useful at this point because it does not add any pertinent information and only delays the necessary procedure.

What type of pneumothorax is presented in this case?
This is a secondary spontaneous pneumothorax because it occurs in a patient who probably has an underlying pulmonary disorder: chronic obstructive pulmonary disease (COPD). Primary spontaneous (or idiopathic) pneumothoraces occur in young, healthy persons with no underlying pulmonary disease. The general classification of pneumothoraces is given in Table 27.1.

Table 27.1. CAUSES OF PNEUMOTHORACES

Classification	Cause
Spontaneous pneumothorax	Primary (idiopathic)
	Secondary
Traumatic	Blunt chest injury
	Penetrating chest injury
Iatrogenic	Thoracentesis
	Central vein catheterization
	Mechanical ventilation
Neonatal	
Catamenial	
Diagnostic	

What clinical features are associated with a primary spontaneous pneumothorax?
Primary spontaneous pneumothoraces occur with an incidence of 6 to 7 per 100,000 men and 1 to 2 per 100,000 women in North America (1). The rupture of a small subpleural bleb within the visceral pleura allows air to escape into the pleural cavity, where it accumulates and collapses the lung. These pneumothoraces are most prevalent in young adults; 85% of patients are younger than 40 years of age. Typically, the patient is a tall, slim 20- to 25-year-old man with a smoking history. Without definite therapy, the recurrence rate is high, estimated at 25% after a first episode, 40 to 50% after a second episode, and more than 60% after a third episode (2, 3).

What is the pathophysiology of subpleural blebs?
The formation of subpleural blebs results from the rupture of apical alveoli. The gradient between the intrabronchial and intrapleural pressures is greater at the lung apices, creating more tension on the walls of the apical alveoli, which leads to their overexpansion and eventual rupture. Once the alveolus ruptures, gas escapes and dissects peripherally along the lobular septa and collects as blebs beneath the visceral pleura. These blebs are generally found at the lung apex, in the superior segment of the lower lobes, and along the fissures. By definition, they are less than 2 cm in diameter.

What alterations of pulmonary physiology are caused by pneumothoraces?
A pneumothorax causes a reduction in pulmonary volumes, lung compliance, and diffusing capacity. Blood shunting through a lung that is poorly ventilated creates a ventilation and perfusion (V/Q) mismatch, and hypoxemia results.

How are secondary spontaneous pneumothoraces defined?
Secondary spontaneous pneumothoraces accompany underlying pulmonary disease. They account for only 20% of spontaneous pneumothoraces overall (80% are primary or idiopathic) and most often are associated with COPD. The mean age of patients is older than 50 years, and as pulmonary functions are compromised, they are more commonly symptomatic (4).

What other diseases are associated with secondary spontaneous pneumothoraces?
Other pulmonary disorders include cystic fibrosis, bullous disease, interstitial diseases (e.g., idiopathic pulmonary fibrosis, sarcoidosis, eosinophilic granuloma), and infectious processes (e.g., pneumonia, tuberculosis, abscesses). Neoplasms, whether primary or metastatic, also may cause a pneumothorax, but this is rare.

Mr. Robinson is seen by the general surgeon on call that day in the emergency department. After reviewing the history, physical examination, and chest radiograph findings, the surgeon proceeds with a tube thoracostomy of the right chest.

What size chest tube should be inserted and where?
The size of a chest tube depends on what type of substance is being drained from the pleural cavity. Generally, a size 20-Fr chest tube is sufficient for pneumothorax. When draining blood, pus, or thick fluid, a large-bore tube (size 28 to 36 Fr) is recommended. The chest tube for a pneumothorax should be inserted in the fifth intercostal space on the midaxillary or anterior axillary line, and it should be directed toward the apex of the pleural cavity. A chest tube for an apical pneumothorax also may be inserted through the anterior chest wall in the second intercostal space on the midclavicular line. A pleural effusion should be drained with a chest tube in the fifth or sixth intercostal space directed posteriorly and inferiorly (5).

Once inserted, should the chest tube have suction?
Suction on a chest tube should be used to ensure optimal drainage of the pleural cavity. Suction is required for pneumothorax when chest radiograph does not show the lung to be completely expanded after tube thoracostomy or if there is a large air leak. Once the lung is completely expanded, suction should be reduced to a minimum or stopped to help seal the air leak.

The chest radiograph taken after Mr. Robinson's chest tube is inserted shows adequate tube placement and a small residual 8-mm pneumothorax at the apex of the right lung field. A moderate-sized air leak from the tube is also shown. The chest tube is placed under water seal drainage, and 20 cm of negative pressure is applied. The patient is admitted to the hospital, and a daily chest radiograph is ordered.

Is chest tube drainage required for all patients with a pneumothorax, and if not, what are the criteria for conservative management?
All patients with a symptomatic pneumothorax need drainage. Some patients who meet specific criteria may be treated with observation alone. These criteria include no symptoms, a pneumothorax less than 20% or 2 cm, and a young and reliable patient (i.e., primary spontaneous pneumothorax). Patients with secondary pneumothorax have much less pulmonary reserve and thus are at higher risk for complications or even death if the pneumothorax progresses rapidly. Conservative management is possible in 15 to 20% of patients overall (2, 6).

When pneumothorax is treated conservatively, how long does resolution take?
The rate of resorption of air from the pleural cavity is estimated to be 1.25% of the volume of the pneumothorax per 24 hours (50 to 70 mL/day). A 2-cm pneumothorax takes up to 3 weeks to resolve completely.

What types of drainage procedures are available?
A spontaneous pneumothorax may be drained by simple needle aspiration using a 16- to 18-gauge needle catheter and a three-way stopcock. However, this procedure is associated with a 50 to 70% failure rate and thus is used very seldom (4). Drainage of the pleural space may be obtained with any of a variety of small-caliber catheters (10 to 16 Fr) to which suction usually can be applied. Although less traumatic on insertion and more comfortable for the patients, these small-bore tubes easily become clogged with fibrin and blood clots. Conventional tube drainage with a 20- to 24-Fr chest tube remains the gold standard because it is safe, effective, and reproducible and is associated with an 80 to 90% success rate in the management of spontaneous pneumothorax (7).

What is a Heimlich valve, and when is its use indicated?
The Heimlich valve is a one-way flutter valve that is connected to the end of a chest tube, eliminating the need for an underwater seal drainage bottle or suction. The valve is designed to let air out of the pleural cavity in the presence of an air leak (8). The valve is ideally suited for outpatient management of uncomplicated spontaneous pneumothorax and for persistent air leaks. It is recommended only for patients whose lungs are fully reexpanded and for reliable patients with adequate pulmonary function. Regular chest radiographs and follow-up are necessary. The chest tube is removed once the air leak has resolved.

What complications are associated with spontaneous pneumothoraces?
Complications include pleural effusion (15%), persistent air leak (10%), tension pneumothorax (5%), hemothorax (3%), pneumomediastinum (2%), and empyema (less than 1%).

How does a hemothorax secondary to a pneumothorax occur?
When a pneumothorax occurs suddenly, adhesions between the parietal and visceral pleura may tear as the lung collapses. These adhesions may contain blood vessels, so when they are torn, bleeding results. Avulsion of a subclavian vein also has been reported in association with a spontaneous pneumothorax. When the hemorrhage is massive or continuous, an exploratory thoracotomy is indicated.

Mr. Robinson's air leak persists for 5 days and eventually seals spontaneously. The chest radiograph shows a well-expanded lung. The chest tube is removed uneventfully, and the patient is discharged from the hospital. Then, 2 weeks after returning home, Mr. Robinson once again develops acute-onset shortness of breath with right-sided chest pain. He is rushed to the hospital, where an emergency department chest radiograph shows complete collapse of his right lung secondary to a pneumothorax. A chest tube is rapidly inserted by the thoracic

surgery resident on call. The patient's shortness of breath markedly improves shortly after the chest tube is placed. Mr. Robinson is admitted to the hospital, and his chest tube is set on 20 cm of suction.

How should Mr. Robinson's problem now be managed?
The patient's spontaneous pneumothorax should be managed the same as the first episode. At this point, surgical therapy should be considered.

What are the indications for surgery in patients with primary and secondary spontaneous pneumothoraces?
These are the indications for surgery:

• Second episode of ipsilateral pneumothorax
• Previous contralateral pneumothorax
• Air leak persisting longer than 7 to 10 days
• Massive air leak preventing adequate lung expansion
• Bilateral simultaneous pneumothorax
• Complications of a pneumothorax (e.g., hemothorax, empyema)
• Indications specific for the underlying pulmonary disorder

Is this patient's occupation an important consideration?
Some occupations carry an inherent risk of pneumothorax. Airline pilots and scuba divers should be managed more aggressively, and surgery should be considered after a first episode. Patients who live far from medical centers also should be managed surgically after an initial episode of spontaneous pneumothorax (4).

What are the objectives of surgical therapy?
The foremost objective of surgery for spontaneous pneumothorax is preventing recurrences. Other objectives include ensuring complete expansion of the lung, treating complications, and managing bronchopleural fistulas.

How are these objectives met?
Surgery for spontaneous pneumothorax consists of resecting the bullous disease at the lung apices (apical bullectomy) and obliterating the pleural space. The pleural space can be obliterated in a number of ways, including parietal pleurectomy (subtotal versus total), mechanical pleurodesis (abrasion), and chemical pleurodesis (e.g., tetracycline, bleomycin, talc, hypertonic glucose) (9, 10).

What type of surgical approach is recommended?
Although the operation can be carried out through a standard posterolateral thoracotomy, most surgeons prefer a miniaxillary thoracotomy in the third intercostal space or a video thoracoscopic (VATS) approach (11–13).

Although Mr. Robinson is doing fine clinically with only a minimal amount of dyspnea at rest and a completely expanded lung on the chest radiograph, his air leak persists for 8 days. Considering that this is his second episode of pneumothorax and his air leak did not seal spontaneously, the patient is seen in consultation by a thoracic surgeon. The surgeon and Mr. Robinson agree that an operation is in his best interest.

What preoperative workup should Mr. Robinson have?
Although this type of operation is not considered major, patients with secondary spontaneous pneumothoraces must be thoroughly screened before surgery. Operability should be assessed, and a cardiac evaluation should be done when indicated. From a pulmonary standpoint, a baseline study of pulmonary function tests (PFTs) should be obtained in all patients with COPD. Chest computed tomography (CT) also is recommended because patients with a history of heavy smoking are at risk for developing a malignancy. CT also may help direct the intervention if areas of bullous disease are found away from the lung apices.

Mr. Robinson's CT shows a 2.5-cm anterior pneumothorax on the right, mild emphysematous changes in both lung fields, no distinct bullae, and no suspicious-looking lesions. His PFTs are as follows: forced expiratory volume in 1 second (FEV_1), 1.5 (38% of predicted); forced vital capacity (FVC), 2.4 (60%); FEV_1/FVC, 62%; and carbon monoxide diffusion in the lung (DL_{CO}), 54%. His workup is otherwise unremarkable.

What type of intervention is best suited for Mr. Robinson?
Although a number of options are available, a VATS approach is best because it allows a thorough inspection of the lung. If specific areas of blebs are found, they should be resected with a stapler. A subtotal pleurectomy or pleural abrasion is performed in most cases. Some surgeons recommend chemical pleurodesis at the time of surgery for secondary spontaneous pneumothoraces. Generally, one chest tube is left in the pleural cavity.

What are the advantages of pleurectomy over pleural abrasion?
The pleurectomy is believed to create a more intense inflammatory reaction and thus better obliteration of the pleural cavity. However, it is associated with a major complication rate of 10% (e.g., hemothorax, fibrothorax, Horner's syndrome) and makes subsequent thoracotomy for unrelated disease more difficult. Pleural abrasion is simpler, more effective, and safer (3% complication rate) (14, 15).

What are the results of surgery for spontaneous pneumothorax?
The standard procedure, consisting of an apical bullectomy with a pleurectomy or pleural abrasion, is highly effective and associated with morbidity below 10%

and a mortality rate of 1 to 2%. The postoperative morbidity and mortality may be significantly higher in patients with COPD. The rate of recurrent pneumothoraces after surgery is reported by a number of surgeons as 1 to 2% for primary spontaneous pneumothorax and 5 to 6% for the secondary type (7, 9, 10, 11).

Mr. Robinson's air leak persists for 2 more days. He is finally taken to the operating room, where he undergoes a VATS apical bullectomy and a subtotal pleurectomy. His chest tube, which shows a minimal air leak on the first postoperative day, is removed 3 days later. The patient is discharged from the hospital after an uneventful postoperative course. Mr. Robinson recovers well from his surgery, and on follow-up visits his radiograph shows a well-expanded lung with no signs of a pneumothorax. Over the years, however, the patient's dyspnea continues to progress, and he now requires inhaled bronchodilators on a regular basis. On two occasions in the past 10 months, he is hospitalized for acute bronchitis and receives antibiotic therapy. He is becoming short of breath even at rest and is no longer able to attend to his regular activities.

How is Mr. Robinson's clinical course described?
Mr. Robinson's evolution is typical of long-standing COPD. Most patients require regular bronchodilators and oral steroids as their dyspnea progresses with time, and hospitalizations for episodes of exacerbated chronic bronchitis become more frequent. More than 50% of patients with end-stage disease become oxygen dependent (16).

What form of COPD is most frequent?
The most frequent type of COPD is emphysema, which affects an estimated two million Americans.

How is emphysema defined?
Emphysema is a condition of the lung characterized by abnormal and permanent enlargement of air spaces distal to the terminal bronchioles accompanied by destruction of their walls and without obvious fibrosis (17).

How is emphysema classified morphologically?
Three subtypes of emphysema have been described: centriacinar, or centrilobular; panacinar, or panlobular; and paraseptal. Centriacinar emphysema develops in the proximal portion of the acinus and is associated with inflammatory destruction of the respiratory bronchioles. This form of emphysema is most common in the upper lung fields and is secondary to tobacco smoking. In panacinar emphysema all portions of the acinus are uniformly destroyed. It diffuses throughout the lung. It has been associated with deficiencies in α_1-antitrypsin. Paraseptal emphysema results from disruption of subpleural alveoli with

the secondary formation of blebs and bullae. These lesions usually are found along the apical segments of the lung and along the fissures, and they are responsible for most episodes of spontaneous pneumothorax (18).

What radiologic features are found on chest radiographs in patients with emphysema?
Common findings include hyperinflation of the lungs, depression or flattening of the diaphragm, vascular deficiency in the parenchyma, bullae, increased intercostal space, increased anteroposterior diameter of the chest, and vertical position of the heart.

What are typical PFT values in a patient with advanced COPD?
PFTs show airflow obstruction (FEV_1 less than 35%), marked thoracic hyperinflation (total lung capacity [TLC] greater than 120%; residual volume [RV] greater than 200%), and altered alveolar gas exchange (DL_{CO} less than 50%).

What is the pathophysiology of respiratory failure in patients with emphysema?
The mechanisms are airflow obstruction, dead space ventilation, compression of normal parenchyma, increase in pulmonary vascular resistance, and respiratory muscle and diaphragmatic dysfunction.

Why does airflow obstruction occur in the emphysematous lung?
In the normal lung, the small bronchi and bronchioles depend on the radial traction forces of the surrounding parenchyma to remain open during expiration. Emphysema destroys the lung tissue and decreases its elastic recoil properties, which in turn causes the small airways to collapse on expiration. Cartilage atrophy in emphysema may render the small bronchi vulnerable to expiratory collapse, also producing airflow obstruction, air trapping, and hyperinflation (19).

What are the objectives of surgery for emphysema?
The primary objective is to improve lung and thoracic function, hence decrease dyspnea, increase exercise tolerance, and improve the quality of life.

What types of surgery can treat emphysema?
Operations for emphysema date to the early 1900s. They include a variety of techniques, most of which are no longer in use. Procedures were developed for the chest wall (costochondrectomy), the diaphragm, the pleura, the nervous system (lung denervation), and the major airways (tracheoplasty). Surgery on the lung itself consists of excision or plication of bullae in patients with bullous lung disease, and volume reduction for patients with diffuse emphysema (20).

What are the objectives of lung volume reduction surgery (LVRS)?
The goals of LVRS for diffuse emphysema are to improve the elastic recoil properties of the lung, correct the chest wall mechanics and respiratory muscle

dysfunction, resect the part of the lung with the most important V/Q mismatch, and improve hemodynamics by decreasing the pulmonary vascular resistance and afterload to the right ventricle.

What patients are candidates for LVRS?
The inclusion and exclusion criteria are given in Table 27.2.

How is LVRS done?
LVRS consists of a unilateral or bilateral lung resection (stapling device versus laser technique) using a standard thoracotomy approach, a median sternotomy, or a VATS. The "functionless" areas of the lung are identified with one-lung ventilation (the emphysematous lung remains hyperinflated). With a stapler, the lung is resected beginning on the anterior surface of the upper lobe, moving toward the apex, and then around and toward the diaphragm. This creates a continuous U-shaped line of excision on the periphery of the lung. A buttress of bovine pericardium is usually applied to the staple line. A pleural tent is developed, and two chests tubes are left in each pleural cavity.

How much lung should be resected?
The exact amount is difficult to define, but generally 20 to 30% of the lung volume on each side is resected.

What are the results and clinical outcome of LVRS for diffuse emphysema?
The outcome of LVRS varies according to the surgical approach used. Results with a VATS-laser technique show only modest improvement. Reports have documented a mean FEV_1 increase of 13 to 18%, a decrease in RV of 11 to

Table 27.2.   SELECTION CRITERIA FOR LUNG VOLUME REDUCTION SURGERY

Inclusion Criteria	Exclusion Criteria
Diagnosis of emphysema	Age >80 years
Disabling dyspnea (grade 3–4/4)	Tobacco use within last 6 months
FEV_1 <35%	Pulmonary hypertension (systolic >45; mean >35)
Residual volume >200%	Resting CO_2 >55 mm Hg
Total lung capacity >120%	Marked obesity or cachexia
Hyperinflated lungs on chest radiograph	Unstable coronary artery disease
Regional heterogeneity of lung perfusion	Dependence on ventilator
Potential for preoperative rehabilitation	Underlying bronchiectasis or chronic bronchitis

FEV_1, forced expiratory volume in 1 second.

14%, an improvement in the partial pressure of arterial oxygen (PaO_2) of 2 to 4 mm Hg, and cessation of oxygen therapy in only 16% of patients. Reports indicate that using a bilateral stapling technique by median sternotomy, surgeons increased FEV_1 by 49 to 96%, decreased RV by 28 to 30%, improved PaO_2 by 8 mm Hg, and eliminated supplemental oxygen therapy in 70% of patients. Results with a bilateral VATS stapling technique are comparable with those of the median sternotomy approach (21–26).

What are the long-term benefits of LVRS?
Although a great number of studies have confirmed the short-term benefits of LVRS, no data on long-term results are available. It generally is believed that over time lung function deteriorates, and the initial benefits of LVRS may be lost.

What are the complication rates associated with LVRS?
The major complication rate ranges from 10 to 40%, and the rate of mortality is reported as 3 to 17%. Air leaks requiring chest tubes for longer than 5 days postoperatively are found in 30 to 48% of patients. Pneumonia has been documented in 9 to 22% of patients and respiratory failure in 2 to 13% (24, 26).

Mr. Robinson, now 58 years old, is severely handicapped by emphysema. He is being followed by a pneumologist who regularly repeats his workup. His PFTs now show FEV_1, 28%; RV, 270%; TLC, 180%; DL_{CO}, 30%; PaO_2 on room air, 51 mm Hg; and PCO_2, 50 mm Hg. After a long discussion with his physician regarding the possibility of LVRS, he decides to go ahead with the preoperative workup. Unfortunately, Mr. Robinson's cardiac evaluation shows moderate right ventricular dysfunction on echocardiogram, and pulmonary hypertension (peak airway pressure is 65/40 mm Hg) is found during his right heart catheterization. These findings rule out LVRS for Mr. Robinson. However, he remains hopeful that a solution for his problem can be found and insists on seeing a lung transplant pulmonologist.

What are the most common indications for lung transplantation?
Lung transplantation is indicated for a variety of diseases. These include COPD (60 to 70% of cases), infections, diseases such as cystic fibrosis (15 to 20%), interstitial lung disease (10 to 15%), and pulmonary vascular disease (5 to 10%) (27).

What are the selection criteria for candidates for lung transplantation?
Selection criteria usually are classified as general and specific (see Table 27.3).

What generally are accepted as contraindications to lung transplantation?
Contraindications to lung transplantation include cachexia, ventilator dependency, other end-organ dysfunction, symptomatic osteoporosis, history of ma-

Table 27.3.   SELECTION CRITERIA FOR
LUNG TRANSPLANTATION

General Criteria	Specific Criteria
Progressive and disabling pulmonary disease	Functional class 3–4/4 (NYHA)
Poor quality of life	Age <55–65 years
No effective medical therapy	Potential for rehabilitation
Life expectancy without transplantation	Phychosocial stability
<12–24 months	No tobacco use >6 months
	No systemic disease (e.g., renal,
	cardiac, hepatic)

NYHA, New York Heart Association.

lignancy, and alcoholism or drug addiction. Some of these criteria vary from one institution to another and according to the underlying pulmonary disease (28).

When should lung transplantation be considered for a patient with emphysema?
The ultimate goals of lung transplantation are to prolong the patient's life and improve the quality of life. A successful transplantation improves a patient's quality of life in more than 85% of cases. Exercise tolerance usually is markedly increased, and supplemental oxygen therapy is discontinued in more than 90% of patients. However, improving survival is more controversial in patients with COPD. Other disease entities have specific guidelines on the indication and timing of the transplantation based on survival data. Emphysema often evolves very slowly over several years when treated with supplemental oxygen, even with end-stage disease (i.e., FEV_1 less than 30%). In this group of patients, 2-year survival rates of 60 to 80% have been reported (29, 30). It generally is accepted that transplantation prolongs the life of COPD patients whose FEV_1 reaches 20%. Patients in the 25% FEV_1 range who have deteriorated rapidly over a short period or who require regular hospitalizations also live longer after transplantation.

What type of transplantation should be performed in a patient with COPD?
A single-lung transplant is sufficient for most patients from a functional and survival standpoint. A double-lung transplant should be considered for emphysema patients younger than 40 years with α_1-antitrypsin deficiencies and for patients with end-stage disease who develop bronchiectasis and have recurrent infections (31).

How often is cardiopulmonary bypass required for transplants in these patients?
Bypass is required for fewer than 4 to 5% of patients with COPD. Patients who do not tolerate one-lung ventilation or who have right ventricular failure and

pulmonary hypertension are at increased risk for requiring cardiopulmonary bypass during the transplantation.

What are the functional results of lung transplantation for COPD?
A number of factors influence the early and long-term functional results after a single- or double-lung transplantation. These factors include native lung dis-

Management Algorithm for Pneumothorax

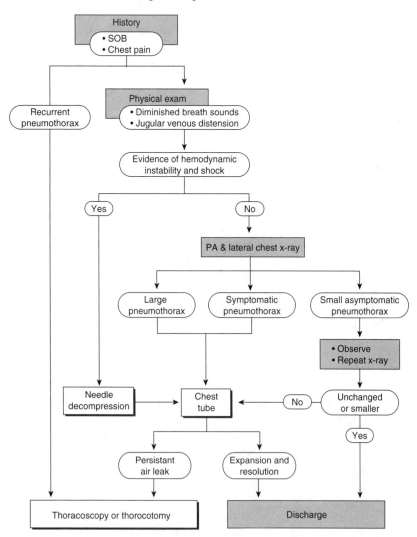

Algorithm 27.1.

ease, overall cardiac function, operative factors (e.g., incisional pain, chest wall restriction, pleural complications), and posttransplant complications. In double-lung transplant recipients, 12 months after the operation the FEV_1 reaches 78% of the predicted value, the DL_{CO} is 76%, and the PaO_2 is within the normal range. After a single-lung transplant, the FEV_1 is found to be in the 50% range for COPD patients and 79% for patients with pulmonary fibrosis, and the DL_{CO} is 60%. In these patients, the PaO_2 is normal, but the alveolar-arterial gradient remains wide. Overall, study of the functional status using the New York Heart Association (NYHA) grades shows 70% of patients class I and 21% class 2 (32).

What are the causes of early and late mortality and overall survival?
In the early postoperative period (up to 30 days), the most frequent cause of death is nonspecific graft failure followed by infection. In the intermediate time (31 days to 1 year), infection is the most common cause of death. After 1 year, bronchiolitis obliterans is responsible for the greatest number of deaths. The operative mortality for a lung transplantation ranges from 5 to 10%. The 1- and 5-year actuarial survival rates are 70% and 50%, respectively. Results in patients with emphysema are significantly better, with 1- and 5-year survival rates of 80% and 60%, respectively. In COPD patients, the outcome is similar whether a single- or double-lung transplant is performed (27).

Mr. Robinson is seen and evaluated by the lung transplant program in his city. He is considered a candidate for transplant and undergoes the full workup. He now requires oxygen 24 hours a day, and his functional status has reached NYHA class 4. To his great relief, no specific contraindications to a lung transplantation are found. Mr. Robinson's name is placed on the patient waiting list for a single-lung transplant. With his blood type, B, he is told, the mean waiting time is 12 to 18 months.

REFERENCES

1. Melton LJ, Hepper NG, Orford KP. Incidence of spontaneous pneumothorax in Olm-stead County, Minnesota: 1950–1974. Am Rev Respir Dis 1979;120:1379–1382.
2. Getz S, Beasley W. Spontaneous pneumothorax. Am J Surg 1983;145:823–827.
3. Gobbell WG, Rhea WG, Nelson IA, et al. Spontaneous pneumothorax. J Thorac Cardiovasc Surg 1963;46:331–345.
4. Beauchamp G. Spontaneous pneumothorax and pneumomediastinum. In: Pearson FG, ed. Thoracic Surgery. New York: Churchill Livingstone, 1995:1037–1054.
5. Miller KS, Sahn SA. Chest tubes: indications, technique, management, and complications. Chest 1987;91:258–264.
6. O'Rourke J, Yee E. Civilian spontaneous pneumothorax. Chest 1989;96:1302–1306.
7. Ferraro P, Beauchamp G, Lord F, et al. Spontaneous primary and secondary pneumothorax: a 10-year study of management alternatives. Can J Surg 1994;37:197–202.

8. Heimlich HJ. Valve drainage of the pleural cavity. Dis Chest 1968;53:282.

9. Singh SV. The surgical treatment of spontaneous pneumothorax by parietal pleurectomy. Scand J Thorac Cardiovasc Surg 1982;16:75–80.

10. Weeden D, Smith GH. Surgical experience in the management of spontaneous pneumothorax. Thorax 1983;38:737–743.

11. Deslauriers J, Beaulieu M, Despres JP, et al. Transaxillary pleurectomy for treatment of spontaneous pneumothorax. Ann Thorac Surg 1980;30:569–574.

12. Cannon WB, Vierra MA, Cannon A. Thoracoscopy for spontaneous pneumothorax. Ann Thorac Surg 1993;56:686–687.

13. Hazelrigg SR, Landreneau RJ, Mack M, et al. Thoracoscopic stapled resection for spontaneous pneumothorax. J Thorac Cardiovasc Surg 1993;105:389–393.

14. Gaensler EA. Parietal pleurectomy for recurrent spontaneous pneumothorax. Surg Gynecol Obstet 1956;102:293–308.

15. Clagget OT. The management of spontaneous pneumothorax. J Thorac Cardiovasc Surg 1968;55:761–762.

16. Maltais F, Bourbeau J. Medical management of emphysema. Chest Surg Clin North Am 1995;5:673–689.

17. American Thoracic Society. Chronic bronchitis, asthma, and pulmonary emphysema. Am Rev Respir Dis 1968;85:762–768.

18. Deslauriers J, Leblanc P. Bullous and bleb diseases of the lung. In: Shields TW, ed. General Thoracic Surgery. 4th ed. Philadelphia: Williams & Wilkins, 1994:907–929.

19. Celli BR. Pathophysiology of chronic obstructive pulmonary disease. Chest Surg Clin North Am 1995;5:623–634.

20. Deslauriers J. A perspective on the role of surgery in chronic obstructive lung disease. Chest Surg Clin North Am 1995;5:575–602.

21. Hazelrigg S, Boley T, Henkle J, et al. Thoracoscopic laser bullectomy: a prospective study with 3-month results. J Thorac Cardiovasc Surg 1996;112:319.

22. Little AG, Swain JA, Nino JJ, et al. Reduction pneumoplasty for emphysema: early results. Ann Surg 1995;222:365–374.

23. McKenna RJ, Brenner M, Gelb AF, et al. A randomized prospective trial of stapled reduction versus laser bullectomy for diffuse emphysema. J Thorac Cardiovasc Surg 1996;111:317–322.

24. Cooper JD, Patterson GA, Sundaresan RS, et al. Results of 150 consecutive bilateral lung volume reduction procedures in patients with severe emphysema. J Thorac Cardiovasc Surg 1996;112:1319.

25. Keenan RJ, Sciurba FC, Landreneau RJ, et al. Superiority of bilateral versus unilateral thoracoscopic approaches to lung reduction surgery. Am J Respir Crit Care Med 1996;153:A268.

26. Miller JI, Lee RB, Mansour KA. Lung volume reduction surgery: lessons learned. Ann Thorac Surg 1996;61:1464–1469.

27. Hosenpud JD, Bennet LE, Keck BM, et al. Registry of the International Society for Heart and Lung Transplantation: fourteenth official report, 1997. J Heart Lung Transplant 1997;16:691–712.

28. Smith CM. Patient selection, evaluation, and preoperative management for lung transplant candidates. Clin Chest Med 1997;18:183–197.

29. Anthonisen NR, Wright EC, Hodgkin JE, et al. Prognosis in chronic obstructive pulmonary disease. Am Rev Respir Dis 1986;133:14–20.

30. Nocturnal Oxygen Therapy Trial Group. Continuous or nocturnal oxygen therapy in hypoxemic chronic obstructive pulmonary disease: a clinical trial. Ann Intern Med 1980;93:391–398.
31. Patterson GA. Indication for unilateral, bilateral, heart-lung and lobar transplant procedures. Clin Chest Med 1997;18:225–230.
32. Williams TJ, Snell GI. Early and long-term functional outcomes in unilateral, bilateral, and living-related transplant recipients. Clin Chest Med 1997;18:245–257.

Melanoma

William P. Reed

Dennis O'Shea is a 45-year-old executive who undergoes a shave biopsy of a mole on the upper part of his right back. He has always had numerous moles scattered over his back and chest but never paid them much attention until his wife noted that one had become somewhat larger than the rest. The pathology report on tissue submitted at the time of the shave biopsy shows a tan to dark brown piece of skin measuring 9 × 5 mm. Microscopic examination shows a benign Spitz nevus extending to the margins of the specimen. Considering the benign nature of the lesion, he is advised that no further therapy is warranted at this time. He seeks a second opinion because several members of his family have died of cancer, and he is concerned that this may be an early sign of malignancy. During physical examination, Mr. O'Shea appears to be a healthy, tanned white man with sandy hair and blue eyes. His vital signs are normal. His lungs are clear. The heart sounds are normal, with no murmurs. His abdomen shows no scars or masses. There is no lymphadenopathy. There is a recent scar over the right scapula that is slightly reddened, with a suggestion of darker pigmentation at the medial margin. He has freckles on the tops of his shoulders and numerous benign-appearing moles scattered over his torso and extremities.

Given this presentation, what is the initial clinical impression?
Any change in a mole or pigmented lesion should be assumed to be malignant melanoma until proven otherwise.

Doesn't the diagnosis of a Spitz nevus prove that this is not a melanoma?
The Spitz nevus has many features in common with melanoma (1–3). Often, the distinction is made on the basis of microscopic features at the depths of the lesion or on the basis of the clinical features. The Spitz nevus tends to be less than 6 mm in diameter, symmetric, and uniform in color, with a progressively benign appearance of cells on histologic examination (maturation) as the deep-

est margin of the lesion is approached. In contrast, melanoma presents with the distinct features of *a*symmetry, *b*order irregularity, *c*olor variegation, and *d*iameter greater than 6 mm (the so-called ABCDs of melanoma). Histologic examination of the lesion shows invasion at the deepest portion.

What is the origin of melanoma?
Melanoma develops from melanocytes, which are pigment-producing cells derived from the neural crest that migrate during fetal development into the skin, eye, central nervous system, and mucous membranes. The most common site of melanoma is the skin, but these tumors can develop in any tissue that contains melanocytes. This cancer comprises approximately 3.5% of malignancies, with 41,000 new cases each year in the United States (4). From the 1930s to the mid-1980s, there was a rapid rise in the incidence of this disease, doubling every 10 years (5). More recent epidemiologic studies suggest that the incidence is leveling off in susceptible populations, perhaps reflecting better attention to preventive measures as the causation becomes clearer (6).

What is the cause of melanoma?
The direct cause is unknown, but there is considerable evidence to suggest that ultraviolet light is the principal carcinogen. Susceptible people are those with pale complexions and reddish hair, who are most prone to skin injury upon exposure to sunlight. An inverse relationship between latitude and incidence of disease has been noted for such persons both in Australia and in North America. Melanoma most commonly occurs on the skin that is left uncovered, such as the back and chest in men and the arms and legs in women.

Is there a sex or race predilection for malignant melanoma? Do these groups differ in prognosis?
A survey of more than 8500 malignant melanoma patients revealed a slight predominance of men (52%) over women (48%) with regard to the total number of cases reported (7). With regard to race, 98% of this group were white. In general, women tend to have a longer survival time than men. In blacks, malignant melanoma tends to occur on the palms, the soles, or beneath the nail plate, and it tends to exhibit an aggressive growth pattern and early metastasis with a poor overall prognosis. The 5-year survival in the black population has been estimated to be as low as 23% (8).

Is there a difference between sexes in the anatomic location of malignant melanoma? Does the location of pigmented lesions offer any prognostic information?
Different patterns of sun exposure lead to a significant difference between men and women with respect to body location of melanoma. Men tend to have more lesions on their trunks, whereas women have more extremity lesions, particularly on the lower limbs. Melanomas in women tend to be thinner, with

less tendency to ulcerate. It is unknown whether this is an inherent feature of the location or is due to easier detectability. As a result, regional lymph node involvement and distant metastasis occur less often in women than in men. Therefore, men with a predominance of trunk lesions have a relatively poor prognosis, whereas women with a predominance of extremity lesions have a relatively good prognosis (5).

Are there any precursor lesions of melanoma?
Yes. The dysplastic nevus syndrome is familial and is believed to be a precursor of malignant melanoma. This syndrome follows a familial pattern and is characterized by a large number of irregularly shaped nevi on the trunk. Those with dysplastic nevus syndrome are believed to have a cumulative lifetime risk of melanoma approaching 100% (9). Giant congenital nevi in children are believed to be premalignant, with a risk of malignancy reported to be as high as 40%.

What specific changes in nevi indicate the need for biopsy?
Any change in size, shape, or color of a nevus, as well as any itching, ulceration, or bleeding, suggests that biopsy should be considered. Changes in size and shape occur in approximately 70% of melanomas. The change in color is usually toward increasing pigmentation; however, amelanotic melanomas do exist. In addition, pigment may fade in some areas (regression) while deepening in others. Ulceration and bleeding are late signs that usually indicate deeply invasive disease (10).

What are the histologic types of cutaneous melanoma? Which have the overall best prognosis and worst prognosis? Which is the most common type?
The histologic types of melanoma and their approximate incidence are as follows: superficial spreading (70%), lentigo maligna (5%), acral lentiginous (10%), and nodular (15%). Both lentigo maligna and superficial spreading melanomas have a relatively good prognosis if they are diagnosed early. These types of melanoma have a prominent horizontal growth phase such that the melanocytes proliferate superficially along the epidermal–dermal junction and only later become locally invasive. For patients with these types of melanoma, changes in size, shape, or color can be detected while the tumor is locally noninvasive. Acral lentiginous tumors also have a prominent horizontal growth component, but they are a bit more invasive than the superficial types. Nodular melanoma develops early deep invasion and tends to metastasize early. This histologic type carries the worst prognosis.

What is the difference between an incisional and excisional biopsy?
An incisional biopsy entails removal of only a portion of the lesion. The size of the incision varies, but the specimen must be large enough to permit an ad-

equate diagnosis. It is best to include the most raised area of the lesion if adequate microstaging is desired. An excisional biopsy entails removal of the entire lesion, leaving only normal tissue at the excised wound edge.

Should an incisional or excisional biopsy be performed?
When possible, an excisional biopsy should be performed. In some areas, such as the face or scalp, excision may not be cosmetically acceptable until a diagnosis of malignancy is established. Incisional biopsy should then be used for initial histologic examination. Punch biopsy can provide a full-thickness sample without the need for suture closure. Superficial skin biopsy by shaving should never be used when melanoma is the suspected diagnosis because this technique may not provide a specimen that is deep enough to extend into the tumor proper. Not only will the diagnosis be missed in such cases, but the partial removal of the upper layers of tumor may interfere with microstaging on subsequent excision.

Why is an excisional biopsy preferable?
An excisional biopsy is preferable because it provides the pathologist with the entire lesion. This allows the deepest extent of the tumor to be determined for microstaging purposes (discussed later). Sometimes, an incisional biopsy permits only a histologic diagnosis and not an accurate determination of the depth of invasion. In addition, excision with adequate margins may obviate further intervention when a thin melanoma or preinvasive lesion is encountered.

Mr. O'Shea notes some itching in addition to the change in size and shape of his mole.

What should the next step be in the management of Mr. O'Shea's mole?
The remaining lesion should be excised.

Biopsy results show a melanoma invasive into the reticular dermis. The thickness of the lesion is 1.4 mm.

How are melanomas staged clinically? What is Mr. O'Shea's stage?
Melanoma is stage I if it is local to the upper dermis, stage II if local to the lower dermis, stage III if invasive into subcutaneous tissue or involving regional nodes, and stage IV if distant metastases are present (11). The information provided indicates that Mr. O'Shea's tumor is at least stage II because the deeper dermis is involved. Nothing is known regarding regional nodes or distant metastatic sites at this point. The thinness of his tumor (less than 1.5 mm) would ordinarily place him in the stage I category, but the prior shave biopsy has removed the upper portion of the tumor, making the Clark's level a more reliable measure of invasion in this instance (discussed next).

What is the microstaging used for melanoma?
The two systems commonly used are the level of skin invasion (Clark's level) and tumor thickness (Breslow's). Both are now incorporated as measures of tumor in the tumor, node, metastasis (TNM) classification system (Table 28.1). Clark's level is based on the anatomic depth of skin to which the tumor invades (12). The levels are as follows:

I   Confined to the dermal–epidermal junction
II   Invading the papillary dermis only
III Extending to the junction of the papillary and reticular dermis
IV   Invading the reticular dermis
V   Extending into subcutaneous tissues

Breslow's microstaging uses an ocular micrometer to measure the thickness of the lesion in millimeters below the granular layer of the epidermis (13). Four levels correlate with increasingly poor prognosis: tumor up to 0.75 mm thick; tumor thicker than 0.75 and up to 1.5 mm thick; tumor thicker than 1.5 and up to 4 mm thick; and tumor thicker than 4 mm.

Is one microstaging system more accurate in predicting survival than the other?
The tumor thickness (Breslow) is a more accurate predictor of survival than is Clark's level of invasion. In studies in which survival was correlated to both tumor thickness and level of invasion, it was found that within each Clark's level there was a wide variation in Breslow thickness and in the associated 5-year survival rates. At various Clark's levels, comparable Breslow measurements were associated with similar 5-year survival rates when matched to thickness. Thus, Breslow thickness appears to be a more consistent prognostic indicator (14). Thickness can be altered by inappropriate removal of the upper portion of a tumor through shave biopsy, however. Under these circumstances, Clark's levels may indicate the true stage when a discrepancy between the two levels is found.

Table 28.1.   MELANOMA MICROSTAGING

Microstage	Characteristics
Tis	Melanoma in situ, not invasive (Clark's level I)
T_1	Tumor 0.75 mm or less thick invading papillary dermis
T_2	Tumor more than 0.75 mm but not more than 1.5 mm thick or invading the papillary–reticular dermal interface (Clark's level III)
T_3	Tumor more than 1.5 mm but not more than 4 mm thick or invading reticular dermis (Clark's level IV)
T_4	Tumor more than 4 mm thick or invading subcutaneous tissue (Clark's level IV) or satellite(s) within 2 cm of primary tumor

Mr. O'Shea's lesion is on his upper back.

Does this location provide any specific prognostic information?
The upper back is part of the so-called BANS area, which includes the upper back, posterior arm, posterior neck, and posterior scalp. It used to be thought that lesions in the BANS area had a poor prognosis because the dermis was thin, allowing for early invasion into the lymphatics. Recent data suggest that this may not be the case (15).

What is the primary treatment of melanoma? What constitutes an adequate margin for these tumors?
Local melanoma can be cured by excision alone. Three prospective studies have established that 2-cm margins are adequate to treat melanomas up to 4 mm thick (16–19). Even narrower margins are adequate for thinner melanomas, as established by a prospective World Health Organization (WHO) study (17). Current recommendations are that in situ tumors (Clark's level I) be excised with 0.5- to 1-cm margins, melanomas less than 1 mm thick be excised with 1-cm margins, and melanomas 2 to 4 mm thick be excised with 2-cm margins. Melanomas that are 1 to 2 mm thick fall into a gray area. The WHO study shows that overall survival is the same whether 1- or 2-cm margins are used, but there is a slightly higher level of local relapse with the narrower margins. It is probably safer to use 2-cm margins whenever possible for such tumors, reserving 1-cm margins for situations in which a local flap or skin graft would be required for closure (20). Margins wider than 2 cm may be appropriate for tumors that extend deeper than 4 mm.

Should the underlying fascia be removed with the specimen?
There is no evidence that removal of the muscular fascia improves local control or long-term survival. Unless the tumor extends to the fascia, there is no reason to include it in the resection.

Should regional lymph nodes be included at the time of initial local excision?
Elective lymph node dissection (ELND) has been proposed as a means of removing microscopic deposits in nodes before they progress to distant disease. The rationale for this procedure is based on the observation that patients with microscopic nodal deposits at the time of node dissection have better survival rates (50%) than patients with gross nodal involvement (15%) (21). A number of retrospective studies also have shown improved survival when ELND is added to local excision for a 1- to 4-mm-thick tumor. Two prospective randomized surgical trials have failed to confirm a survival benefit for ELND, however (22, 23). The most recent trial, the Intergroup Melanoma Surgical Trial, did show that ELND was beneficial for certain subgroups, namely patients who were 60 years of age or younger with 1- to 2-mm-thick tumors that had not

ulcerated. For patients with these characteristics, ELND appears to improve survival by 10% at 5 years ($p < .005$) (23). For other patients, ELND actually may lower survival.

Are there any drawbacks to ELND?
Expected complications after axillary dissection include wound infections (11%), wound separation (3.5%), and lymphedema (3%). The resulting disability may add 21 to 30 days to the time lost from work for surgical treatment of melanoma. For inguinal node dissection, complications occur in as many as 50% of patients, including wound infections (21%), wound separation (20%), and lymphedema (21%) (23).

Mr. O'Shea is a 45-year-old man with an intermediate-thickness nonulcerated melanoma of the upper back.

Which nodal basin should be dissected to provide him with the benefits of ELND?
Lesions of the upper back may metastasize to the cervical or axillary nodal basin. If the lesion is near the midline, either side or both sides may drain the primary site. To determine which basin is most likely to contain nodal metastases, preoperative lymphatic mapping (i.e., lymphoscintigraphy) can be carried out by injecting ^{99}Tc-labeled albumin or sulfur colloid in the subcuticular space around the tumor and scanning the patient to determine the nodal basins draining the tumor-bearing area.

Is there any way to limit the complications of dissection in the patients who have involved nodes?
Studies now under way are addressing whether intraoperative lymphatic mapping by tumor injection of isosulfan blue (Lymphazurin), a vital blue dye, or ^{99}Tc–sulfa colloid to identify the first draining node (sentinel node) allows a limited sampling to replace full node dissection in patients without nodal metastasis. Pilot studies indicate that fewer than 2% of patients with negative sentinel nodes according to these tests, will develop recurrent tumor in undissected nodal basin.

Suppose Mr. O'Shea had a 2- to 3-cm firm node palpated in his right axilla. Is there any reason to perform an axillary dissection, considering the poor prognosis of stage III disease?
Surgical removal is still the most effective treatment for regional nodal metastases. Survival rates as high as 40% at 10 years can be achieved with node dissection alone when only one node is affected. With two to four positive nodes, survival drops to 26%; with five or more positive nodes, survival drops to 15%.

Are effective adjuvant treatments available to patients with positive nodes?
Until recently, no systemic therapy had shown a significant survival advantage for patients with melanoma. Recombinant interferon (IFN-α_{2b}) has been

shown to improve the survival of node-positive stage III patients when given at maximally tolerated intravenous and subcutaneous doses for 1 year after node dissection (24).

Mr. O'Shea undergoes wide excision of his melanoma and an axillary node dissection. He accepts interferon treatment postoperatively but gives up after the first month because of toxicity. Six months later he has progressive symptoms of crampy abdominal pain. Physical examination is unremarkable except for heme-positive stool on rectal examination.

What is the diagnosis?
Along with the usual causes of gastrointestinal blood loss, metastatic melanoma in the small bowel must be considered. This is a common site for metastatic disease. Other common sites are the liver, lungs, brain, skin, and bone.

Is there a role for surgery in the treatment of metastatic disease? Is systemic therapy effective?
With rare exceptions, resection of metastatic disease is palliative. Patients may benefit from resection of metastatic lesions that are symptomatic if the patients' overall condition warrants intervention. Gastrointestinal metastases that produce obstruction or significant hemorrhage fit this category. Long survivals, up to 20 years, have occasionally resulted from removal of a solitary gastric or intestinal metastasis. Survival after resection of brain metastases combined with radiation also appears better than survival after radiation alone. A number of nonsurgical approaches to widespread disease, including chemotherapy, immunotherapy, and irradiation, have provided only temporary and inconsistent results.

Suppose Mr. O'Shea's melanoma was deeper than 4 mm and just above his left knee on the anterior thigh. Does this location suggest any additional therapeutic modality?
Patients with advanced extremity lesions may be candidates for regional hyperthermic perfusion. This treatment entails tourniquet isolation of the extremity and cannulation of the vessels supplying the affected limb. Chemotherapeutic agents (usually melphalan) are infused at temperatures up to 40°C for at least 1 hour through an extracorporeal membrane oxygenation system. A large number of patients have received this treatment; however, no unifying criteria for treatment have been established, which makes it difficult to draw conclusions. At best, it may be fair to say that local chemotherapy results in local or regional control for a limited amount of time.

Are there noncutaneous forms of melanoma?
Yes, primary melanomas of the mucous membranes occur mainly in the head and neck and in the vulva or vagina. A study of 47 patients older than 27 years

indicates that head and neck tumors are the most common (43%), followed by the vulva (30%) and vagina (15%). Other sites include the anorectum (6%) and the esophagus (2%). The overall 5-year survival rate of these patients was less than 25%) (25).

Management Algorithm for Suspicious Nevus

Algorithm 28.1.

How does melanoma of the anorectum typically present?
Unfortunately, anorectal melanoma usually presents with rectal bleeding, which is a sign of advanced and locally invasive disease.

What is the general prognosis of patients with anorectal melanoma?
Because of the occult nature of anorectal melanoma, it may go undetected, resulting in locally advanced invasive disease. Abdominoperineal resection has been attempted with poor survival rates, less than 10%, at 5 years. Fortunately, this form of melanoma is rare, accounting for fewer than 1% of all primary melanomas.

Should a patient with a history of melanoma receive an ophthalmologic evaluation?
Yes. Both primary and metastatic ocular melanomas have been described. These lesions usually arise from the choroidal layer, and as with cutaneous melanoma, if they are recognized and treated early, the prognosis is relatively good.

Thorough workup of Mr. O'Shea did not reveal any metastatic melanoma, and his abdominal symptoms resolved without intervention. He is discharged with a follow-up appointment a month later.

REFERENCES

1. Reed RJ, Ichinose H, Clark WH, et al. Common and uncommon melanocytic nevi and borderline melanomas. Semin Oncol 1975;2:119–147.
2. Weedon D, Little JH. Spindle and epithelioid cell nevi in children and adults: a review of 211 cases of the Spitz nevus. Cancer 1977;40:217–225.
3. Paniago-Pereira C, Maize JC, Ackerman AB. Nevus of large spindle and/or epithelioid cells (Spitz's nevus). Arch Dermatol 1978;144:1811–1823.
4. Landis SH, Murray T, Bolden S, et al. Cancer statistics 1998. CA Cancer J Clin 1998; 48:6–29.
5. Balch CM, Soong SJ, Multon GW, et al. Changing trends in cutaneous melanoma over a quarter century in Alabama, USA, and New South Wales, Australia. Cancer 1983; 52:1748–1753.
6. Korsary CL, Ries LAG, Miller BA, et al. SEER Cancer Statistics Review, 1973–1992. Tables and graphs. NIH Pub 96–2789. Bethesda, MD: National Cancer Institute, 1995 (abstract).
7. Balch CM, Soong SJ, Shaw HM, et al. An analysis of prognostic factors in 8500 patients with cutaneous melanoma. In: Balch CM, Houghton AN, Milton GW, et al., eds. Cutaneous Melanoma. 2nd ed. Philadelphia: Lippincott, 1992:165–187.
8. Balch CM et al. Management of cutaneous melanoma in the United States. Surg Gynecol Obstet 1984;158:311–318.
9. Greene MH, Clark WH, Tucker MA, et al. Acquired precursors of cutaneous malignant melanoma. The familial dysplastic nevus syndrome. N Engl J Med 1985;312:91–97.
10. Langley RGB, Fitzpatrick TB, Sober AJ. Clinical characteristics. In: Balch CM,

Houghton AN, Sober AJ, et al., eds. Cutaneous Melanoma. 3rd ed. St. Louis: Quality Medical, 1998:82–101.

11. Fleming ID, Cooper JS, Hanson DE, et al., eds. AJCC Cancer Staging Manual. 5th ed. Philadelphia: Lippincott-Raven, 1997:163–167.

12. Clark W Jr, From L, Bernardino E, et al. The histogenesis and biologic behavior of primary human malignant melanomas of the skin. Cancer Res 1969;29:705–727.

13. Breslow A. Thickness, cross-sectional areas and depth of invasion in the prognosis of cutaneous melanoma. Ann Surg 1970;172:902–908.

14. Vollmer RT. Malignant melanoma: a multivariate analysis of prognostic factors. Pathol Annu 1989;24:383–407.

15. Stadelmann WK, Rapaport DP, Soong SJ, et al. Prognostic, clinical and pathologic features. In: Balch CM, Houghton AN, Sober AJ, et al., eds. Cutaneous Melanoma. 3rd ed. St. Louis: Quality Medical, 1998:15–35.

16. Veronesi U, Cascinelli N. Narrow excision (1 cm margin): a safe procedure for thin cutaneous melanoma. Arch Surg 1991;126:438–441.

17. French Cooperative Group. In: Balch CM, Houghton AN, Sober AJ, et al., eds. Cutaneous Melanoma. 3rd ed. St. Louis: Quality Medical, 1998:143.

18. Balch CM, Urist MM, Karakousis CP, et al. Efficacy of 2 cm surgical margins for intermediate-thickness melanomas (1–4 mm): Results of a multi-institutional randomized surgical trial. Ann Surg 1993;218:262–267.

19. Karakousis CP, Balch CM, Urist MM, et al. Local recurrence in malignant melanoma: long-term results of the multi-institutional randomized surgical trial. Ann Surg Oncol 1996;3:446–452.

20. Reintgen DS, Albertini J, Miliotes G, et al. The accurate staging and modern day treatment of malignant melanoma. Cancer Res Ther Control 1995;4:183.

21. Veronesi U, Adamus J, Bandiera DC, et al. Inefficacy of immediate node dissection in stage I melanoma of the limbs. N Engl J Med 1997;297:627–630.

22. Sim FH, Taylor WF, Pritchard DJ, et al. Lymphadenectomy in the management of stage I malignant melanoma: a prospective randomized study. Mayo Clin Proc 1986;61:697–705.

23. Balch CM, Soong SJ, Bartolucci AA, et al. Efficacy of an elective regional lymph node dissection of 1 to 4 mm thick melanomas for patients 60 years of age and younger. Ann Surg 1996;224:255–263.

24. Kirkwood J, Strawderman MH, Ernstoff MS, et al. Interferon alfa-2b adjuvant therapy of high-risk resected cutaneous melanoma. Eastern Cooperative Oncology Group Trial EST 1684. J Clin Oncol 1996;14:7–17.

25. Iversen K, Robins RE. Mucosal malignant melanomas. Am J Surg 1980;139:660–664.

CHAPTER
29

Burn Injury

Larry L. Shears II and Andrew B. Peitzman

During a severe thunderstorm, the home of the Joneses is struck by lightening. The house catches fire, trapping Lucy Jones and her infant son, Thomas. Luke Jones, who was about to enter the house, is thrown to the ground unconscious after sustaining a high-voltage electric shock. A neighbor witnessing the event pulls Mrs. Jones and Thomas from the burning home and smothers their smoldering clothes with a blanket. Mrs. Jones has obvious burns on most of her torso and upper extremities. Thomas has burns on both upper extremities. Paramedics arrive quickly.

Which of these patients would benefit from an urgent transfer to a trauma center equipped with an established burn unit?

All three. The American Burn Association has established guidelines indicating whose patients' outcomes are most likely to be improved by treatment in a burn unit (1). These guidelines include the following:

1. Second- and third-degree burns involving more than 10% of body surface area (BSA) in patients younger than 10 or older than 50 years of age
2. More than 20% BSA burned in a patient of any age
3. Full-thickness burns over more than 5% BSA
4. Burns to face, hands, feet, or perineum that may result in cosmetic or functional disability
5. High-voltage electric shock
6. Suspected inhalation injury
7. Significant chemical burns
8. Significant burns in patients with severe premorbid disease

In assessing these three patients, what are the initial priorities in their acute medical management?

All trauma patients, regardless of age or mechanism of injury, should undergo a rapid assessment of the ABCs—airway, breathing, and circulation. Although severe injuries can be distracting, failure to address the ABCs places patients at risk. In addition, all burn patients trapped in a closed space are at risk for carbon monoxide poisoning and should be treated immediately with 100% humidified oxygen. Carbon monoxide has an affinity for hemoglobin that is 200 times that of oxygen. This shifts the oxyhemoglobin dissociation curve to the left, reducing the ability of hemoglobin to deliver oxygen to the peripheral tissues (2). Administering 100% oxygen helps overcome the competitive binding for hemoglobin by carbon monoxide. Upper airway edema can progress rapidly, resulting in complete airway obstruction. Therefore, early intubation is essential if inhalation injury is suspected.

Upon arrival to the local trauma center, Mrs Jones becomes acutely agitated, confused, and combative. Her vital signs are as follows: pulse, 98 beats per minute; blood pressure, 148/89 mm Hg; and respiratory rate, 28 breaths per minute.

What is the most likely cause of her confusion?
Hypoxia, carbon monoxide poisoning, and hemodynamic instability all can alter the mental status of a burn trauma patient. Inhalation injury, the most common cause of death in burn patients, can be due to direct inhalation of superheated air, water vapor, toxic chemicals, or a combination thereof. Many patients with inhalation injury rapidly develop extensive oropharyngeal edema, which can quickly close a previously patent airway.

What physical findings suggest inhalation injury?
Inhalation injury should be assumed in all burn patients until proven otherwise. A history of burn injury in an enclosed space, facial burns, singed facial hair, hoarseness, coughing, wheezing, and carbonaceous sputum all suggest inhalation injury. These findings should prompt bronchoscopy to evaluate for upper airway erythema or edema. The bronchoscopy should be performed with an endotracheal tube over the scope to allow rapid nasotracheal intubation if the airway is inadvertently lost. Visibly reddened and ulcerated mucosa is a reliable indicator of infraglottic airway injury. Also, ^{133}Xe lung scans can provide insight into any significant injury at the level of the alveoli (3). [133]Xe is injected intravenously but readily diffuses across the alveolar capillary membrane. The alveolar clearance of ^{133}Xe is delayed in patients with significant alveolar injury. This test does not quantify the alveolar injury, but it is a qualitative marker of significant infraglottic injury.

What physical findings and objective data suggest carbon monoxide poisoning?
Cherry-red skin, hypoxemia, mental status changes, and persistent acidosis are findings consistent with carbon monoxide poisoning. Patients suspected of having carbon monoxide poisoning immediately should be administered 100%

oxygen. Hyperbaric therapy in patients with severe carbon monoxide toxicity may prevent the long-term sequela of neurologic injury. In general, levels above 20% are associated with neurologic symptoms. Levels above 60% commonly result in death. The normal carboxyhemoglobin level is below 5% for nonsmokers and below 10% for smokers. It is important to remember that carbon monoxide negates the reliability of pulse oximetry.

Describe the course of inhalation injury.
Initially, patients develop acute pulmonary insufficiency secondary to carbon monoxide poisoning, tracheobronchitis, bronchospasm, tracheobronchial edema, and atelectasis. Pulmonary edema develops hours to days after the injury. Pneumonia usually occurs 5 to 10 days after the injury.

Mrs. Jones is intubated uneventfully. She is found to have burns with blisters over the anterior and posterior portions of her chest and abdomen. Her left thigh appears pale and firm and is insensate.

How is the severity of burns evaluated?
Burns are classified as superficial, partial, or full thickness. They can worsen over time, eventually progressing to a full-thickness injury.

Superficial burns (first-degree burns) are erythematous without blistering and are associated with pain that usually resolves over 48 to 72 hours. Sunburn is an example of a superficial burn.
Partial-thickness burns (second-degree burns) involve the entire epidermis and variable layers of dermis. The skin is painful and erythematous, with blisters. Because dermal appendages are still present with these injuries, spontaneous healing may occur in a matter of weeks.
Full-thickness burns (third-degree burns) involve the entire dermis and epidermis, destroying all dermal appendages. Therefore, no reepithelialization occurs in full-thickness injuries. They appear leathery and are not painful. Healing requires debridement and skin grafting.

What percent of Mrs. Jones's body was burned?
Mrs. Jones had burns on 54% of her body. The calculation of burned BSA is estimated with the *rule of nines,* a method of determining the percent of involved BSA: the head and arms contribute 9% each, the front and back of the torso contribute 18% each, and each lower extremity contributes 18%. The perineum contributes 1%. In children, the head is disproportionately larger than in adults and thus the rule of nines is not applicable (4).

Thomas has erythematous changes and blistering around his left arm and hand. His entire back is similarly involved.

What percent of his body was burned?
Thomas has burns on 27% of his body.

Despite being intubated, it becomes difficult to ventilate Mrs. Jones. The monitor on the ventilator keeps indicating elevated peak airway pressures. Her blood gas reveals a pH of 7.21, a P_{CO_2} of 58, and a P_{O_2} of 65.

What is the likely reason for the difficulty in ventilating Mrs. Jones?
Mrs. Jones is burned over much of her trunk. Circumferential burns on the trunk can be life-threatening. The eschar does not expand as normal skin would. In addition, the accumulation of edema fluid and swelling further compresses the chest cavity. Urgent release of the constricting band is accomplished by use of longitudinal escharotomy. Because the eschar is the result of a full-thickness injury, escharotomy is painless and can be performed at the bedside. Incisions are made bilaterally along the anterior axillary line extending from the clavicle to the costal margin. These incisions are joined by a transverse escharotomy at the level of the costal margin. Escharotomies are most often required to relieve compartment syndromes in extremities suffering circumferential burns. Without urgent escharotomy, these limbs are at risk for irreversible ischemic injury.

After Mrs. Jones's respiratory problems are completely addressed, the nurse tending her addresses the need for intravenous fluids.

How much fluid should Mrs. Jones receive?
The most commonly used formula to assess a burn patient's fluid requirement during the first 24 hours is based on the Parkland formula. Using this formula, 4 mL of crystalloid per kilogram of body weight multiplied by the percentage of BSA with second- and third-degree burns is delivered over the first 24 hours. Half of the volume is delivered over the first 8 hours and the remainder over the remaining 16 hours. Isotonic salt solutions, such as lactated Ringer's, are recommended to replace the high sodium losses in burn patients. Glucose-containing solutions should be avoided because burn patients are often hyperglycemic and glucose intolerant. Hyperglycemia resulting from such large-volume infusions may induce a rapid diuresis secondary to glucose spilling in the urine. Remember that these formulas produce only an estimate of the volume that may be required. The rate of the fluid infusion must be sufficient to maintain adequate intravascular volume as evidenced by end organ perfusion. This is most easily assessed by monitoring a patient's urine output. In adults, urine output should be at least 0.5 mL/kg body weight; in children weighing less than 30 kg, output should be at least 1 mL/kg body weight.

Do fluid requirements change after the initial resuscitation?
Yes. Capillary integrity is restored after 24 hours, allowing colloids to remain in the vascular space; 5% colloid solutions are often used. A colloid administered at 0.3 to 0.5 mL/kg per percent burned BSA in conjunction with clinical monitoring is a good starting point. Clinical monitoring should include hourly assessments of urine output and, in patients with questionable cardiac function, pulmonary artery catheters.

After Mrs. Jones's cardiopulmonary status is stabilized, her wounds are addressed.

How should her burn wounds be managed initially?
Once the patient is hemodynamically stable, the burn wounds should be cleaned with a mild topical antimicrobial agent either at the bedside or, if possible, in a heated bath. Blisters are gently debrided. Once the patient has complete fluid resuscitation and the pulmonary status is stabilized, a vigorous excision of eschars and a skin-grafting program should be initiated. This approach is used to limit the metabolic effects of the burn injury and to reduce the risk of developing wound sepsis. Areas of full-thickness injury should be fully excised and grafted or covered with any of various types of gauze dressings, biologic dressings, or both. These dressings are used to stimulate granulation tissue to prepare for eventual skin grafting. Once an acceptable granulation bed is obtained, the patient can be taken to the operating room for definitive skin grafting.

What types of topical antimicrobial agents are used on burn patients, and what are their advantages and disadvantages?
Topical antimicrobial agents in burn wounds significantly decrease the occurrence of invasive burn wound infections and improve the survival rates for these patients. They are as follows (5):

Sodium mafenide acetate (Sulfamylon) penetrates eschars well and has the broadest spectrum of activity against *Pseudomonas*. However, it inhibits carbonic anhydrase and can induce significant metabolic acidosis and hyperventilation. Also, it is painful when applied.
Silver sulfadiazine (Silvadene) is bacteriostatic but lacks the penetrating ability of sodium mafenide acetate and can also result in neutropenia. Unlike sodium mafenide acetate, silver sulfadiazine is not painful when applied.
Silver nitrate solution 0.5% is also bacteriostatic, but it discolors the skin and causes hyponatremia and hypochloremia.
Povidone iodine (Betadine), despite its antiseptic activity, is seldom used on burn wounds because of its excessive drying of the eschar.

What are the most common organisms cultured in burn wounds, and how are invasive wound infections identified?
Burn wounds are quickly colonized by several organisms, including *Staphylococcus aureus*, Streptococcus, *Pseudomonas aeruginosa*, *Escherichia coli*, Enterococcus, and *Candida albicans*. Invasive wound infection is determined by full-thickness biopsy. Quantitative cultures are performed on the tissue. More than 10^5 organisms per gram of tissue is diagnostic of an invasive infection. Systemic antibiotics have no role in treating wound colonization because the drugs do not penetrate into the eschar. However, systemic antibiotics are warranted for invasive wound infections. Broad-spectrum agents that cover gram-positive and gram-negative organisms should be used until culture findings return to normal.

Should burn patients receive tetanus prophylaxis?
Yes. All burn wounds should be considered contaminated. Therefore, tetanus prophylaxis is mandatory except for patients immunized within the preceding 12 months. If the patient has had a booster within the preceding 10 years, tetanus toxoid is usually adequate. If the patient has not been previously immunized, the patient should be treated with tetanus immunoglobulins as well as with the standard immunization.

Mrs. Jones undergoes extensive debridement of her eschars and is in the intensive care unit (ICU) on a ventilator.

What effect does her injury have on her normal resting metabolic rate?
Burn injuries induce the most pronounced hypermetabolic responses of all injuries. Energy requirements for burn patients increase by 1.5 to 2 times the normal rate in patients with burns covering greater than 50% BSA. This hypermetabolic response is manifested by hyperventilation, increased oxygen consumption, tachycardia, fever, weight loss, and negative nitrogen balance. These manifestations commonly result in difficulty in extubating the patient, increasing the susceptibility to infection and retarding the wound healing process. Optimal calorie-nitrogen ratios in burn patients vary from 100:1 to 150:1 to achieve a positive nitrogen balance (6).

What is the best way to provide nutrition to the burn patient?
Many burn patients develop an ileus, necessitating parenteral nutrition. However, this form of nutrition is fraught with infectious complications and complications associated with line placement. Therefore, when possible, enteral nutrition is preferred.

Mrs. Jones undergoes successful surgical debridement of deep second-degree burns and successful debridement and skin grafting of her third-degree burns. Her hemodynamic status stabilizes, her organ

perfusion is good, she is receiving adequate nutrition, and her ventilatory requirements are decreasing.

What are the principles of wound care now that healing has begun?
Nongrafted burn sites require daily gentle care. Hypothermia and hemodynamic instability during wound care should be prevented, as should the inevitable pain and pyrogenic response associated with daily wound care. Therefore, analgesics and antipyretics are essential.

How can scarring be minimized?
Early excision and skin grafting of deep dermal burns initiates epithelialization, minimizes collagen deposition, and provides a barrier to infection. Burn wounds that have not been grafted have a higher population of fibroblasts and myofibroblasts and correspondingly greater amounts of collagen deposition. Wound contracture is also proportional to the quantity of myofibroblasts in the wound.

How do pressure dressings reduce hypertrophic scarring?
Pressure dressings with elastic (Ace) bandages and later with fitted garments minimize hypertrophic scarring. Although the precise mechanism is unclear, pressure applied to a wound minimizes edema, reduces the relative number of myofibroblasts in the wound, and decreases total collagen synthesis. The pressure must be applied continuously and used until the wound matures.

Like his wife, Mr. Jones is transferred to the local burn unit. During transfer, Mr. Jones regains consciousness and is hemodynamically stable. His wounds consist of an entrance site in the left forearm and a large exit site in his right lower leg. Both sites are smaller than 10 cm.

Has Mr. Jones suffered significant burn injury?
Yes. Electrical injuries produce significant damage that may show only minimal exterior skin involvement. However, the underlying muscle and organs may be severely injured. Tissue injury is most evident in muscle and nerve tissue. Early surgical debridement is necessary to remove dead tissue and open fascial compartments. Extremities involved in electric shock injuries are at high risk for compartment syndromes due to the extensive damage to the underlying tissue. Fascial compartment pressures greater than 30 mm Hg require fasciotomy. Additionally, a high proportion of electric shock burns are associated with significant blunt trauma from falls. A thorough history from emergency medical technicians and other rescue personnel is important.

Low-voltage electric shock is classified as less than 1000 volts. This type of injury is likely to occur at home or in the office. High-voltage injuries (more than

Management Algorithm for Burn Injury

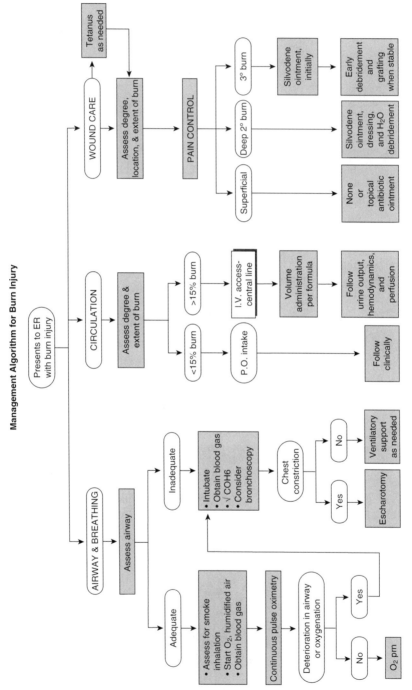

Algorithm 29.1.

1000 volts) occur outdoors and involve power lines and equipment (7). High-voltage current passes indiscriminately through any body tissue and can cause severe tissue destruction and coagulation necrosis.

Do standard fluid requirement formulas apply for patients with severe electric shock injury? No. The degree of tissue injury is unpredictable with electric shock burns. Standard formulas for fluid resuscitation may be used as a starting estimate, but monitoring to ensure adequate systemic perfusion is essential.

Mr. Jones's urine is noted to be very dark. What may be the significance of this finding? The energy contained by the electric charge is dissipated in the skin in the form of heat. Heat necrosis in muscle can result in the destruction of large amounts of muscle and the release of detrimental amounts of myoglobin. Myoglobin can precipitate in the collecting tubules of the kidneys and ultimately cause renal failure. Patients suspected of having myoglobinuria should be aggressively hydrated to maintain an induced diuresis in excess of 1 mL/kg per hour to help clear the pigment load. Mannitol and other diuretics can also be used to facilitate the diuresis. Sodium bicarbonate can be given systemically in an attempt to alkalinize the urine, as myoglobin precipitates more readily in acidic fluids.

Mr. Jones requires fasciotomy of both his forearm and right leg, after which pulses and perfusion are restored. His entrance and exit wounds heal with local wound care, and the fasciotomy sites are skin grafted uneventfully.

REFERENCES

1. American College of Surgeons Committee on Trauma. Injuries due to burns and cold. In: Advanced Trauma Life Support Program for Doctors. Chicago: American College of Surgeons, 1997:346.
2. Stewart RD. The effect of carbon monoxide to humans. Ann Rev Pharmacol 1975; 15:409.
3. Goodwin CW, Finkelstein JL, Madden MR. Burns. In: Schwartz S, Shires T, Spencer F, eds. Principles of Surgery. 6th ed. New York: McGraw-Hill, 1994:242–243.
4. American College of Surgeons Committee on Trauma. Injuries due to burns and cold. In: Advanced Trauma Life Support Program for Doctors. Chicago: American College of Surgeons, 1997:341.
5. McManus WF, Pruitt BA Jr. Thermal injuries. In: Feliciano DV, Moore EE, Mattox KL, eds. Trauma. 3rd ed. Stanford, CT: Appleton & Lange, 1996:943–945.
6. Demling RI. Burns: after the first postburn week. In: Wilmore DW, Brennan MF, Harken AH, et al., eds. Care of the Surgical Patient. New York: Scientific American 1989;3:5–6.
7. Goodwin CW, Finkelstein JL, Madden MR. Burns. In: Schwartz, Shires, Spencer, eds. Principles of Surgery. 6th ed. New York: McGraw-Hill, 1994:263.

Trauma: Initial Assessment

Bruce J. Simon

Corey Smith, a 28-year-old man, is brought in by the volunteer ambulance squad after he is involved in a motor vehicle collision. He is clearly unconscious and does not open his eyes or respond to verbal or physical stimuli. He has obvious facial abrasions and contusions. Mr. Smith is in a cervical collar, and an intravenous line connected to a bag of lactated Ringer's solution has been inserted. His breathing is shallow and spontaneous at 22 breaths per minute.

What helpful information can the ambulance crew provide?
Information on the mechanism of injury is useful because the mechanism may correlate with the type and severity of the injuries. If vital signs are abnormal at the scene, serious injury should be suspected. Evidence of depressed level of consciousness immediately after the accident indicates a possible closed head injury. Patients with a loss of consciousness lasting more than 5 minutes have an increased likelihood of significant head injury even if they are mentating normally on admission (1).

The squad reports that the patient was not in a seat restraint when he drove into a telephone pole at high speed. The front of the car was heavily damaged, and there was no air bag. At the scene, the patient's blood pressure was 170/90 mm Hg and his heart rate was 110 beats per second. He was unconscious and totally unresponsive to pain, and his Glasgow Coma Scale score was 3. A significant quantity of blood was lost at the scene from a forearm laceration.

What is the Glasgow Coma Scale, and what is its significance in evaluation of trauma patients?
The Glasgow Coma Scale (2) (Table 30.1) is an objective measure of level of consciousness in patients with head trauma. It grades three indicators of neurologic performance: motor, verbal, and eye-opening responses. It has prognostic value at time of admission and provides a common base for different ex-

Table 30.1.   GLASGOW COMA SCALE

Indicator	Score
Eye opening	
Spontaneous	4
To voice	3
To pain	2
None	1
Verbal response	
Oriented	5
Confused	4
Inappropriate words	3
Incomprehensible words	2
None	1
Motor response	
Obeys command	6
Purposeful movement (pain)	5
Withdraw (pain)	4
Flexion (pain)	3
Extension (pain)	2
None	1
Total GCS points	3–16

Reprinted with permission from Michael DB, Wilson RF. Head injuries. In: Wilson RF, Walt AJ, eds. Management of Trauma: Pitfalls and Practice. Baltimore: Williams & Wilkins, 1996:173–202.

aminers to evaluate changes in the neurologic examination over time. The normal (and maximum) score is 15; the minimum score is 3. A Glasgow Coma Scale score of 8 or less indicates coma.

What basic therapeutic interventions and initial monitoring procedures are appropriate for all patients with major trauma?
All trauma patients should receive a balanced salt solution, usually lactated Ringer's solution, through two large-bore intravenous cannulas placed in a peripheral vein. If airway control is not indicated, high-flow oxygen should be delivered via mask. Patients should be immobilized until injuries to the axial skeleton are ruled out. Baseline monitoring consists of cardiac rhythm measurement, noninvasive blood pressure measurement, pulse oximetry, and capnography if the patient is intubated. Pulse oximetry by monitoring oxygen saturation and pulse amplitude via the toes or fingers (3) may warn of pulmonary or cardiovascular deterioration before the condition becomes clinically evident. Capnography measures the carbon dioxide tension in expired air. A sudden decrease in the tension may suggest mechanical problems in the airway or hypoventilation (4).

As Mr. Smith is being moved to the trauma room stretcher, he is connected to cardiac and blood pressure monitors and a pulse oximeter. His blood pressure is 120/90 mm Hg, his heart rate is 105 beats per minute, and the arterial oxygen saturation is 99% with a 100% nonrebreathing oxygen mask.

What principles guide the initial assessment in trauma patients?
Trauma patients are assessed through a protocol of primary and secondary surveys. The primary survey follows an ABCDE sequential protocol in which immediately life-threatening problems are treated as they are identified and in order of their level of threat to the patient (Table 30.2) (5).

Airway is always addressed first regardless of the type of injuries. By definition, a patient who can talk has a patent airway. Signs of possible airway obstruction include agitation, stridor, decreased breath sounds, and evidence of increased airway resistance such as respiratory retractions and accessory muscle breathing. An unconscious patient must be presumed to have an occluded airway, in which case the oropharynx must be suctioned for debris, an oral airway placed, and the airway then definitively controlled.
Breathing is assessed by auscultation, percussion, and visualization of the chest wall to determine respiratory rate and depth. The goal of breathing is to provide adequate oxygenation and ventilation, which are assessed by signs such as cyanosis and altered mentation and from information provided by pulse oximetry. However, a person with inadequate breathing mechanics manifests inadequate oxygenation or ventilation only as a late event. Early appreciation of the signs of breathing difficulty help lead to timely intervention. Conditions that may impair breathing include tension pneumothorax, flail chest, pulmonary contusion, and hemothorax.
Circulation is best assessed by level of consciousness and pulse. Full, slow, and regular pulses indicate normovolemia, whereas rapid, thready pulses may indicate hypovolemia. Absent central pulses usually indicate profound hypo-

**Table 30.2.   SEQUENTIAL PROTOCOL FOR PRIMARY
SURVEY OF TRAUMA PATIENTS**

A	**Airway** with cervical spine control
B	**Breathing** and ventilation
C	**Circulation** with hemorrhage control
D	**Disability:** neurologic status
E	**Exposure** and environmental control

Reprinted with permission from American College of Surgeons (ACS). Advanced Trauma Life Support Program for Physicians: Instructor Manual. Chicago: ACS, 1993:21.

volemia with impending death if rapid resuscitation is not undertaken. Capillary refill and skin color may also be useful indicators. A person with pink skin is rarely severely hypovolemic, whereas an ashen color characterizes hemorrhage. Bleeding is controlled during the assessment of circulation. **Disability** of the neurologic system is evaluated by means of the Glasgow Coma Scale score and by testing whether the patient moves all extremities. **Exposure** is assessed by removal of all of the patient's clothing, usually by cutting. Because injured persons have impaired thermoregulatory ability, the patient is covered with warm blankets and the ambient temperature is increased to prevent hypothermia.

Should Mr. Smith's airway be controlled, and if so, how?
Although Mr. Smith's pulmonary function is adequate, his mental status is severely depressed, and his airway should be controlled. Those who have Glasgow Coma Scale scores of 8 or less or who are not following commands (Glasgow Coma Scale motor score less than 6) are at risk for respiratory failure. The airway may be obstructed by the flaccid tongue, or progression of intracranial injury may cause the patient to stop breathing. The preferred method of intubation is via the orotracheal route following rapid-sequence anesthesia induced with any of a variety of pharmacologic combinations while a team member maintains in-line cervical spine control. Initially, an oral airway is placed and the patient is preoxygenated with a bag-valve-mask unit. The neck should not be hyperextended, but rather the jaw-lift thrust maneuver should be used to expose the airway. Nasotracheal intubation can be used, but it is contraindicated in this case because of external facial injury. Fractures of the cribriform plate may result in a nasotracheal tube being misguided into the cranial vault. If endotracheal intubation fails, surgical cricothyroidotomy through the cricothyroid membrane is indicated.

Mr. Smith is intubated, and endotracheal positioning of the tube is checked by auscultation and capnography as the primary survey continues. During the assessment of the circulation, brisk arterial bleeding from a deep laceration on his right forearm is noted. Mr. Smith remains normotensive but has tachycardia.

When should bleeding be treated and by what method?
External hemorrhage identified during the initial assessment should be controlled with pressure. Probing deep wounds with clamps outside the operating room is unproductive and may make definitive treatment more difficult. Tourniquets only impede venous drainage and are contraindicated.

How is the degree of hemorrhage assessed? How is appropriate resuscitation performed?
Clinical degrees of hemorrhage are assessed by a grading scale of I to IV, as follows (6) (Table 30.3):

Table 30.3.   ESTIMATED FLUID BLOOD LOSSES BASED ON PATIENT'S INITIAL PRESENTATION

	DEGREE OF HEMORRHAGE			
Parameter	Class I	Class II	Class III	Class IV
Blood loss (mL)	Up to 750	750–500	1500–2000	>2000
Blood loss (% blood volume)	Up to 15%	15–30%	30–40%	>40%
Pulse rate (beats/min)	<100	>100	>120	>140
Blood pressure	Normal	Normal	Low	Low
Pulse pressure	Normal or high	Low	Low	Low
Respiratory rate (breaths/min)	14–20	20–30	30–40	>35
Urine output (mL/hr)	>30	20–30	5–15	Negligible
CNS, mental status	Slightly anxious	Mildly anxious	Anxious and confused	Confused and lethargic
Fluid replacement (3:1 rule)	Crystalloid	Crystalloid	Crystalloid and blood	Crystalloid and blood

Adapted with permission from American College of Surgeons (ACS). Advanced Trauma Life Support Program for Physicians: Instructor Manual. Chicago: ACS, 1993:21.

Class I hemorrhage produces physical findings (loss of 15% of blood volume) that are very subtle. There may be a slight delay in capillary refill and mild tachycardia to less than 100 beats per minute, which is often mistaken for the effects of fear and pain. Blood pressure, pulse pressure, and urine output remain unchanged. Patients with class I hemorrhage should be resuscitated with a balanced crystalloid solution, such as lactated Ringer's solution, three times the volume of estimated blood loss to allow for the distribution volume of crystalloid in the extracellular space.

Class II hemorrhage (loss of 15 to 30% of blood volume) also produces mild clinical signs. Patients have a constellation consisting of mildly delayed capillary refill time, unchanged or minimally increased pulse pressure, mild tachycardia, and tachypnea. Most patients with class II hemorrhage require blood transfusion.

Classes III and IV hemorrhage produce signs that are clearly apparent as life threatening, with profound alterations in perfusion. Class III is loss of 30 to 40% of blood volume, and class IV, loss of more than 40% of blood volume. Patients are cold, constricted, tachycardic, and hypotensive, and their mentation is profoundly altered. All patients with class III or class IV hemorrhage require blood transfusion. The volume of blood transfused should be in excess of the calculated value, because bleeding must be presumed to continue during resuscitation. All class IV and some class III hemorrhages are immediately life threatening, and patients must receive readily available type-specific blood or universal donor blood to avoid delays for cross-matching.

Mr. Smith has a class II hemorrhage, and he is initially resuscitated with crystalloid solution; a transfusion with type-specific cross-matched blood has also been ordered. His heart rate decreases to 90 beats per minute, and the primary survey is continued. The neurologic assessment (disability) reveals that he can move all four extremities and that his response to painful stimuli is purposeful, but he does not follow commands. His eye-opening response is negative and he does not attempt to speak. His Glasgow Coma Scale score is 7. He is fully disrobed and is found to have left chest wall and sternal contusions in addition to the laceration of the right forearm, which has stopped bleeding actively. His right lower leg is angulated and pulses are absent in the right foot, which is slightly pale. He is covered with warm blankets to prevent the rapid development of hypothermia, a certainty in immobilized injured patients, and the ambient temperature is increased to 32 to 35°C.

What are the major presumptive diagnoses at this time?
The persistent alteration in mentation suggests a closed head injury. This group of injuries includes such focal mass lesions as subdural and epidural hematomas and more diffuse processes, such as brain contusions and diffuse axonal or shear injury, caused by sudden deceleration. The chest wall and sternal contusions suggest intrathoracic injury. The deformity of the right lower leg points to a likely fracture of the tibia and fibula. No pulse is felt in the foot, and there may be associated vascular injury.

What therapy is indicated for patients with blunt trauma and suspected head injury? What are the appropriate diagnostic tests?
Brain injury is the leading cause of morbidity and death in patients with blunt trauma (2). The injured brain loses autoregulation, or the ability to maintain a normal cerebral blood flow, leading to variations in cerebral perfusion. Increased pressure in the cranial vault from mass lesions or diffuse edema may contribute to decreased perfusion (7–9). Although there is no treatment for primary head injury, secondary injury can be prevented by scrupulous maintenance of cerebral perfusion. Particular attention must be paid to maintaining euvolemia and normotension pending definitive diagnosis and treatment. Mild hyperventilation to a partial carbon dioxide pressure of 30 to 35 torr or end-tidal carbon dioxide pressure of 25 to 30 torr should be maintained; this induces intracerebral alkalosis and mild vasoconstriction and may offer benefit by decreasing intracranial

pressure (1). As soon as the patient is stable, computed tomography (CT) of the head should be obtained. Laboratory tests should be performed to rule out other causes of altered mentation, such as hypoglycemia and substance intoxication. Dextrose (50% water) and naloxone may be administered empirically. Because the physical examination is unreliable in the setting of altered mentation, additional diagnostic tests will be needed to rule out intraabdominal injury.

What are the components of the secondary survey?
The secondary survey includes the following assessments:

1. A full physical examination, including a rectal examination and for women, a pelvic examination. A Foley catheter should be inserted after the rectal examination. Gastric decompression should be achieved orally to avoid the possibility of cranial penetration resulting from facial fractures and unidentified basilar skull fractures (10).
2. A basic radiologic assessment in cases of blunt trauma, including radiographs of the chest and pelvis. A lateral cervical spine radiograph is indicated if there are signs or symptoms of cervical spine injury or if the patient has altered mentation, has distracting injuries, or has received analgesia (11).
3. Continuing assessments of the patient's stability and neurologic status.

What are the contraindications for passing a urethral catheter in a trauma patient?
A rectal examination should be performed before placement of a urinary catheter in men. A high-riding prostate gland felt during the rectal examination, blood at the urethral meatus, or a penile or periscrotal hematoma may indicate urethral rupture. If any of these findings are present, a urethrogram should be done before a urinary catheter is placed. This should be followed by a cystogram to assess the integrity of the bladder after the catheter is placed. In unstable patients, a suprapubic catheter may be placed in the bladder by percutaneous techniques, and genitourinary evaluation is delayed.

How and when should Mr. Smith's right leg fracture be treated?
Fractures may cause long-term disability if not properly treated, but they are not life-threatening injuries. They are initially addressed during or after the secondary survey, when life-threatening problems have been corrected and the patient has been stabilized. Fractures are placed in a splint or on traction, as appropriate, for later definitive treatment. Adequate analgesia should be used for fracture reduction unless cardiovascular instability contraindicates use of opioids. Vascular compromise with long-bone fractures may be due to kinking of the blood supply, direct vascular injury, or compartment syndrome. Compartment syndrome is compression of the nerve or blood supply within fascial compartments because of either accumulation of blood or edema. With most closed fractures, pulses that were absent return after the fracture is reduced in

this manner. If this is the case, at many centers further evaluation for vascular injury is deferred with good results. If the pulse does not resume, vascular injury may be evaluated by angiography. Compartment syndrome can be assessed by measuring compartment pressures with a special device, or fasciotomy can be performed on a presumptive basis. Setting priorities between treatment of a threatened extremity and correction of life-threatening injuries in the trauma patient with multiple injuries requires experience and judgment.

During the secondary survey, preparations are being made to perform the basic radiographic studies. Mr. Smith meanwhile has an episode of hypotension, with his blood pressure dropping to 80/40 mm Hg and a heart rate of 120 beats per minute; the pulse is thready. Arterial oxygen saturation remains 99%. He receives another blood transfusion, and his blood pressure increases to 95/60 mm Hg.

What is shock?
Shock is an abnormality of the circulatory system that results in a state of inadequate perfusion and oxygen delivery at the tissue and cellular level. Shock is manifested by several findings relating to the affected organ systems. These include peripheral vasoconstriction and tachycardia as the earliest findings, a narrowed pulse pressure, altered sensorium, oliguria, and metabolic acidosis. Hypotension is a late finding in shock because homeostatic mechanisms maintain blood pressure until volume loss is greater than 30%. Any trauma patient who has vasoconstriction and tachycardia should be considered to be in shock until proven otherwise (6).

What are the types of shock commonly identified in trauma patients, and how are they differentiated?
The types of shock seen in trauma include the following:

Hypovolemic shock, which is caused by blood loss, is the most common form of shock seen in trauma (12).
Traumatic shock, a variant of hypovolemic shock in blunt trauma, may also entail the release of tissue substances that exert additional detrimental effects on organ function.
Cardiac compressive shock is consequent to pericardial tamponade or tension pneumothorax. It is associated with distended neck veins, which indicate high cardiac filling pressures.
Neurogenic and **septic shock** constitute the distributive forms of shock because alterations in vasomotor tone result in pooling of blood in the peripheral circulation. Neurogenic shock occurs after spinal cord injury and is caused by bradycardia and pooling of blood consequent to sympathetic denervation. It is remarkable in that patients are warm and pink, which indicates

a low peripheral vascular resistance. In septic shock, vasomotor failure results from inflammatory substances and other mediators released as a result of the infection process. Septic shock often complicates the later hospital course after major injury but is rarely seen immediately after the injury.

Cardiogenic shock is rare in acute trauma. It may occur as a consequence of ischemic myocardial injury, which may be caused by prolonged hypovolemia, hypoxia, or preexisting coronary artery disease. Table 30.4 (12) summarizes the major features of the different forms of shock.

How is hypotension evaluated and treated?
The first step in evaluating unexpected deterioration in a patient's condition is always a reassessment of the ABCs. The integrity of the airway and breathing should be reevaluated as in the primary survey, with renewed attention to life-threatening injuries that may have been missed. The degree of any hemorrhage should be quantified, and resuscitation should be renewed. Control of external bleeding should be reconfirmed.

What are the possible causes of Mr. Smith's hypotension?
Mr. Smith has multiple injuries, and he may have unknown injuries. The major causes of hypotension in patients with blunt trauma are hypovolemic shock caused by external or internal blood loss and cardiac compressive shock resulting from tension pneumothorax or pericardial tamponade. Neurogenic shock is unlikely if spinal function is intact. In the absence of impending brainstem herniation, head trauma per se is not a cause of hypotension. Severe arterial hypoxemia may cause hypotension via cardiac ischemia, but Mr. Smith's oxygen saturation remains at 99%.

How is tension pneumothorax diagnosed and treated? Should the diagnosis be confirmed with a chest radiograph?
Tension pneumothorax occurs when an injury causes a one-way valve air leak from the lung or the chest wall. Air leaks into the pleural space on inspiration, but on expiration the air does not reenter the lung, so it rapidly accumulates in the thorax. Positive pressure collapses the lung and compresses the mediastinum. This compromises venous return, circulation, and pulmonary function. Tension pneumothorax is diagnosed by unilateral absence of breath sounds, neck vein distention, respiratory distress, arterial desaturation, and signs of hypoperfusion such as tachycardia and late cyanosis. Not all of these signs may be present, and a high index of suspicion should be maintained. Intubated patients may have increased airway resistance that manifests as difficulty in ventilation. Tension pneumothorax is immediately life-threatening, and if suspected, it should be treated without radiographic confirmation. Immediate decompression is achieved by passing a 14- or 16-gauge needle into the thorax through the second intercostal space in the midclavicular line. This vents positive pressure and alleviates cardiac compromise.

Table 30.4.   CHARACTERISTICS OF SHOCK STATES

	Types of Shock			Distributive	
	Cardiogenic	Cardiac compressive	Hypovolemic or traumatic	Septic	Neurogenic
Skin perfusion	Pale	Pale	Pale	Pink	Pink
Urine output	Low	Low	Low	Low	Low
Pulse rate	High	High	Normal	High	Low
Blood pressure	Normal	Low	Normal	Low	Low
Neck veins	Distended	Distended	Flat	Flat	Flat
O$_2$ consumption	Low	Low	Low	Low	Low
Cardiac index	Low	Low	Low	High	Low
Filling pressures	High	High	Low	Low	Low
SVR	High	High	High	Low	Low

SVR, systemic vascular resistance. Modified with permission from Holcroft JH. Emergency care: Shock. In: Wilmore DW, Brennan MF, Harken AH, et al., eds. ACS Care of the Surgical Patient. New York: Scientific American, 1989;1:1–30.

Needle decompression should be followed by conventional tube thoracostomy in the lateral fifth intercostal space to treat the remaining simple pneumothorax.

How is cardiac tamponade diagnosed and treated?
Cardiac tamponade occurs when bleeding within the rigid fibrous pericardial sac compresses the heart and prevents cardiac filling. This results in low cardiac output and hypotension, so-called cardiac compressive shock. Tamponade is suggested classically by any of the following findings:

Beck's triad: arterial hypotension, muffled heart sounds, and elevated central venous pressure manifesting as distended neck veins
Pulsus paradoxus: a decrease of systolic blood pressure of more than 10 mm Hg on inspiration
Kussmaul's sign: an increase in central venous pressure with inspiration during spontaneous breathing
Pulseless electrical activity in the trauma patient

Any of these findings may be absent. Pulsus paradoxus and Kussmaul's sign are rarely detected in acute trauma. Furthermore, tamponade is often mistaken for left-sided tension pneumothorax, which is more common and which also causes distended neck veins. These entities can be differentiated by hyperresonance over the hemithorax or with tension pneumothorax, by empiric treatment of tamponade if chest tube placement is unproductive. Cardiac tamponade is immediately treated by fluid resuscitation to increase cardiac filling pressures. Pericardiocentesis may not be diagnostic or effective because of the presence of clotted blood, and all patients subjected to pericardiocentesis should have exploratory thoracotomy for cardiac injury as soon as possible (13). Pericardiocentesis with a needle is rarely helpful in a trauma patient, so it is not recommended.

The ABCs of the primary survey are reassessed. Mr. Smith has decreased breath sounds on the left side, and the respiratory therapist notes difficulty in ventilation. The neck veins are slightly distended. Needle thoracentesis is performed, and this results in rapid return to normal blood pressure and pulse rate and quality. A tube thoracostomy is placed in the left fifth intercostal space, yielding a moderate air leak. Mr. Smith's condition seems to have stabilized, and the secondary survey is completed. A nasogastric tube and urinary catheter are placed and basic trauma radiographs obtained. The chest radiograph reveals multiple left-sided rib fractures and a well-positioned thoracostomy tube. The mediastinal silhouette is abnormally wide. The radiograph of the pelvis reveals an open-book type of pelvic fracture with a widened pubic symphysis and sacroiliac joints. The cervical spine radiograph is normal. A comminuted fracture of the tibia and fibula is

revealed from a radiograph of the right femur. The fracture is manually reduced, and this leads to return of pulses and improvement in color and warmth of the foot. A posterior splint is placed. Mr. Smith remains stable, but there is no neurologic improvement.

What is the significance of a wide mediastinum on chest radiographs in patients with blunt trauma?
Traumatic aortic transection at the level of the ligamentum arteriosum may occur because of rapid deceleration. Fixation of the descending aorta and relative mobility of the aortic arch produce stress that tears the aorta. Most patients die immediately, but those in whom the aortic bleed is contained as a mediastinal hematoma may survive to reach medical care. Such patients are neither unstable nor symptomatic, but free rupture may cause sudden death. The most common radiographic indicator of aortic transection is a wide mediastinum. Other signs that may be present include the following:

• Obliteration of the aortic knob
• Deviation of the trachea to the right
• Pleural cap (an indication of extrapleural hematoma)
• Elevation and shift to the right of the right main stem bronchus
• Depression of the left main stem bronchus
• Deviation of the esophagus (nasogastric tube) to the right
• Obliteration of the aortopulmonary window
• A normal radiograph, which does not rule out a transected aorta

The gold standard for diagnosis of aortic transection is aortography. Dynamic CT is another acceptable modality. Transesophageal echocardiography may be used for rapid diagnosis in the operating room or intensive care unit.

The assessment of Mr. Smith's injuries includes the following: multiple rib fractures with tension pneumothorax that has been treated with needle decompression and tube thoracostomy; an open-book pelvic fracture; possible closed head injury; and possible aortic transection. Serious injuries that are not life threatening include right arm laceration and closed right tibia and fibula fracture.

How is life-threatening injury assessed after a trauma patient is stabilized?
CT of the head must be obtained immediately, and aortic injury must be ruled out by any of the imaging modalities described earlier.

Before he is taken for CT, Mr. Smith's systolic blood pressure drops again to 80 mm Hg, and the diastolic blood pressure is not audible. His heart rate is 120 beats per second. There is no arterial desaturation and he is easy to ventilate. The initial assessment is rapidly repeated. The tube thoracostomy is in good position and there are bilateral breath sounds. There is a small air leak, as expected. The neck veins are collapsed and the trachea is in midline position. Crystalloid infusion is given, but the response is only partial.

What is the cause of the recurrent hypotension? What is the significance of a partial response to resuscitation?
With other causes ruled out, the most likely cause of recurrent hypotension in this patient is hypovolemic shock consequent to ongoing hidden blood loss. The partial response to crystalloid resuscitation indicates profound hypovolemia or loss of red cell mass. Failure to respond to crystalloid infusion or recurrent hypotension indicates continuing blood loss at a significant rate and is a definite indication to transfuse type-specific or universal donor blood immediately (6) (Table 30.5).

What are the possible sites of blood loss in trauma patients?
Sites of significant blood loss include the following:

- One or both pleural spaces
- Peritoneal cavity
- Pelvic fracture causing a retroperitoneal hematoma

Table 30.5. RESPONSES TO INITIAL FLUID RESUSCITATION

	Rapid Response	Transient Response	No Response
Vital signs	Return to normal	Transient improvement; recurrence of drop in blood pressure, rise in heart rate	Remain abnormal
Estimated blood loss	Minimal (10–20%)	Moderate, ongoing (20–40%)	Severe (>40%)
Need for more crystalloid	Low	High	High
Need for blood	Low	Moderate to high	Immediate
Blood preparation	Type and cross-match	Type specific	Emergency release
Need for surgery	Possible	Likely	Highly likely
Surgical consultation	Yes	Yes	Yes

Fluid resuscitation consists of 2 L Ringer's lactate in adults, 20 mL/kg Ringer's lactate in children, over 10–15 min.
Reprinted with permission from American College of Surgeons (ACS). Advanced Trauma Life Support Program for Physicians: Instructor Manual. Chicago: ACS, 1993;3:75–94.

• Other retroperitoneal injuries
• Long bone fractures, particularly a fracture of the femur, in which two units of blood may accumulate in each thigh unnoticed
• Severe contusion to muscular and subcutaneous tissues (soft tissue hematomas)
• Missed external injuries with underestimated losses into linens, dressings, and onto the floor

How is the site of bleeding determined?
All of the possible sites must be assessed. Hemothorax should be checked for with a repeated chest radiograph. The patient should be quickly reexamined for external bleeding and expanding hematomata of the lower extremities or soft tissues. This process of elimination points to the abdomen (peritoneal cavity) and fractured pelvis (retroperitoneum) as the likely sites of bleeding.

What are the options for evaluating abdominal injuries? Which modality is most appropriate for this patient?
The modalities for evaluating the abdomen include diagnostic peritoneal lavage or ultrasonography in the trauma room and CT. Ultrasonography performed by surgeons trained in it is supplanting peritoneal lavage in most centers, as it is similarly accurate and is noninvasive (14). Both stable and unstable patients may be evaluated for abdominal blood by ultrasonography if equipment is readily available in the trauma room. Diagnostic peritoneal lavage is slightly more sensitive than ultrasonography and requires minimal equipment, but it is invasive and remains nonspecific. It involves passing a catheter through a small incision in the abdomen, followed by aspiration of fluid and irrigation with saline solution. The presence of gross blood or an irrigation return containing more than 100,000 red cells per cubic millimeter indicates significant shed blood in the abdomen. CT is sensitive and is the most specific modality, but it is time consuming and entails moving the patient to the radiology suite. CT is contraindicated for a patient who is or has been hemodynamically unstable. Patients with evidence of blood loss who show signs of peritoneal irritation (e.g., rebound tenderness) should be taken promptly to the operating room for laparotomy without further diagnostic tests. Other patients may be initially evaluated with ultrasonography. Unstable patients with positive results from ultrasonography should also undergo prompt laparotomy. Unstable patients with equivocal ultrasonography results may be further assessed with a peritoneal lavage. Other sites of bleeding should be sought for unstable patients with definitively negative ultrasonography results. Stable patients with positive ultrasonography results may safely have further evaluation by CT, which is more specific than ultrasonography and which may assist in the nonoperative management of certain injuries (14). A patient such as Mr. Smith, whose condition is unstable, should be evaluated in the trauma room by ultrasonography or by a peritoneal lavage if ultrasonography is not available.

Mr. Smith undergoes ultrasonography, and a large amount of fluid is revealed in Morrison's pouch. He continues to be borderline hypotensive, with a blood pressure of 95/40 mm Hg despite the ongoing blood transfusion. It is now known that the sites of blood loss are the abdomen and most likely the retroperitoneum as a result of his pelvic fracture.

How should a patient such as Mr. Smith be treated next?
An exploratory laparotomy should be performed to control abdominal bleeding. The presumed pelvic fracture bleeding should be treated concurrently. Pelvic fractures, such as Mr. Smith's, bleed from torn sacral veins at the sacroiliac joints and from arterial branches of the hypogastric arteries. Treatment usually entails placement of an external orthopaedic fixator device in the operating room. By compressing the pelvis, the external fixator reduces the fracture and decreases bleeding from the sacral veins. At many centers, iliac angiography is performed to embolize bleeding branches of the hypogastric arteries with coils, synthetic gel, or autologous clot. Mr. Smith is taken to the operating room, where an external fixator is applied while exploratory laparotomy is performed. His spleen is lacerated, and there is approximately 2 L of blood in his abdomen. Splenectomy is performed. He is markedly hypotensive during the operation, but eventually his condition is stabilized in the operating room. During the operation, transesophageal echocardiography rules out aortic injury. With support from the anesthesia staff and with rapid control of bleeding, Mr. Smith is restored to a warm, nonacidotic, euvolemic state. After the operation, he is taken to the angiography room, where bleeding in several branches of the left hypogastric artery is controlled by angiographic gel embolization. Because his condition remains stable, he is transported to the CT unit for assessment for closed head injury. A minimal subdural hematoma is identified, with moderate local edema and no midline shift. Mr. Smith is taken to the intensive care unit for ongoing monitoring and care.

What are the options for managing splenic injury?
Splenic injury ranges from grade I to grade IV (15), with grade I being a small subcapsular hematoma and grade IV being a deep laceration of the hilar vessels or a ruptured intraparenchymal hematoma. CT is needed for grading of splenic injuries. To preserve the benefits of the intact spleen for cell-mediated immunity, all grades of injury may be initially managed nonoperatively in select patients (16). The major requirement is that the patient be hemodynamically stable without evidence of major ongoing blood loss, as monitored by hematocrit, vital signs, and physical examination. An ongoing decrease in the hematocrit value or a worsening examination indicate unsuccessful nonoperative management, and immediate surgery is dictated. As mentioned earlier, unstable patients such as Mr. Smith would not be transported for CT or for any nonoperative

management. In such persons, the appropriate course of action is to identify the abdominal bleeding by ultrasonography or peritoneal lavage and to perform immediate surgery. At many centers, patients with neurologic trauma or multisystem injury are not considered candidates for nonoperative management.

What are the options for managing a splenic injury operatively? Is splenectomy the appropriate procedure for Mr. Smith?
Surgical options for managing an injured spleen are splenectomy and repair, also known as splenorrhaphy. Techniques of splenorrhaphy include partial splenectomy, suture repair, and use of various mesh wraps. Splenorrhaphy is more time consuming than splenectomy and is not completely reliable in ensuring hemostasis. It is contraindicated in patients who are unstable in the operating room or who have multiple intraabdominal injuries. For a patient such as Mr. Smith, who is highly unstable in the operating room and who has multiple serious injuries, a rapid splenectomy is the appropriate procedure. He will need vaccination against pneumococcal and *Haemophilus influenzae* infection before hospital discharge.

What are the ongoing risks created by the patient's head injury?
Secondary cerebral injury may occur from decreased cerebral blood flow caused by the loss of autoregulation, brain edema, or enlarging mass lesions (2). Measures to normalize intracranial pressure that were instituted presumptively in the trauma room should be continued. These include the maintenance of mild hyperventilation and hyperosmolarity with diuretics or osmotic agents. Euvolemia must also be maintained in the trauma patient. Thus, patients should not be dehydrated; a state of euvolemic hyperosmolarity must be maintained. Coagulation parameters should be monitored frequently and normalized, and corrective action must be taken at the first signs of disseminated intravascular coagulation. Patients with closed head injury and profoundly altered mentation cannot be monitored with a neurologic examination. In such patients, the intracranial pressure (ICP) should be continuously monitored. Because the cerebral perfusion pressure in the injured brain is equal to the difference of mean arterial blood pressure and ICP, the ICP should be lowered to normal levels. If this is not possible, arterial blood pressure may have to be increased to supranormal levels with vasopressors. Follow-up CT should be performed if possible, and enlarging surgical mass lesions should be removed. The cerebral metabolic demand for oxygen may be lowered by the induction of barbiturate coma and/or hypothermia, although any benefit of these techniques is unproven.

Mr. Smith's condition remains stable, and he shows improvement for the first 24 hours. However, on the second hospital day, his fluid requirement to maintain blood pressure increases. The urine output decreases, and urinalysis reveals sediment. A meticulous search for

bleeding sites is unproductive. A pulmonary artery catheter is passed to assess volume and cardiac function; the results reveal high cardiac output, normal pulmonary capillary wedge pressure, and low systemic vascular resistance. The arterial oxygenation level decreases, and the chest radiograph shows patchy infiltrates indicating adult respiratory distress syndrome. The urinary sediment is compatible with a diagnosis of acute tubular necrosis. Liver enzymes are mildly elevated, and prothrombin time is prolonged. The platelet count decreases to 75,000 per cubic millimeter.

What do these findings indicate?
These findings indicate multisystem organ failure, the cause of which is poorly understood but that is probably multifactorial. The major contributors may be direct ischemic injury to organs and the systemic inflammatory response syndrome (SIRS).

What is SIRS?
Formerly called sepsis syndrome, SIRS is now known to be initiated by stresses that do not involve infectious agents. These include ischemic insult, pancreatitis, burns, and trauma. The organ injury and the sepsis type of high-output hemodynamics of SIRS that Mr. Smith has may be caused by inflammatory mediators, such as cytokines and kinins, released from damaged tissues. Cytokines are protein mediators that are produced at the site of injury and by various cells throughout the body. Their concentration is very low, but they are critical determinants of the response to injury and infection (17). These substances include tumor necrosis factor, interleukins, and interferons. Cytokines regulate immune, cardiovascular, and metabolic responses to injury in a complicated cascade that amplifies the response to injury for an extended period after the initial insult. They act both locally and systemically and may also activate conventional endocrine mechanisms (17) (Table 30.6). It is postulated that exaggerated production of or response to cytokines may produce both the hemodynamic manifestations of septic shock and the refractory catabolic state and tissue wasting seen in severe injury and infection.

What is the treatment for SIRS? What are future treatment possibilities?
The alleviation of persisting causes, such as infection, ischemia, shock, and any necrotic tissue, offers the best hope for treating multisystem organ failure. Beyond this, the treatment for SIRS is supportive care only. Organ function is supported by mechanical ventilation, inotropic agents, dialysis, correction of coagulopathy, and nutritional support. A number of natural inhibitors of cytokines have been identified, and very likely there are more. A disturbance of the complex balance between cytokines and their natural inhibitors may be responsible for the deleterious effects of cytokines in SIRS. In addition, selective

Table 30.6.   BIOLOGIC ACTIVITIES OF SELECT CYTOKINES

	Tumor Necrosis Factor	Interleukin-1	Interleukin-2	Interleukin-6
Immune system				
Neutrophils	↑Bone marrow release ↑Margination ↑Transendothelial passage ↑Activation	↑Bone marrow release ↑Influx to site of injury ↑Transendothelial passage	Leukocytosis	
Monocytes	↑Blood monocyte differentiation ↑Activation ↑Cytotoxicity	↑Blood monocyte differentiation ↑Activation		
Lymphocytes	↑Lymphokine production	↑T-cell activation ↑Lymphokine production	↑T-cell proliferation ↑Cytotoxicity ↑Lymphokine synthesis Eosinophilia Organ infiltration	↑Differentiation ↑B-cell proliferation ↑Cytotoxicity
Eosinophils	Activation of eosinophils			
Cardiovascular system	Hypotension Shock ↑Vascular leak	? Hypotension	↑Vascular leak ? Hypotension	
Metabolic effects	Anorexia Weight loss Fever	Anorexia Weight loss Fever	? Fever	Fever
Hepatic	↑Lipogenesis ↑Amino acid uptake ↑Acute-phase protein synthesis ↓Albumin synthesis	↑Acute-phase protein synthesis ↓Albumin synthesis		↑Acute-phase protein synthesis

continued

Table 30.6. BIOLOGIC ACTIVITIES OF SELECT CYTOKINES—*Continued*

	Tumor Necrosis Factor	Interleukin-1	Interleukin-2	Interleukin-6
Skeletal muscle	↓ Resting membrane potential	↑ Nitrogen loss		
		↓ Myofibrillar protein mRNA		
	↑ Amino acid loss			
	↑ Myofibrillar protein mRNA			
	↑ Hexose transporters			
	↓ Cellular glycogen			
	↑ Lactate production			
Lipid	Inhibition of lipoprotein lipase	Inhibition of lipoprotein lipase		
	↓ Free fatty acid synthesis			
	↑ Lipolysis			

Reprinted with permission from Fong Y, Lowry S. Trauma: cytokines and cellular response to injury and infection. In: Wilmore DW, Brennan MF, Harken AH, et al., eds. ACS Care of the Surgical Patient. New York: Scientific American, 1996;4:1–25.

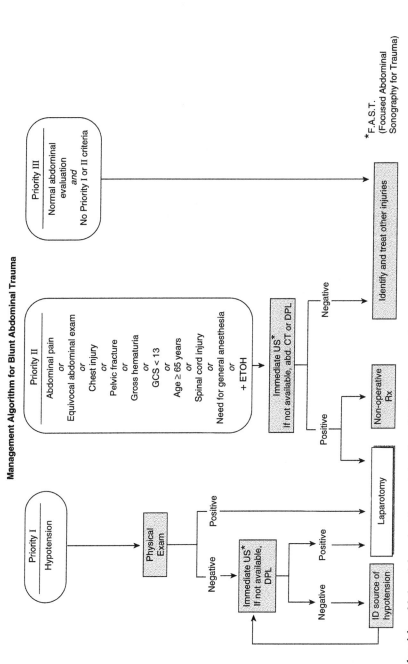

Algorithm 30.1.   Adapted with permission from McElveen TS, Collin GR. The role of ultrasonography in blunt abdominal trauma: a prospective study. Am Surg 1997;63:184–188.

antibodies against many cytokines are available. Inhibitors and antibodies may have a clinical role in limiting cytokine activity and thus preventing death from multisystem organ failure in trauma and other life-threatening conditions.

REFERENCES

 1. Miller SM. Management of central nervous system injuries. In: Capan LM, Miller SM, Turndorf H, eds. Trauma: Anesthesia and Intensive Care. Philadelphia: Saunders, 1985:207.
 2. Michael DB, Wilson RF. Head injuries. In: Wilson RF, Walt AJ, eds. Management of Trauma: Pitfalls and Practice. Baltimore: Williams & Wilkins, 1996:173–202.
 3. Taylor MB, Whitman JG. The current status of pulse oximetry. Anesthesia 1986;1:943.
 4. Wilson RF. Post traumatic pulmonary insufficiency. In: Wilson RF, Walt AJ, eds. Management of Trauma: Pitfalls and Practice. Baltimore: Williams & Wilkins, 1996:894.
 5. American College of Surgeons. Advanced Trauma Life Support Program for Physicians: Instructor Manual. Chicago: ACS, 1993:21.
 6. American College of Surgeons. Advanced Trauma Life Support Program for Physicians: Instructor Manual. Chicago: ACS, 1993;3:75–94.
 7. Maull KI. Alcohol abuse: its implications in trauma care. South Med J 1982;75:794.
 8. Walls RM. Rapid-sequence intubation in head trauma. Ann Emerg Med 1993;22:1008.
 9. Woster PS, LeBlanc KL. Management of elevated intracranial pressure. Clin Pharm 1990;9:762.
10. American College of Surgeons. Advanced Trauma Life Support Program for Physicians: Instructor Manual. Chicago: ACS, 1995.
11. American College of Surgeons. Advanced Trauma Life Support Program for Physicians: Instructor Manual. Chicago: ACS, 1997.
12. Holcroft JW. Shock. In: Willmore DW, Brennan MF, Harken AH, Holcroft JW, Meakins JL, eds. Care of the Surgical Patient. New York: Scientific American, 1989: 1–12.
13. Stephenson LW, Wilson RF. Thoracic trauma: heart. In: Wilson RF, Walt AJ, eds. Management of Trauma: Pitfalls and Practice. Baltimore: Williams & Wilkins, 1996: 343–360.
14. McElveen TS, Collin GR. The role of ultrasonography in blunt abdominal trauma: a prospective study. Am Surg 1997;63:184–188.
15. Moore EE et al. Organ injury scaling: spleen, liver, kidney. J Trauma 1989;29: 1664–1666.
16. Cogbill TH et al. Nonoperative management of blunt splenic trauma: a multicenter experience. J Trauma 1989;29:1312–1317.
17. Fong Y, Lowry S. Trauma: cytokines and cellular response to injury and infection. In: Wilmore DW, Brennan MF, Harken AH, et al., eds. ACS Care of the Surgical Patient. New York: Scientific American, 1996;4:1–25.

Renal Transplantation

Robert L. Madden

David Novak is a 37-year-old man who has a 1-year history of end-stage renal disease resulting from glomerulonephritis. He has been maintained on hemodialysis. He recently asked his nephrologist about the possibility of obtaining a kidney transplant, and she referred him to the local transplant center for evaluation as a candidate for transplantation.

What criteria must a patient meet to receive a renal transplant?
Potential recipients must have near-end-stage renal failure (creatinine clearance less than 20 mL/minute) or end-stage renal failure (be dialysis dependent). Contraindications to transplantation include active infection, HIV infection, cancer (patients may be considered for a transplant if they have been disease free for more than 2 years after treatment), severe medical disease (e.g., chronic obstructive pulmonary disease, inoperable coronary artery disease), or history of noncompliance with medications (1).

What does a pretransplant evaluation entail?
Patients referred for transplantation are usually assessed by a multidisciplinary team consisting of personnel from nephrology, transplant surgery, social work, and psychiatry, as well as nurse coordinators. A thorough medical evaluation is performed with emphasis on identifying conditions that could complicate the posttransplant course. Potential problems such as gallstones, genitourinary abnormalities, cardiopulmonary disease, infection, cancer, peptic ulcer disease, periodontal disease, noncompliance, psychosocial concerns, and other issues are addressed (1). Financial issues must also be discussed, because although the hospitalization and surgery costs are usually covered by third-party payors, the costs for immunosuppressive medications ($10,000 to $15,000 per year) are reimbursed for only a limited period after transplantation.

During his pretransplant evaluation, Mr. Novak mentions that his mother, sister, and a close friend have all volunteered to donate a kidney.

What are the sources of donor kidneys and how do they compare?
At present, the only sources of kidneys for transplantation are living donors and cadavers. Xenotransplantation is not yet clinically feasible. At most transplant centers, kidneys from living donors are preferred to those from cadaveric donors for several reasons:

1. A living donor kidney allows the recipient to bypass the lengthy waiting list for cadaveric organs. Of the approximately 50,000 people awaiting transplantation in the United States, two-thirds are for a kidney transplant. The waiting period can range from 6 months to 4 years (median, 2 years), depending on blood type, because only about 5,500 cadaveric donors are available per year (2, 3).
2. The rate of immediate function is higher with living donor kidneys than with cadaveric kidneys. This translates into shorter hospital stays, fewer diagnostic procedures, less immunosuppression, and lower costs.
3. Many patients with chronic renal insufficiency can be transplanted before initiating dialysis.
4. If a living donor kidney is used whenever possible, a cadaveric kidney can be received by a patient for whom no living donor is available; each living donor kidney adds to the pool available for.transplantation. Successful renal transplantation enhances the patient's rehabilitation and over time is more cost-effective than dialysis.
5. The survival of transplanted living donor kidneys is higher than that of cadaver kidneys, a strong argument for using living donor kidneys (4, 5).

What are the criteria applied to selection of a suitable living kidney donor?
For successful transplantation, the living kidney donor must have a compatible ABO blood type and be free of HIV infection. Other criteria for living donation vary among transplant centers. Some centers do not perform living donor transplantation because of the risk to an otherwise healthy person. Most centers, however, use living donors because of the low rate of donor complications (major morbidity, 0.23%; mortality, 0.03%) and the advantages. All centers that perform living donor kidney transplants perform a thorough medical and nephrologic evaluation of potential donors. In general, renal disease, severe medical problems, cancer, infection, or psychosocial issues can preclude living kidney donation. If more than one potential donor for a given patient is found to be medically suitable, tissue typing determines the preferred donor (4, 5).

What determines tissue compatibility?
Tissue compatibility between a donor and a recipient (assuming ABO blood group compatibility) is determined primarily by their respective genomes. In humans, a cluster of genes called the major histocompatibility complex (MHC) resides on the short arm of chromosome 6. These genes encode membrane-

bound cell-surface glycoproteins known as human leukocyte antigens (HLA) that are present on a wide variety of cells in the body. Early in transplantation research scientists discovered that if donor and recipient animals differed with respect to the genes in their MHC, a strong rejection reaction occurred rapidly. If they were identical with respect to their MHC genes (HLA-identical), rejection was slow and weak. If the animals were identical with respect to the entire genome, no rejection occurred. From these experiments, it was concluded that differences in HLA antigens between individuals were the *major* determinants of histocompatibility. If the HLA antigens were identical, a mild rejection could still occur because of differences at other genetic loci that produced *minor* histocompatibility differences (6).

How is tissue compatibility assessed before transplantation?
Before transplantation, blood is drawn from a potential donor or recipient for determination of the HLA antigens. This is tissue typing. The clinically relevant HLA antigens are HLA-A, HLA-B, and HLA-DR. Each of these antigens has a variety of subtypes based on allelic differences of the particular MHC genes in the individual (e.g., HLA-A has subtypes HLA-A1, HLA-A2, and so on). The amino acid sequence of different HLA subtype antigens can differ by as little as a single amino acid. Each individual inherits one set of these three antigens (a haplotype) from each parent and therefore has a tissue typing report that lists six HLA antigens (e.g., HLA-A1, A2; HLA-B3, B4; HLA-DR5, DR6). Although this concept is somewhat controversial in the transplant community, the closer the HLA match between the donor and the recipient, the better the survival of the kidney. HLA matching is used to determine order of preference of potential donors for a given recipient when all other donor factors are equivalent (6).

Can an unrelated close friend be a living donor?
Although the practice is not universal, many transplant centers are actively encouraging living unrelated kidney donation when no related donor is available. One of the most common unrelated transplants is between spouses. Transplants between close friends are also performed, but it is incumbent on the transplant center to ensure that the motive for donation is altruistic. Donation for financial gain is illegal in the United States. Living unrelated donation provides additional kidneys for transplantation, and these kidneys have been shown in recent studies to have better survival than cadaveric kidneys (7).

Unfortunately, none of Mr. Novak's potential living donors is tissue compatible, and his name is added to the cadaveric kidney waiting list.

How are cadaveric kidneys distributed in the United States? What is the waiting list?
The U.S. government employs an organization called the United Network of

Organ Sharing (UNOS) to oversee the distribution of cadaveric organs. UNOS divides the United States into 11 regions. Within each region, a number of local organ procurement organizations (OPO) are responsible for identifying potential organ donors, obtaining consent for donation, managing the donor prior to donation, preserving the organs, and shipping them to the appropriate transplant centers (8). UNOS maintains a national computerized waiting list that includes the names of all patients awaiting cadaveric organ transplantation in the United States. When an organ becomes available, UNOS generates a list of prospective recipients ordered on the basis of blood type, waiting time, and HLA match. The transplant center offers the organ to persons on the list in order of priority until the organ is placed. In general, organs are first offered locally, then regionally, and then nationally. An exception to this rule is when a kidney is found to match all six HLA-antigens with a recipient; in such a case, the kidney is transported to that center regardless of location. This exception is made because survival with these six-antigen match, or zero-mismatch, kidneys is considerably higher than those matching fewer than six antigens (8).

Meanwhile, a 23-year-old man is drinking beer with his friends when the pick-up truck in which they are riding hits a bump in the road and swerves sharply to the right. The young man loses his grip and falls from the back of the truck. He suffers a severe closed head injury and is transported by ambulance to the local trauma center. Despite resuscitation and support, massive cerebral edema results in herniation of the brainstem. The intensive care nurse queries whether the patient's condition is consistent with brain death.

What is brain death and how is it confirmed?
The diagnosis of brain death has evolved over the past 40 years and remains a source of controversy today. Human death has been described as an irreversible loss of the capacity for consciousness and breathing, both of which are functions of the brainstem. Brainstem death therefore can be considered the core of brain death, and this concept is used in the clinical diagnosis of brain death. Before a patient can be considered brain dead, certain conditions and exclusions must be met. The patient must be ventilator dependent and comatose, and the cause must be firmly established. Reversible causes of a nonfunctioning brainstem, such as hypothermia, drug intoxication, severe hypoxia, hypotension, and metabolic disturbances, must be ruled out. Once these preconditions and exclusions have been satisfied, a clinical diagnosis of death can be made on the basis of established criteria of the absence of brainstem reflexes and the presence of apnea. The tests are performed twice, usually 2 to 12 hours apart. Any uncertainty precludes the diagnosis, and the patient is observed. After death has been established, the patient can be

transferred to the operating room for organ donation. Although their role is controversial, electroencephalogram, cerebral angiography, and radioisotopic scans are sometimes used for confirmation; however, they are not required for the diagnosis of death (9).

How is the suitability for organ donation of a brain-dead patient determined?
The suitability for organ donation of a brain-dead patient should be determined by the organ procurement coordinator from the OPO together with a transplant surgeon. These coordinators are trained not only in the identification and management of cadaveric donors but more importantly, in approaching family members and obtaining consent for donation. In general, all brain-dead patients with no incurable transmissible disease should be considered for donation.

A neurologist and an intensivist examine the patient and find no brainstem reflexes. During the apnea test, he fails to breathe spontaneously, confirming absence of brainstem activity. The local OPO is notified, and a coordinator arrives promptly to review the chart. She identifies the patient as an acceptable donor and obtains his family's consent for multiple organ and tissue donation. The patient is maintained on mechanical ventilation and inotropic support over the next 5 hours, until he is transported to the operating room for organ procurement. In the operating room, the donor's heart, lungs, liver, pancreas, and kidneys are removed by three transplant teams. After removal of the solid organs, technicians procure corneas, bone, and skin. The cadaver is transferred to the hospital morgue and then to the funeral home, where an open-casket service is held. Except for immediate family, none of the visitors paying their last respects could discern that the patient had been an organ donor.

In what order are organs removed, and how are they preserved?
The life-saving organs are removed first, the order being heart, lungs, and liver. The organs that improve the quality of life, the pancreas and kidneys, are procured next. Organ preservation is accomplished by in situ flushing. The cadaver is opened with a midline incision from the sternal notch to the symphysis pubis, and the organs are dissected. Large cannulae are introduced into the aorta and preservation solution (University of Wisconsin [UW]) at 4°C is rapidly infused to flush out the blood and preserve the intraabdominal organs. A different solution is used concomitantly for the heart and lungs. The ventilator is disconnected, and each organ is removed by the appropriate transplant team. The intraabdominal organs are most commonly simply stored at 4°C in UW solution and transported in coolers. Kidneys are occasionally stored on a perfusion pump machine, a practice that many surgeons believe prolongs the viability of the organs. Kidneys can be stored up to 72 hours (10).

Mr. Novak is third on the UNOS computer-generated waiting list. The first patient is found to have a positive cross-match, and the second has an infected diabetic foot ulcer. Therefore, the kidney is offered to Mr. Novak.

What is a cross-match?
If a potential transplant recipient has been exposed to human tissues, for example, blood transfusions, previous transplants, or pregnancies, that recipient may develop antibodies against certain human antigens. If antibodies directed at antigens on the kidney are circulating in the recipient at the time of transplant, the antibodies attack the endothelium of the newly transplanted kidney and kill the kidney within a few hours of transplantation. This is called hyperacute rejection. To prevent such an event, a cross-match is performed by testing serum from the recipient against lymphocytes from the donor. If antibodies are present, the cross-match is positive and the transplant should not be performed.

Mr. Novak is taken to the operating room and placed under general anesthesia. A right lower quadrant oblique incision is made in the abdomen. The peritoneal cavity is avoided and the retroperitoneum is opened. The lymphatic vessels crossing the external iliac vessels are ligated and divided. While the kidney is kept cold with ice packs, end-to-side anastomoses are performed between Mr. Novak's external iliac artery and vein and the donor renal artery and vein, respectively. The vascular clamps are removed, and the kidney turns pink. An opening is created in the urinary bladder and the donor ureter arising from the transplanted kidney is implanted with an antireflux technique. Total operative time is 2.5 hours, and cold ischemic time (time the kidney was preserved outside of a body) is 29 hours. After a short stay in the recovery room, Mr. Novak is transported to the transplant ward. His urine output is approximately 30 mL per hour.

How much urine should a newly transplanted kidney produce? What factors reduce the urine output?
During the transplant operation, recipients are commonly given mannitol, furosemide, and 3 to 5 L of intravenous fluid. A kidney with good function responds to these maneuvers with a vigorous urine output of up to 1 L per hour. Other than technical problems, such as a thrombosed renal vessel or an obstructed ureter, a common cause of early renal dysfunction is acute tubular necrosis (ATN). During preservation, ischemic damage occurs slowly within the kidney, with the tubules being the most sensitive structures. After a kidney has been preserved for more than 24 to 30 hours, the incidence of ATN rises. If the ATN is mild, the renal dysfunction may last only a few hours to days,

but if it is severe, it can persist for weeks and may necessitate the continuation of dialysis. Rejection, drug toxicity, hypovolemia, and technical problems are other factors that can also impede renal function (10).

About 8 hours after he leaves the operating room, Mr. Novak's urine output increases, and his serum creatinine level decreases to 8.7 mg/dL from a pretransplant level of 9.5 mg/dL. His new kidney continues to function well, and his Foley catheter is removed on the third postoperative day. He is discharged on the fifth day with a creatinine level of 4.2 mg/dL. His maintenance immunosuppressive medications include cyclosporine, mycophenolate mofetil, and a rapidly tapering dose of corticosteroids. He also takes drugs to prevent viral, bacterial, and fungal infections. He is initially followed in the transplant clinic three times per week.

Why is immunosuppressive therapy necessary? How long must it be continued?
After transplantation, the recipient's immune system recognizes the donor kidney as foreign and without intervention will destroy it. This process is rejection. There are three kinds of rejection: hyperacute, acute, and chronic. To prevent acute and chronic rejection, medication is given to suppress the immune system. These potent immunosuppressive drugs are initiated before transplantation and must be taken for the remainder of the recipient's life. Although some of these medications can be tapered over time, current knowledge of the immune system is not advanced enough to enable the complete cessation of immunosuppressive drugs.

What cellular processes underlie rejection?

Hyperacute rejection has been described earlier. It is caused by preformed antibodies in the recipient that are directed at antigens on the donor kidney.
Acute cellular rejection most commonly occurs during the first 3 months after transplantation. It is mediated by the cellular arm of the immune system. Through a variety of mechanisms, $CD4^+$ (helper) T lymphocytes are presented with fragments of donor antigen bound to HLA-class II molecules and are stimulated with interleukin-1 (IL-1) from antigen-presenting cells. These T cells become activated, proliferate, and secrete IL-2. In response, $CD8^+$ (cytotoxic) T lymphocytes are activated to proliferate and destroy the kidney. Nonspecific killing cells, such as macrophages and neutrophils, can also be recruited. As the process continues, B lymphocytes differentiate into plasma cells, which produce antibodies directed at the kidney (11). Recipients must have maintenance immunosuppression to counteract these events.
Chronic rejection, an insidious process of unclear causation involving both cellular and humoral components of the immune system, affects some re-

cipients despite compliance with immunosuppressive medications. There is no successful therapy for this form of rejection, and it often leads to loss of the transplanted organ.

What are the types of immunosuppressive drugs? How do they work, and what are the side effects?

Corticosteroids were one of the first clinically relevant immunosuppressive agents, and they are still an integral part of regimens. The actions of steroids are multiple and complex. They have widespread antiinflammatory effects and suppress the cellular activity and cytokine secretion of many cell types in the immune system. Specifically, they are known to inhibit the secretion of IL-1, which decreases activation of CD4$^+$ T cells. The side effects of steroids (growth retardation, impaired healing, bone disease, cataracts, diabetes, weight gain) are numerous and well known, but they have decreased in frequency because steroid doses have been greatly reduced after the introduction of newer immunosuppressive agents (12).

Azathioprine (Imuran), a derivative of 6-mercaptopurine, was first used in clinical transplantation in 1963 and became a mainstay of immunosuppression for the next 30 years. Being an antimetabolite, this drug inhibited both DNA and RNA synthesis in rapidly dividing cells, such as T cells, during acute cellular rejection. However, azathioprine also caused bone marrow suppression, and its use was limited by this toxicity (12).

Mycophenolate mofetil (MMF) (CellCept) is a more effective and specific drug that has recently become available for clinical use, and it has replaced azathioprine at many transplant centers. MMF inhibits inosine monophosphate dehydrogenase and thereby blocks the de novo pathway of purine synthesis. Most cells can use a salvage pathway for purine synthesis, but lymphocytes depend on the de novo pathway. In recent worldwide trials, MMF significantly reduced rejection rates at a dose that was associated with minimal toxicity. Some gastrointestinal side effects were noted, but bone marrow suppression was rare (13). However, MMF costs up to $5000 per year.

Cyclosporine (CsA) (Sandimmune or Neoral) is the mainstay of most renal immunosuppressive regimens. It was isolated from a soil fungus and introduced into clinical trials in 1978. It binds a cytosolic isomerase, cyclophilin, and ultimately inhibits IL-2 production at the level of transcription. This results in a marked diminution of CD4$^+$ T-cell activation and proliferation, which in turn inhibits the production of cytotoxic T cells. It is given orally twice a day, and most centers adjust the dose according to trough levels. Numerous clinical toxicities limit the dose of CsA, which can cause acute and chronic nephrotoxicity. It is also responsible for hypertension, hirsutism, tremor, diabetes, and as with all immunosuppressive medications, increased susceptibility to infection and malignancy. Drug interactions are also numerous, and any medication that is metabolized through the hepatic cytochrome P-450 enzyme pathway can drastically alter the blood levels of CsA (12). Like MMF, it costs up to $5000 per year.

Tacrolimus (Prograf, FK506) is another widely used immunosuppressive agent that is given instead of CsA. Its mechanism of action and toxicity profile are similar to those of CsA, but tacrolimus is more potent. It is also given twice a day, and the dose is based on trough levels. Although some centers use tacrolimus for renal transplants, it is more commonly used for liver transplants.

Other immunosuppressive agents include compounds such as rapamycin, 15-deoxyspergualin, brequinar, and leflunomide. They are being investigated in animal and human trials but are not yet available for widespread clinical use.

What is the dosing regimen for immunosuppressive drugs?
There are numerous ways to administer immunosuppressive medications after organ transplantation, and each transplant center has its own protocols. In the United States, renal transplant recipients are commonly maintained on a triple therapy regimen of CsA, azathioprine or MMF, and corticosteroids. Relatively high doses of these drugs are given initially to prevent early rejection, but with time the doses are tapered to prevent long-term toxicities. Some centers use induction therapy with the monoclonal antibody OKT-3 or a polyclonal anti-lymphocyte globulin and delay the introduction of CsA. Overall, the exact nature of the immunosuppressive protocol is less important than the outcome with respect to patient and organ survival and complications. The outcomes of each transplant center are published for public scrutiny each year, and centers whose results fall below established standards are reviewed by UNOS.

Over the ensuing few days, Mr. Novak's creatinine decreases to 1.5 mg/dL. On the 12th postoperative day, however, he complains of some malaise and swelling in his ankles. His temperature is 37.7°C, his weight has increased by 3 kg, and his serum creatinine level is 2.3 mg/dL. On examination, his kidney appears to be enlarged, and he has bilateral pretibial edema.

What is the differential diagnosis of Mr. Novak's clinical presentation? What diagnostic tests should be performed?
Many types of problems can cause kidney dysfunction (10) (Table 31.1). The differential diagnosis includes prerenal causes such as dehydration or inadequate perfusion (technical vascular complications, myocardial infarction), urinary obstruction or leak, transplant pyelonephritis, ATN, drug toxicity, recurrence of initial renal disease, de novo renal disease, and rejection. An accurate diagnosis is imperative, because misdiagnosing an infection as rejection and treating with increased immunosuppression can prove fatal. The diagnosis is based on clinical

Table 31.1.   CAUSES OF RENAL DYSFUNCTION
AFTER RENAL TRANSPLANTATION

Prerenal
  Hypovolemia
  Hypotension
    Myocardial infarction, congestive heart failure
    Medication
  Decreased perfusion secondary to mechanical factors
    Renal artery stenosis or thrombosis
    Arterial anastomotic technical error
    Thrombosis of renal artery branch or polar artery
    Proximal iliac artery stenosis or thrombosis
    Renal artery embolus
    Renal vein thrombosis
Renal
  Acute tubular necrosis
    Prolonged cold ischemia (preservation)
    Prolonged warm ischemia (during transplant)
    Donor factors
      Hypotension
      Vasopressors
      Warm ischemia
  Rejection
    Hyperacute
    Accelerated acute
    Acute
    Chronic
  Drug toxicity
    Cyclosporine or tacrolimus nephrotoxicity
    Allergic interstitial nephritis
    Other nephrotoxic medications
  Infection
    Transplant pyelonephritis
    Cytomegalovirus infection
  Donor factors
    Preexisting renal disease
    Advanced age
  Hemolytic uremic syndrome/thrombotic thrombocytopenic purpura
  Recurrence of recipient renal disease
  De novo recipient renal disease
  Lymphoproliferative disease/lymphoma
Postrenal
  Obstruction
    Urinary catheter (blood clot)
    Ureteral (lymphocele, ischemic stenosis, urolithiasis, ureteroneocystostomy
      technical error)
    Bladder (prostatic hypertrophy, neurogenic)
    Urethra (stricture)
  Urinary leak
    Ureter/pelvis injury
    Ureteroneocystostomy leak

and laboratory information. Prerenal causes can often be ruled out by physical examination. Doppler ultrasonography can assess arterial and venous blood flow and rule out obstruction. A urinalysis can reveal pyuria or show casts that are consistent with a diagnosis of ATN. CsA levels, if drastically elevated, can be assessed and lowered if necessary. If the diagnosis cannot be established, a biopsy must be performed. Biopsy is the gold standard of diagnosis, although it is not 100% accurate. Most biopsies are now performed percutaneously with ultrasound guidance.

How is rejection manifested? How is it diagnosed?
Rejection can result in a variety of signs and symptoms, depending on severity. Malaise, low-grade fever, weight gain, edema, decreased urine output, kidney enlargement and tenderness, and hypertension can occur. Laboratory measures include an increase in creatinine levels and blood urea nitrogen and a decrease in platelets. A histologic examination of biopsy specimens may reveal the renal interstitium to contain lymphocytic infiltrates, but the hallmark of acute rejection is tubulitis (lymphocytic inflammation of the renal tubules) with or without vasculitis (14).

How is rejection controlled?
As with immunosuppressive protocols, treatment regimens for acute rejection vary by center. Most centers initially treat with high-dose corticosteroids, and approximately 75% of rejection episodes resolve. For steroid-resistant cases, OKT-3 is frequently used. OKT-3 is a murine monoclonal antibody that is specific for the pan-T-cell marker CD3. It is an activating antibody that causes T cells to release multiple cytokines. Side effects include nausea, vomiting, fever, chills, tremors, headache, diarrhea, and if the patient is fluid overloaded, pulmonary edema. OKT-3 is given once a day, and the cytokine release side effects abate after the second to third dose. Most steroid-resistant rejections can be successfully treated with OKT-3, but ongoing rejection requires other forms of rescue therapy. In rare instances, antirejection therapy is discontinued and kidney loss is accepted to avoid the complications (infection or malignancy) of the therapy (10).

After biopsy, Mr. Novak is diagnosed with acute cellular rejection and is successfully treated with a 3-day course of pulse methylprednisolone 1 g per day followed by an oral recycling of prednisone. His symptoms resolve and his creatinine level returns to 1.5 mg/dL. He returns to work and leads a productive life free from dialysis.

How long do transplanted kidneys last?
It is impossible to predict how long an individual kidney will last. Statistically, a first-time cadaveric kidney transplant recipient has an 80 to 85% chance of retaining the kidney for 1 year and a 40 to 45% chance of retaining it for 10 years,

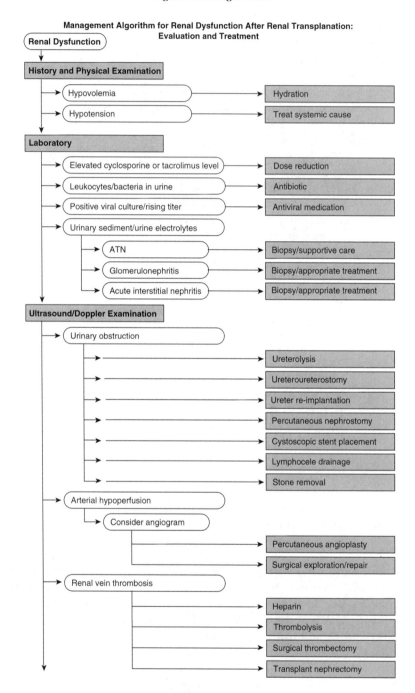

Management Algorithm for Renal Dysfunction After Renal Transplanation: Evaluation and Treatment

Renal Dysfunction

History and Physical Examination

- Hypovolemia → Hydration
- Hypotension → Treat systemic cause

Laboratory

- Elevated cyclosporine or tacrolimus level → Dose reduction
- Leukocytes/bacteria in urine → Antibiotic
- Positive viral culture/rising titer → Antiviral medication
- Urinary sediment/urine electrolytes
  - ATN → Biopsy/supportive care
  - Glomerulonephritis → Biopsy/appropriate treatment
  - Acute interstitial nephritis → Biopsy/appropriate treatment

Ultrasound/Doppler Examination

- Urinary obstruction
  - → Ureterolysis
  - → Ureteroureterostomy
  - → Ureter re-implantation
  - → Percutaneous nephrostomy
  - → Cystoscopic stent placement
  - → Lymphocele drainage
  - → Stone removal
- Arterial hypoperfusion
  - Consider angiogram
    - → Percutaneous angioplasty
    - → Surgical exploration/repair
- Renal vein thrombosis
  - → Heparin
  - → Thrombolysis
  - → Surgical thrombectomy
  - → Transplant nephrectomy

Algorithm 31.1A.

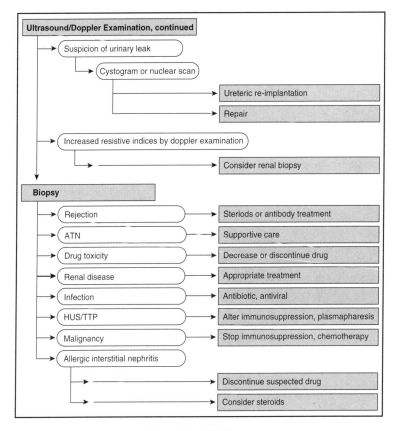

Algorithm 31.1B.

on the basis of current data (15). Results with living donor kidneys are better, with 10-year kidney survival rates as high as 80% for HLA-identical siblings. Recipients can lose their kidneys to a variety of causes, such as acute and chronic rejection, recurrent or de novo renal disease, and drug toxicity. The addition of newer, more specific immunosuppressive agents should improve survival.

REFERENCES

1. Kasiske BL, Ramos EL, Gaston RS, et al. The evaluation of renal transplant candidates: clinical practice guidelines. J Am Soc Nephrol 1995;6:1–34.
2. United Network of Organ Sharing Bulletin 1997;2:issue 5. Richmond, VA: UNOS.
3. Harper AM, Baker AS. The UNOS OPTN waiting list: 1988–1995. In: Cecka JM, Terasaki PI, eds. Clinical Transplants 1995. Los Angeles: UCLA Tissue Typing Laboratory, 1995:69–84.

4. Cosimi AB. The donor and donor nephrectomy. In: Morris PJ, ed. Kidney Transplantation: Principles and Practice. Philadelphia: Saunders, 1994:56–70.
5. Bia MJ, Ramos EL, Danovitch GM, et al. Evaluation of living renal donors: the current practice of U.S. transplant centers. Transplantation 1995;60:322–327.
6. Abbas AK, Lichtman AH, Pober JS. Cellular and molecular immunology. Philadelphia: Saunders, 1994:96–114.
7. Terasaki PI, Cecka JM, Gjertson DW, et al. High survival rates of kidney transplants from spousal and living unrelated donors. N Engl J Med 1995;333:333–336.
8. Smith CM, Ellison MD, eds. UNOS 1996 annual report: the U.S. scientific registry of transplant recipients and the organ procurement and transplantation network. Richmond, VA: UNOS.
9. Pallis C. Brainstem death: the evolution of a concept. In: Morris, ed. Kidney Transplantation: Principles and Practice. Philadelphia: Saunders, 1994:71–85.
10. Rawn JD, Tilney NL. The early course of a patient with a kidney transplant. In: Morris, ed. Kidney Transplantation: Principles and Practice. Philadelphia: Saunders, 1994:167–178.
11. Abbas AK, Lichtman AH, Pober JS. Cellular and molecular immunology. Philadelphia: Saunders, 1994:337–355.
12. Flye MW. Immunosuppressive therapy. In: Flye, MW, ed. Principles of Organ Transplantation. Philadelphia: Saunders, 1989:155–175.
13. Keown PA, Hayry P, Mathew T, et al. A blinded, randomized clinical trial of mycophenolate mofetil for the prevention of acute rejection in cadaveric renal transplantation. Transplantation 1996;61:1029–1037.
14. Solez K, Roy AA, Hallgrimur B, et al. International standardization of criteria for the histologic diagnosis of renal allograft rejection: the Banff working classification of kidney transplant pathology. Kidney Int 1993;44:411–422.
15. Cecka JM, Terasaki PI. The UNOS scientific renal transplant registry. In: Cecka JM, Terasaki PI, eds. Clinical Transplants 1995. Los Angeles: UCLA Tissue Typing Laboratory, 1995:1–18.

Mechanical Ventilation

K. Francis Lee

Mechanical ventilation may be provided via two modes: *negative pressure* and *positive pressure*. Iron lungs and cuirass ventilators use negative-pressure ventilation, in which the patient's entire body is encased in a stiff chamber. By intermittently applying negative pressure to the chest wall, the lungs expand similarly to natural breathing. This method is seldom used today because it is cumbersome and fraught with mechanical failures. The development of endotracheal intubation and positive pressure ventilation has made mechanical ventilation a cornerstone of surgical therapy.

INDICATIONS

Although unique to each clinical situation, the indications for mechanical ventilation, in general, are as follows:

- Failure to oxygenate; partial pressure of oxygen (PO_2) less than 50 mm Hg on high oxygen-delivery content, resulting in tachypnea or respiratory distress
- Failure to ventilate leading to progressive hypercapnia: PO_2 less than 50 mm Hg associated with moderate-to-severe acidosis, pH less than 7.3, and acute mental status changes
- Compromised airway control with impending hypoventilation or apnea (e.g., closed head injury or stroke)

Common clinical situations that require ventilatory support include adult respiratory distress syndrome (ARDS), severe acute pulmonary diseases (e.g., pulmonary edema, bronchospasm), aspiration pneumonia, inhalation tracheobronchial injury, severely depressed mental status, compromised airway protection, severe chest trauma, and impending cardiopulmonary arrest.

DEFINITIONS AND VENTILATORY SETTINGS

Various respiratory parameters may be confusing to surgical students. The following are definitions of commonly used ventilatory settings. Generally, the fractional concentration of oxygen in inspired gas (F_iO_2) and positive end-expiratory pressure effect changes in PO_2. The parameters that alter minute ventilation (e.g., tidal volume, rate, and pressure support ventilation) effect changes in the partial pressure of carbon dioxide (PCO_2).

RATE OR MODE

In intermittent mandatory ventilation (IMV), the patient receives a mandatory preset rate of mechanical ventilation in addition to what the patient breathes on his or her own. The mandatory mechanical ventilation and the patient's spontaneous breathing are not synchronized. The initial setting is usually 10 breaths per minute.

In synchronized intermittent mandatory ventilation (SIMV), a preset rate of ventilation is delivered in synchrony with the patient's own breathing pattern. A preset rate of 10 delivers only 10 breaths per minute in synchrony with the patient's own breathing, even if the patient is taking 30 breaths per minute. (Compare with assisted control ventilation, next.)

In assisted control ventilation (ACV), each breath initiated by the patient triggers the mechanical ventilator to deliver the tidal volume. A preset rate of 10 delivers at least 10 ventilatory breaths per minute if the patient is breathing at less than that rate. However, if the patient is breathing at 30 breaths per minute, ACV provides 30 assisted breaths per minute.

In pressure support ventilation (PSV), each breath initiated by the patient triggers the mechanical ventilator to deliver a variable flow of air into the lungs until the inspiratory pressure reaches a preset value. The actual assisted volume provided by the respirator depends on the preset pressure, lung compliance, and the patient's inspiratory efforts. This mode has been designed to diminish the work required by the patient to breathe and is useful for patients with weaning difficulties.

VOLUME PARAMETER

Tidal volume (TV) is usually calculated as 12 to 15 mL/kg per breath.
Minute ventilation is the TV multiplied by the respiratory rate per minute.

PRESSURE PARAMETERS

Peak inspiratory pressure (PIP) is the peak pressure achieved in the respirator-lung circuit during inspiration. When tidal volume is preset, PIP depends on lung compliance. In stiff lungs, even a small tidal volume may result in high PIP. A PIP greater than 50 cm H_2O is associated with barotraumatic pneumothorax.

Peak negative inspiratory pressure is the peak negative pressure generated by the patient's own breathing. It is used as an index of the patient's ability to breathe on his or her own following extubation.

Positive end-expiratory pressure (PEEP) is the pressure in the respirator-lung circuit at end expiration. Increased PEEP raises functional residual capacity by distending small patent alveoli (those with less than 10 cm H_2O) and by recruiting collapsed alveoli (those with more than 10 cm H_2O). Alveolar oxygen exchange improves, and PO_2 increases. PEEP is generally used in cases of suboptimal oxygenation (e.g., ARDS; pulmonary edema; severe pneumonitis, as in AIDS-related *Pneumocystis pneumonia;* and severe chronic obstructive pulmonary disease). A PEEP of more than 15 cm H_2O can be used to institute tamponade of intrathoracic bleeding following thoracic surgery. As a disadvantage, the cardiac output is known to fall with increasing PEEP because of decreased venous return, right ventricular dysfunction, and decreased left ventricular distensibility. Barotraumatic pneumothorax is also a known complication of PEEP therapy.

Continuous positive airway pressure (CPAP) keeps the inspiratory airway pressure above atmospheric pressure without increasing the work of breathing, while PEEP is applied to the patient's spontaneous breathing. CPAP maintains improved functional residual capacity, improved lung compliance, and a subjective sensation of breathing better. CPAP is therefore helpful in weaning patients who have been chronically dependent on a respirator.

INSPIRATION-EXPIRATION RATIO

The inspiration-expiration (I/E) ratio is the ratio of the inspiratory time to expiratory time of each ventilatory cycle. The physiologic I/E ratio is 1:2.

VENTILATION TYPES

Volume control. The amount of ventilation is preset by tidal volume, so that regardless of the state of the patient's pulmonary mechanics, a known volume of air is delivered into the patient's lungs. Depending on the lung compliance, the inspiratory pressure may vary. In normal lungs, large tidal volumes result in normal peak inspiratory pressure. However, in stiff lungs (e.g., in patients with ARDS), a small tidal volume may result in a high peak inspiratory pressure, resulting in barotrauma or pneumothorax.

Pressure control. This is also known as volume-variable mode. The inspiratory pressure is preset, and enough volume is delivered into the lungs until the set pressure is met, at which point the mechanical ventilator ceases to deliver air. The actual tidal volume depends on lung compliance and the preset inspiratory pressure. The tidal volume is variable, but the advantage is that dangerously high inspiratory pressures can be avoided in patients with stiff lungs.

High frequency. This mode is effective in patients with bronchopleural fistula. High-frequency jet ventilation may provide adequate ventilatory support for a short term while maintaining a relatively low mean airway pressure. This mode also has been used with variable results in the treatment of patients with severe ARDS or refractory respiratory failure whose need for pressure-controlled ventilation has been pushed to the limit.

OXYGEN THERAPY

The F_iO_2 is the fraction of oxygen in the air delivered to the patient.

WEANING FROM VENTILATORY SUPPORT

The goal of weaning is to have the patient breathe at ventilatory settings consistent with extubation. The usual parameters are: F_iO_2, 40%; IMV rate, less than 6 per minute; PEEP, 5 cm H_2O; PSV, 5 cm H_2O. The patient is usually weaned down to these ventilatory settings while the PO_2 and PCO_2 levels are observed to be within the acceptable range. When the patient's ventilatory status nears that of extubation, a set of weaning parameters are obtained to assess the patient's likelihood of successful extubation. The weaning parameters are negative inspiratory force, less than -20 cm H_2O; vital capacity, more than 15 mL/kg; respiratory rate, less than 25 per minute; spontaneous tidal volume, more than 5 mL/kg; and adequate mentation and respiratory comfort. The decision to wean and extubate a patient is foremost a clinical judgment. No predetermined set of criteria may suffice to replace individual consideration.

APPENDIX

2

Hemostasis and Coagulation Disorders

Cornelius M. Dyke

OVERVIEW OF HEMOSTASIS AND FIBRINOLYSIS

The body's intrinsic control of hemorrhage necessitates a complex interplay between clot formation and lysis. Clot formation is essential to maintain hemostasis when vessel injury occurs, yet uncontrolled clot formation results in thrombosis and the ischemic complications thereof. Hemostasis may be considered to occur in three steps: blood vessel vasoconstriction, platelet activation and aggregation, and the formation of the insoluble fibrin clot. These three manifestations of the hemostatic response occur in unison to arrest bleeding. When a blood vessel is injured, local factors produced by platelets and endothelial cells result in an intense vasoconstrictive response that effectively reduces the rate of ongoing blood loss. The disruption of the endothelial barrier also exposes underlying tissue factor in the vessel wall, resulting in potent platelet activation and aggregation, as well as activation of the extrinsic pathway of the coagulation system (Fig. A2.1). The net result is the conversion of fibrinogen, a soluble plasma protein, into fibrin, an insoluble protein, which when cross-linked results in a stable clot. Simultaneously with clot formation, the fibrinolytic system is geared up to control and limit this process, preventing disseminated clot formation (Fig. A2.1).

Antithrombin III and the protein C and S system are the two dominant anticoagulant systems that prevent uncontrolled thrombosis. Antithrombin III binds to thrombin and activated factor X, inhibiting their procoagulant functions. (This reaction is powerfully potentiated by heparin, which makes heparin an effective anticoagulant.) Proteins C and S work together as cofactors to inhibit activated factors V and VIII, limiting thrombin formation.

NORMAL PLATELET FUNCTION

Platelets are the first, middle, and last line of defense against hemorrhage, and they contribute to every aspect of hemostasis and blood vessel repair after injury. Platelets from the initial platelet plug spread over the area of vessel injury and attract and promote migration of other platelets and inflammatory cells. In doing so, they create a dynamic scaffold for fibrin cross-linking and clot stabilization,

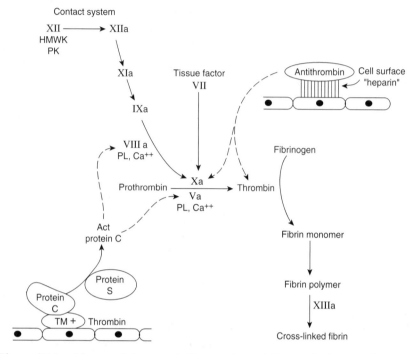

Figure A2.1. The coagulation cascade illustrates how soluble proteins interact when triggered to form an insoluble clot.

and they modulate the remodeling process of the vessel wall. Thrombin is an especially potent stimulant for platelet activation, causing a change in platelet glycoprotein receptors that up-regulates their adhesiveness.

Two platelet membrane glycoprotein receptor complexes, the glycoprotein Iv–factor IX-V complex and the glycoprotein Iib-IIIa complex, are important for platelet adhesion and aggregation. The glycoprotein Ib complex, which is constitutively expressed on the platelet membrane, mediates initial adhesion of the platelet to the injured vessel wall via its interaction with von Willebrand factor, a protein associated with the subendothelial matrix. The importance of the glycoprotein I receptor to platelet adhesion is illustrated in Bernard-Soulier syndrome, a rare genetic disorder resulting in a dysfunctional glycoprotein I receptor on the platelet plasma membrane. Patients with Bernard-Soulier syndrome have platelets that respond normally to platelet agonists and activation but not to thrombin. These patients have significantly impaired platelet adhesion.

After initial platelet contact with subendothelial proteins (e.g., tissue factor) and subsequent activation, the platelet releases granules containing serotonin, epinephrine, thrombin, adenosine diphosphate, and thromboxane. These substances cause local vasocontriction, increase capillary permeability, and are potent chemoattractants, causing cellular migration of inflammatory cells and other platelets. The initial platelet plug is stabilized through interactions between another platelet glycoprotein complex expressed on the plasma membrane: that is, the glycoprotein IIb-IIIa receptor, causing high-affinity binding with fibrin, von Willebrand factor, and other platelet receptors. This results in a firm, sticky, solid clot of platelets and coagulation proteins covering the site of vessel injury. Without activation of the glycoprotein IIb-IIIa complex, mature clot formation does not occur. This is remarkably demonstrated in patients with Glanzmann's thrombasthenia, a condition caused by a point mutation that results in a congenitally defective glycoprotein IIb-IIIa receptor. People with this disorder have a normal platelet count and normal initial adhesion; however, platelet aggregation is completely impaired, resulting in a clinically significant bleeding disorder. The dependence on the glycoprotein IIb-IIIa receptor for platelet aggregation and clot stabilization is clinically important. Several drugs that are available or are in clinical trials block this receptor selectively and inhibit platelet function in patients with acute coronary syndromes or who have had coronary angioplasty. Other indications are likely to follow.

PREOPERATIVE EVALUATION OF THE COAGULATION SYSTEM

The preoperative hemostatic assessment of the surgical patient should raise three questions:

- Are there any preexisting coagulation abnormalities?
- What corrections should be made?
- What are the intraoperative and postoperative transfusion requirements likely to be?

A careful history and physical examination are the most important components of the preoperative assessment of the coagulation system in the surgical patient; they are more important than a routine battery of coagulation tests. A congenital bleeding diathesis is elicited by careful questioning about bruising ability, prolonged bleeding from minor cuts or shaving, frequent nosebleeds, or arthralgias. The physical examination is important in confirming these findings. A medication history is particulary important, because many medications affect the coagulation system (Table A2.1).

Routine laboratory testing ("coag screen") is not cost effective and adds little information about patients who have no evidence of coagulation defects on history or physical examination and who are undergoing surgery in which blood loss is expected to be minimal. Laboratory testing is useful in patients who may have a coagulation defect or whose potential for intraoperative bleeding is high.

Table A2.1. COMMON MEDICATIONS
AFFECTING HEMOSTASIS

Medication	Mechanism	Severity of Effect
Warfarin	Inhibits vitamin K–dependent factors (i.e., Factors II, VII, IX, X)	Severe
Heparin	Potentiates antithrombin III	Severe
Aspirin	Inhibits platelet aggregation	Moderate to severe
Nonsteroidal antiinflammatory drugs	Inhibits platelet aggregation	Moderate
Ca^{2+} channel blockers	Inhibits platelet aggregation	Mild
GP IIb, IIIa inhibitors	Inhibits platelet aggregation	Severe

Ca^{2+}, calcium; GP, glycoprotein.

ORDERING BLOOD PRODUCTS

Blood typing and screening are usually performed for patients who may, but are unlikely to, need transfusion (e.g., before a routine colectomy). When antibodies in the patient's blood sample are detected, donor blood lacking those antibodies is identified in case it is needed. Although antigens may be present in the blood that is set aside, they usually do not cause a serious hemolytic reaction. A type-and-cross-match order completely cross-matches donor and recipient blood and makes available compatible blood cells. Partially cross-matched blood transfusions use blood that is ABO type specific, Rh matched, and tested for acute phase reactants without cross-matching lesser antigens. These transfusions are used in emergencies and are slightly safer than type-specific blood only. The last choice for emergency transfusion (limited to exsanguination) is the use of type O Rh-negative blood. Hemolytic reactions from antibodies in the plasma may occur (a form of graft-versus-host disease) when non–cross-matched O-negative blood is used.

AUTOLOGOUS BLOOD TRANSFUSION

Selected patients electively scheduled for surgery may donate their own blood preoperatively for planned transfusion during the operation. Self (autologous) blood donation is frequently used by patients undergoing elective operations who have a high risk of bleeding, including those undergoing prostatic resection and major orthopaedic surgery. The obvious benefit is the elimination of the infectious complications of donor blood transfusion (Table A2.2). Candidates for predonation of blood are patients without significant cardiopulmonary or neurologic disease who have a hemoglobin level greater than 11 g/dL. Patients may donate 2 to 3 units of blood in the weeks preceding surgery, with

Table A2.2.   ESTIMATED RISK OF BLOOD TRANSFUSION PER UNIT

Reaction or Adverse Event	Incidence
Minor allergic reaction	1:100
Fatal hemolytic reaction	1:600,000
Viral hepatitis (A, B, C, or D)	1:50,000
HIV infection	1:500,000

the last donation no later than 3 days before the operation. Patients take supplemental iron to enhance red blood cell production in the bone marrow. The use of erythropoietin to stimulate red blood cell production and allow more voluminous blood donation has been described, but it is not necessary in patients who are stockpiling only 2 or 3 units.

TRANSFUSING BLOOD PRODUCTS

Before transfusing blood or blood products, careful identification of the patient is mandatory. Human clerical error is the most common cause of blood transfusion reactions. Although there are infectious complications of blood transfusion, careful and universal testing has ensured a safe blood supply in the United States (Table A2.2). Normal saline is used with packed red blood cells to decrease the viscosity of the transfused blood. Calcium-containing solutions are not appropriate because they may induce clotting; hypoosmolar solutions are not used because they may induce cell lysis. Blood is filtered through a 170-μ filter to remove aggregates and cellular debris. Smaller filters may be used to remove white blood cells and thereby reduce febrile reactions that may occur with transfusion; however, the cost utility of this has been questioned. Blood should be warmed prior to transfusion in the operating room or when large quantities are needed.

Major signs of a transfusion reaction include flushing, hypotension, urticaria, hemoglobinuria, back pain, pruritis, chills, and fever. Obviously, in the anesthetized patient, these signs and symptoms are not apparent. Excessive bleeding and coagulopathy are a common sign of a transfusion reaction intraoperatively.

INTRAOPERATIVE BLOOD SALVAGE

When significant amounts of intraoperative bleeding occurs, blood may be scavenged from the operative field with suckers, washed, and the red blood cells returned to the patient. The hematocrit of this washed red blood cell volume is approximately half that of a unit of blood from the blood bank. However, it does have the advantage of being autologous. Intraoperative blood salvage is not appropriate in all patients. Patients with active infections or sepsis and those with cancer undergoing localized resection are not candidates for intraoperative blood scavenging because of the risk of spread of infection or tumor. Similarly, patients in whom significant bleeding and blood transfusion is unlikely do not justify the additional cost of the equipment to scavenge, wash, and retransfuse red blood cells "just in case."

ADJUNCTS TO HEMOSTASIS

Electrocautery (the Bovie) is ubiquitous in surgical practice today. Developed by William Bovie, a physicist, and Harvey Cushing at Johns Hopkins University, electrocautery dessicates tissue and locally destroys body proteins, creating an intense stimulus for thrombosis and heat-welding small blood vessels. Normal coagulation is needed for effective use.

Thrombin and collagen may be used topically on raw surfaces to stimulate coagulation and platelet adherence and activation. When used in sheets or pads, local tamponade may also contribute to hemostasis. Numerous commercial varieties are available. Gelatin foam is also used as a local hemostatic agent, and although it has no procoagulant effect, it soaks up blood and plasma, increasing its size, which exerts a local tamponade effect, and concentrating plasma proteins at the site of bleeding. Fibrin glue may be used to create an instant clot at a specific site. Fibrin glue is created by mixing fibrinogen in one syringe and calcium and thrombin in another; a fibrin clot is formed when these ingredients are mixed. However, the ingredients must be kept separate until used because the reaction is instantaneous.

Surgical Nutrition

Jeannie F. Savas

The nutritional status of a patient may be poor because of inadequate intake, poor absorption, or an increased metabolic state, such as is seen with sepsis or recent surgery. The nutritional assessment should begin with the history and physical examination. Specifically, has there been weight loss, diarrhea, vomiting, dysphagia, anorexia, or steatorrhea? Has the patient had surgery or a medical condition that is associated with malabsorption or malnutrition? Many surgical patients are unable to eat because of recent abdominal surgery, bowel obstruction, ileus, pancreatitis, or alteration of mental status. All of these factors should be considered in determining whether a patient is at risk for malnutrition. The physical examination may reveal cachexia, abdominal distention, jaundice, poor skin turgor, edema, or dermatitis. Calculations such as the Harris-Benedict equation estimate the nutritional needs. Nonspecific laboratory tests that may be clues to malnutrition include serum albumin, transferrin, total protein, liver function tests, total lymphocyte count, and prealbumin. A 24-hour urine specimen for nitrogen can evaluate whether a patient is in positive or negative nitrogen balance. The respiratory quotient (R/Q) is an accurate means of determining the adequacy of and proper balance of protein, carbohydrate, and fat calories in the diet. However, this test is difficult unless the patient is ventilator dependent.

Indications for supplementation include no intake for more than 5 days, inadequate intake, inadequate absorption, and a hypermetabolic state that renders the patient in negative nitrogen balance. The route of supplementation should then be decided. Enteral nutrition if possible is preferred. This may be accomplished orally or via a nasogastric or nasojejunal tube. If long-term supplementation is expected, a gastric or jejunal tube should be placed either endoscopically or surgically. Oral or gastric routes should be used only for patients not at high risk for aspiration. Common complications of enteral feeding are tube dislodgment or dysfunction, abdominal distention, and diarrhea. The latter two can usually be avoided by beginning with a diluted formula and advancing the amount slowly as tolerated. Sometimes the addition of kaolin pectin or antimotility agents is necessary once infection is excluded. Enteral nutrition is beneficial to maintain mucosal integrity and prevent bacterial translocation even if parenteral supplementation is also required to meet the patient's nutritional needs. Special formulas are available for patients with diabetes, renal failure, hepatic failure, and ileus or malabsorptive states.

If enteral nutrition is not an option (e.g., bowel obstruction, severe ileus, bowel ischemia, or malabsorptive state), parenteral nutrition should be instituted. If short-term or partial supplementation is necessary, it may be achieved via a peripheral venous catheter. If long-term or complete supplementation is needed, the patient must have a central venous catheter despite the risk of sepsis, glucose intolerance, and catheter-related complications. There are special formulations for patients with renal or hepatic failure. All patients need to be monitored for glucose intolerance, electrolyte imbalances, hypophosphatemia, and cholestasis.

The amount and type of supplementation a patient requires should be periodically assessed with routine laboratory tests, measurement of nitrogen balance, and/or the quotient. As a guideline, the nonstressed person needs 25 kcal/kg per day. Stresses such as sepsis, tumor, trauma, burns, multiple illnesses, and/or recent surgery may increase these needs by 50 to 400%. Underfeeding a patient produces a catabolic state and an inability to heal or fight infection. Overfeeding a patient may result in carbon dioxide retention and ventilator dependence.

Occasionally, a patient who is nutritionally depleted needs surgery, such as for cancer. If possible, supplementation should be given until the patient is in positive nitrogen balance to diminish the perioperative morbidity and mortality.

Surgical patients are often at risk for malnutrition. Start feeding and/or supplementing patients at risk as soon as possible, and frequently reassess the adequacy of nutrition. Feed enterally whenever possible, even if parenteral nutrition is also required to meet the patient's needs. Consider placing a feeding tube at the time of surgery in patients at risk. Remember that stress, such as trauma, surgery, or sepsis, greatly increases the metabolic needs of the patient.

Surgical Instruments

A. Kocher clamp
B. Straight hemostat
C. Needle holder
D. Crile clamp
E. Curved hemostat
F. Kelly clamp

G. Tonsil forceps
H. Right-angle clamp
I. Army-Navy retractor
J. Deaver retractor
K. Small and medium
   Richardson retractors

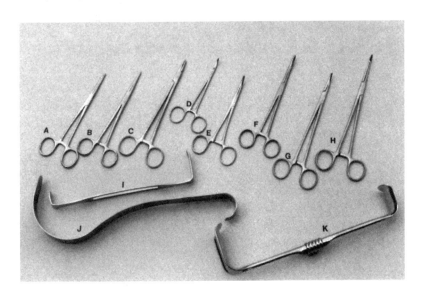

A. Sponge forceps
B. Babcock clamps
C. Allis clamps
D. Towel clips
E. Simm's scissors
F. Pott's scissors
G. Metzenbaum scissors
H. Straight Mayo scissors
I. Curved Mayo scissors

J. Scalpel (No. 10 blade)
K. Scalpel (No. 11 blade)
L. Scalpel (No. 15 blade)
M. Adson forceps with teeth
N. Brigham forceps with teeth
O. Debakey forceps
P. Ring forceps

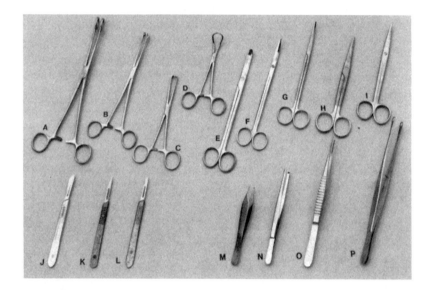

Index

Page numbers in italics denote figures; those followed by a t denote tables.